THE CIBA COLLECTION OF MEDICAL ILLUSTRATIONS

VOLUME I

A Compilation of Paintings on the
Normal and Pathologic Anatomy of the

NERVOUS SYSTEM

With a Supplement on
THE HYPOTHALAMUS

Prepared by
FRANK H. NETTER, M. D.

With a foreword by

JOHN F. FULTON, M. D.

Sterling Professor of the History of Medicine
Yale University School of Medicine

Commissioned and published by

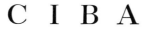

C I B A

OTHER PUBLISHED VOLUMES OF
THE CIBA COLLECTION OF MEDICAL ILLUSTRATIONS
By
FRANK H. NETTER, M.D.

REPRODUCTIVE SYSTEM

UPPER DIGESTIVE TRACT

LOWER DIGESTIVE TRACT

LIVER, BILIARY TRACT AND PANCREAS

ENDOCRINE SYSTEM AND SELECTED METABOLIC DISEASES

HEART

KIDNEYS, URETERS, AND URINARY BLADDER

(See page 168 for additional information)

FIRST PRINTING, 1953
SECOND PRINTING, 1955
THIRD PRINTING, 1957
FOURTH PRINTING, 1958
FIFTH PRINTING, 1962
SIXTH PRINTING, 1964
SEVENTH PRINTING, 1967
EIGHTH PRINTING, 1968
NINTH PRINTING, 1972
TENTH PRINTING, 1974
ELEVENTH PRINTING, 1975
TWELFTH PRINTING, 1977

ISBN 0-914168-01-0

LIBRARY OF CONGRESS CATALOG NO.: 53-2151

PRINTED IN U.S.A.

ORIGINAL PRINTING BY COLORPRESS, NEW YORK, N.Y.
COLOR ENGRAVINGS BY EMBASSY PHOTO ENGRAVING CO., INC., NEW YORK, N.Y.
OFFSET CONVERSION BY THE CASE-HOYT CORP., ROCHESTER, N.Y.
TWELFTH PRINTING BY THE CASE-HOYT CORP., ROCHESTER, N.Y.

FOREWORD

In the early texts of anatomy the central nervous system of human beings was seldom adequately depicted because, although the art of embalming was known, this procedure was rarely used for the preservation of the brain and spinal cord. The result was that by the time the anatomist or the pathologist came to expose the brain, it was generally soft and disintegrated and not well suited for anatomical study. The first adequate illustrations of cerebral structure are those found in the *Fabrica* of Andreas Vesalius, published in 1543. His plates representing the nervous system show many of the major structures, but the sulci are flattened and the hemispheres themselves have the appearance of being more or less collapsed. However, Vesalius had depicted the major gross structures of the human brain, including the cerebellum, the cerebral ventricles, and the majority of the cranial nerves.

It was discovered later that the cerebral ventricles had been much more clearly portrayed some years earlier in the manuscript notebooks of Leonardo. He injected the ventricular system with wax and, on macerating the surrounding cortical tissue, he emerged with an accurate cast of the ventricles which he had drawn in his notebook; but unfortunately these excellent drawings did not become public property for nearly four centuries.

There were many other anatomists in the sixteenth century who made anatomical illustrations of various parts of the central nervous system — Eustachio, whose plates of the cranial nerves, including the vagus, represent a conspicuous advance over the Vesalian portrayal of corresponding structures. And then the Florentine Guidi, better known as Vidius (the Latin form of his name), grandson of Ghirlandajo, made good use of the artistic talent which he inherited and published an illustrated anatomical and also a surgical text. Vidius' contemporary, Costanzo Varolio, in 1573, issued a monograph on the optic nerves which contains a plate illustrating the base of the brain that was more accurate than anything before him and was only matched by the celebrated plate which Thomas Willis issued in 1674 in his *Cerebri anatome*. The latter plate, showing the vascular circle which still bears Willis' name, was designed by the young Christopher Wren, who had learned the art of injection of blood vessels in London while working as an assistant in the anatomical theatre of Sir Charles Scarborough. Wren introduced the new technique at Oxford, and I have always suspected that it was Wren rather than Willis who discovered the arterial circle.

In the seventeenth and eighteenth centuries there were a number of other notable illustrations of the brain and spinal cord in monographs such as those of Vieussens (1685) and Ridley (1695). In the eighteenth century the most remarkable plates of the nervous system were the colored portrayals of Jan Ladmiral and Jacques Fabian Gautier d'Agoty. The color process employed by these artists, although they claimed it as their own invention, was probably that of the German Le Blon, since they had both worked with him as assistants.

There was little progress in anatomical illustration of the nervous system during the nineteenth century, although note should be made of the plates published by Charles Bell who was as much artist as he was anatomist and of whom it is generally said that he colored his anatomical plates by hand. Those of Cruveilhier should also be mentioned. His plates depicting tumors of the central nervous system are as fine as anything that had appeared before or has been published since.

With the advent of the modern period, hand coloring has largely disappeared and in its place we have the three-color process employed by the German anatomists such as Spalteholtz. The present volume, composed of the beautiful plates of Dr. Frank H. Netter, makes use of every modern device to present the structural relations of the nervous system with care and precision. At a time when a high value is placed on visual aids as an accompaniment to the written word in the educational process, these exquisite and highly accurate illustrations commend themselves to all who are either teaching or learning the functions of the nervous system. Although there have been a number of artists throughout medical history who have achieved lasting acclaim for the excellence of their work even though they were not themselves physicians, this collection of drawings well illustrates the happy result of artist and physician being combined in one person. Dr. Netter's knowledge of function cannot but lend clarity to his plates.

The legends and descriptions to the illustrations as provided by Doctors Kaplan, Kuntz and von Bonin of course do not substitute for a textbook but are comprehensive and yet masterpieces of conciseness. Both illustrations and text together are quite obviously the result of a most cheerful and successful cooperation. The consultant experts have left their imprint also on the pictures and in the method of demonstrating a variety of details, since one may readily recognize traces of their own scientific contributions in their respective fields.

One common source of confusion to students — the position of the Island of Reil — is beautifully resolved in one of Dr. Netter's diagrams to be found in Plate 17. His portrayal of the Circle of Willis in Plate 16 is probably the clearest that one will find in any modern anatomical text. His diagram of the relations of the cerebellum in Plate 44 is also highly illuminating and the diagram in Plate 72 of the innervation of the female genital system is excellent.

These are but a few selections from a work of consistently high quality. Ciba Pharmaceutical Company, in offering this new volume in their series of anatomical illustrations, adds another to their enviable list of contributions to the progress and the history of medicine.

JOHN F. FULTON, M.D.

New Haven, March, 1953

PREFACE TO THE TENTH PRINTING

When the ninth printing of Volume 1 of THE CIBA COLLECTION OF MEDICAL ILLUSTRATIONS was completed in 1972, it was hoped that a proposed revision would eliminate the need for yet another printing. In the last two years, however, the unprecedented and increasing requests for this book, the demand on Dr. Netter's time for artwork, and the monumental task of concisely revising Volume 1 have combined to make this, the tenth printing, necessary.

As with previous printings, Volume 1 remains essentially unchanged. A supplement on the hypothalamus with its own index comprises pages 145-168, following the regular index. Prepared with the collaboration of Dr. W. R. Ingram and edited by the late Dr. Ernst Oppenheimer, this section first appeared in the July-August 1956 issue of CIBA CLINICAL SYMPOSIA. It was added to Volume 1 during the third printing. The color scheme used to identify the various hypothalamic nuclei in the supplement is different from that used for the same nuclei represented on pages 76 and 77. This obvious difference should present no confusion for the reader.

Minor inconsistencies which had been called to our attention by our readers have been corrected. In particular, a variation between pages 58 and 72 in the nomenclature of the thalamic nuclei has been rectified, and a revision of the text on page 154 to correct a disparity with the illustration on the same page has been completed.

The major change instituted for the tenth printing was a modernization of production methods. Like the recently completed Volume 6 and the third printing of Volume 3 Part II of THE CIBA COLLECTION OF MEDICAL ILLUSTRATIONS, this reprint of Volume 1 was produced by offset on a higher grade, whiter, nonglare paper using conversions from the original engravings. The conversion process provided an opportunity to correct a certain amount of color "drift" which had occurred from printing to printing as a result of changes in ink and paper since the original publication. Color proofs were compared to the original artwork, thus making this printing more faithful to Dr. Netter's original paintings in color, detail, and esthetic value than any version since the first.

Gratitude must be expressed to those persons whose painstaking work brought this reprinting of Volume 1 successfully to completion. In the Medical Education Division of CIBA Pharmaceutical Company, Miss Louise Stemmle and Mrs. Helen Sward, as always, reliably and with exacting preciseness proofread every illustration and page. Mr. Pierre Lair, as Production Manager, directed the overall project and assisted in the color evaluation. Appreciation is also due Mr. Gary Meicht, under whose direction all color conversions and corrections were produced, and the numerous other skilled craftsmen of The Case-Hoyt Corporation whose commitment to fine printing was so necessary for this endeavor.

Robert K. Shapter, M.D., C.M.

PREFACE TO THE ELEVENTH PRINTING

At the time the tenth printing of Volume 1 of THE CIBA COLLECTION OF MEDICAL ILLUSTRATIONS was completed in 1974, work on a revision of this book was already in progress. It was hoped that supplies of the tenth printing would have lasted until publication of the revision. However, because demand for *Nervous System*—the most popular volume of the CIBA COLLECTION series—continued to grow beyond our expectations, it has become necessary to reprint the work. This eleventh printing remains unchanged, except for correction of a minor error on page 76.

It is fitting that a special note of appreciation be accorded Miss Louise Stemmle, who is retiring as Production Editor

of the Medical Education Division, CIBA Pharmaceutical Company. Miss Stemmle's contributions to both Volume 5 and Volume 6 of the CIBA COLLECTION have been significant and essential. Even the volumes of the series that were originally published prior to her association with the CIBA COLLECTION bear the mark of her dedicated and painstaking work. The conversion process from letterpress to offset, which was necessary for our continuous reprinting schedule, could not have been completed without Miss Stemmle's diligent checking and rechecking of 1,984 pages and 1,584 illustrations. We will miss her.

Robert K. Shapter, M.D., C.M.

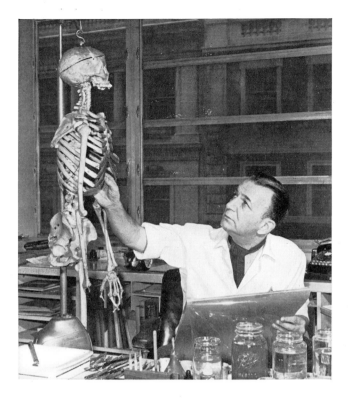

THE ARTIST

Many readers of the CIBA COLLECTION have expressed a desire to know more about Dr. Netter. In response to these requests this summary of Dr. Netter's career has been prepared.

Frank Henry Netter, born in 1906 in Brooklyn, New York, received his M.D. degree from New York University in 1931. To help pay his way through medical school and internship at Bellevue, he worked as a commercial artist and as an illustrator of medical books and articles for his professors and other physicians, perfecting his natural talent by studying at the National Academy of Design and attending courses at the Art Students' League.

In 1933 Dr. Netter entered the private practice of surgery in New York City. But it was the depth of the depression, and the recently married physician continued to accept art assignments to supplement his income. Soon he was spending more and more time at the drawing board and finally, realizing that his career lay in medical illustration, he decided to give up practicing and become a full-time artist.

Soon, Dr. Netter was receiving requests to develop many unusual projects. One of the most arduous of these was building the "transparent woman" for the San Francisco Golden Gate Exposition. This 7-foot-high transparent figure depicted the menstrual process, the development and birth of a baby, and the physical and sexual development of a woman, while a synchronized voice told the story of the female endocrine system. Dr. Netter labored on this project night and day for 7 months. Another interesting assignment involved a series of paintings of incidents in the life of a physician. Among others, the pictures showed a medical student sitting up the night before the osteology examination, studying away to the point of exhaustion; an emergency ward; an ambulance call; a class reunion; and a night call made by a country doctor.

During World War II, Dr. Netter was an officer in the Army, stationed first at the Army Institute of Pathology, later at the Surgeon General's Office, in charge of graphic training aids for the Medical Department. Numerous manuals were produced under his direction, among them first aid for combat troops, roentgenology for technicians, sanitation in the field, and survival in the tropics.

After the war, Dr. Netter began work on several major projects for CIBA Pharmaceutical Company, culminating in THE CIBA COLLECTION OF MEDICAL ILLUSTRATIONS. To date, five volumes have been published and work is in progress on the sixth, dealing with the urinary tract.

Dr. Netter goes about planning and executing his illustrations in a very exacting way. First comes the study, unquestionably the most important and most difficult part of the entire undertaking. No drawing is ever started until Dr. Netter has acquired a complete understanding of the subject matter, either through reading or by consultation with leading authorities in the field. Often he visits hospitals to observe clinical cases, pathologic or surgical specimens, or operative procedures. Sometimes an original dissection is necessary.

When all his questions have been answered and the problem is thoroughly understood, Dr. Netter makes a pencil sketch on a tissue or tracing pad. Always, the subject must be visualized from the standpoint of the physician; is it to be viewed from above or below, from the side, the rear, or the front? What area is to be covered, the entire body or just certain segments? What plane provides the clearest understanding? In some pictures two, three, or four planes of dissection may be necessary.

When the sketch is at last satisfactory, Dr. Netter transfers it to a piece of illustration board for the finished drawing. This is done by blocking the back of the picture with a soft pencil, taping the tissue down on the board with Scotch tape, then going over the lines with a hard pencil. Over the years, our physician-artist has used many media to finish his illustrations, but now he works almost exclusively in transparent water colors mixed with white paint.

In spite of the tremendously productive life Dr. Netter has led, he has been able to enjoy his family, first in a handsome country home in East Norwich, Long Island, and, after the five children had grown up, in a penthouse overlooking the East River in Manhattan.

ALFRED W. CUSTER

ACKNOWLEDGMENTS

Ciba Pharmaceutical Company expresses its most sincere appreciation to Ernst Oppenheimer, M.D., Richard H. Roberts, M.D., William T. Strauss, M.D., J. Harold Walton, M.D., Miss Ruth S. Godwyn, Messrs. James R. Beattie, George L. Cantzlaar, Alfred W. Custer, John N. Kolen, and Paul W. Roder, who participated in the development of this volume.

INTRODUCTION

For many years the teaching of the anatomy, physiology, and pathology of the nervous system was conducted in an atmosphere of academic discipline. It was the custom to capture the imagination of the medical student with the more striking natural phenomena and the more dramatic pathologic manifestations, even though their clinical incidence lagged far behind the importance that was accorded them in the lecture hall. Such stress on minutiae tended to lend to this field a character of remoteness in the mind of the student. By the same token the general practitioner and the nonneurologic specialist, pressed for time while meeting the demands of a busy practice, have been relatively impatient with the labyrinthine complications of neurology and have, as a consequence, left the full command of this body of information to specialists in neurology and neurosurgery.

Allowing for recent advances in medical education and for the increasing recognition of neurologic factors in all kinds of illness, the present group of illustrations is offered as a leavening agent. To the end that the intricacies of the nervous system may be more easily comprehended, the most important and clinically useful facts are herein "compressed" and so arranged that one can readily refer to the plates and their accompanying text when confronted by a neurologic problem. The index is designed to further this aim and to anticipate the needs and reference habits of any reader.

The backbone of this collection is, of course, generally accepted information. While minute details and controversial theories have been avoided, this was not done at the expense of accuracy or completeness. Clinical significance has been the guiding principle. In many instances certain anatomic structures are either deliberately omitted or deemphasized in order to stress points that have broader clinical application.

A section on the anatomy of the spine is included instead of being reserved for another volume covering bones and ligaments in general, because an understanding of spinal anatomy is fundamental to a proper appreciation of spinal cord injuries, the compression effects of spinal tumors, the significance of intervertebral herniations, and numerous other clinical conditions. It is for this same reason that a practicing neurosurgeon was chosen as collaborator in selecting and discussing the illustrations concerned with anatomy of the spine. The descriptive text by Dr. Abraham Kaplan in three sections — "Anatomy of the Spine," "The Central Nervous System," and "Pathology of the Brain and Spinal Cord" — exemplifies again the principal aim of this atlas, to serve the practicing physician and the student in their efforts to understand the underlying reasons and conditions of diseases and clinical syndromes.

In view of the considerable individual variations of the spine, the prominence of the tubercles and processes, etc., efforts have been made to portray an average form and to illustrate all the processes so that they might be easily recognized and remembered. The plates show not only the detailed configuration of the individual vertebrae but also the manner in which these articulate. The principal ligaments were also included in such a way as to illustrate their functions, the structures which they bind together, and the motility permitted by them. Different viewing angles are used to foster complete understanding.

In the plates illustrating the basic anatomy of the brain and the spinal cord, the physician will doubtless recognize that a great many details have been omitted. This was done deliberately. The complexity of the central nervous system is such that one must be guided by the fundamental requirements of simplicity if effectiveness in presentation is to be achieved. Only as much of the gross anatomy has been selected as was thought necessary to provide a clear apprehension of the principles developed in the sections dealing with functional neuro-anatomy and, to a degree, the autonomic nervous system.

(*continued*)

The task of pictorializing functional neuro-anatomy was undertaken with a great deal of trepidation. The complexity of the subject certainly is unsurpassed by any other topic from the standpoint of both the teacher in the field as well as the graphic medical artist. Of necessity, the illustrations in this section are almost entirely schematic. In general, controversial points are by-passed, but it would be vain to hope that differences of opinion would not arise on some details.

In the preparation of the chapter illustrating functional neuro-anatomy, I was fortunate to have had the most valuable and enjoyable cooperation of Dr. Gerhardt von Bonin. His profound knowledge and proficiency in teaching continuously aroused my admiration.

The next section, "The Autonomic Nervous System," presented difficulties, particularly from the graphic point of view, because of the enormous and diverse ramifications. Controlling at least to some extent the function of nearly every organ of the body, this system has a significant interest for every physician, may he be an obstetrician, a gastroenterologist, an endocrinologist, cardiologist, or pharmacologist.

The literature that has accumulated relative to the autonomic system is so voluminous that the practicing physician or student generally cannot afford the time to read even in cursory fashion this tremendous mass of information. The material in this atlas tries to fulfill a need for a simplified, but fairly comprehensive presentation of the subject.

This task, with all its inherent problems, was facilitated through the devoted efforts of Dr. Albert Kuntz. He has for many years been active in this field, and has added a great deal to the knowledge of the autonomic nervous system by his own scientific contributions. His concise explanatory text should guarantee that this chapter will serve fully its intended purposes.

The first ten plates portray the overall morphology of the autonomic nervous system; its functional relation and its manner of distribution to the various body systems. The illustration which analyzes the autonomic nervous system from the point of view of adrenergic and cholinergic nerve endings, should be of particular interest because this field of study is presently receiving ever-increasing attention.

The second group of ten plates in the section deals with the autonomic innervation of specific organs. In these, schematic treatment was resorted to almost exclusively, since this seemed to be the most practical way to sort out the widely disseminated and detailed neuronal ramifications.

The illustrations comprising the last section, "Pathology of the Brain and Spinal Cord," are exemplary rather than specific. Admittedly, it would have been relatively easy to pad the section with pictures of the many varieties of meningiomas, spinal fractures, and cerebral hemorrhages. Instead, a trial has been made to portray, insofar as possible, the *typical* appearance of each condition along with its more important modifications, to achieve overall coverage of a subject rather than a detailed study of any of its aspects. These presentations are intended to serve as "visual definitions" of meningocele, meningomyelocele, syringomyelocele, and the other conditions. The text which accompanies the plates compresses into a few words the generally recognized etiology, symptomatology, diagnostic findings, and therapeutic indications.

Every artist thrives on appreciation, understanding and encouragement. In this respect I have been doubly fortunate. First, the warm reception which the medical profession has accorded my pictures has been a wonderful source of satisfaction to me. Second, more personal and close at hand, has been the inspiring personality of Dr. Ernst Oppenheimer. His understanding of the things I was trying to do, his appreciation of what I had done, and his encouragement to do more were a constant assurance that I was not alone. In addition, his vision of the scope and value of this atlas and his many co-ordinating activities in its behalf have been vital factors in the project.

FRANK H. NETTER, M.D.

CONTENTS

Section I

ANATOMY OF THE SPINE

with descriptive text by

ABRAHAM KAPLAN, M.D., F.A.C.S., D.N.S.

Clinical Professor of Neurosurgery
New York Polyclinic Medical School and Hospital
New York, N. Y.

PLATE I

GENERAL CONFIGURATION

The spinal column consists of 33 vertebrae joined together by multiple ligaments and intervening cartilages. There are seven cervical, twelve thoracic, five lumbar, five sacral vertebrae (the last five fused as one) and one coccygeal vertebra, a fusion of four small vertebrae. Occasionally when an extra lumbar vertebra is present it is usually compensated for by one vertebra less in the thoracic region. Mobility of the vertebrae in the cervical, thoracic and lumbar region is relatively free as compared with those in the sacrum and coccyx which are usually fixed. As a rule, the spinal column in the female is four or five inches shorter than in the male.

Viewed from the side, the cervical curve is convex forward, the thoracic curve convex backward, most prominent at the level of the seventh thoracic vertebra and the lumbar curve, most accentuated in the female, is convex forward, ending at the lumbosacral angle. The pelvic curve is concave downward from the lumbosacral angle to the tip of the coccyx. Viewed from the rear, a slight

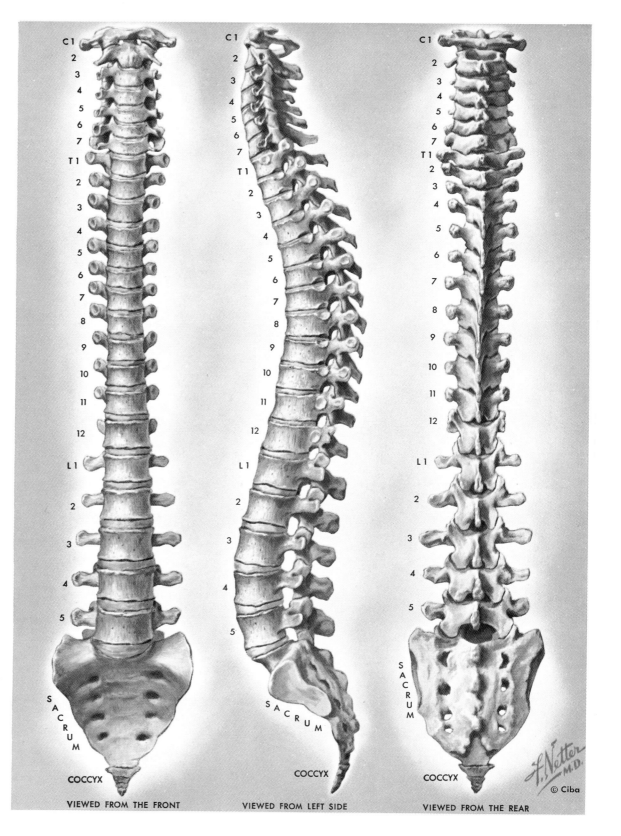

VIEWED FROM THE FRONT   VIEWED FROM LEFT SIDE   VIEWED FROM THE REAR

lateral curvature of the trunk to the right can be observed because most people are right-handed. From the second cervical vertebra to the first thoracic the bodies of the vertebrae gradually increase in width. They decrease in width with the next two or three vertebrae and then again their width steadily increases as far down as the lumbosacral angle. The oval-shaped intervertebral foramina are smallest in the cervical region and gradually increase in size as they approach the lowest lumbar vertebrae. Through these foramina pass the spinal nerves. Viewed from the rear, the spinal column shows the spinous processes in the midline. They are bifid from the second to the sixth cervical vertebrae and these run almost in a horizontal direction. The spines in the thoracic region are described in Plate 6, page 26. In the lumbar region,

the spines are practically horizontal. On either side of each spinous process are the laminae which form shallow grooves for muscle layers, and lateral to these laminae are the articular facets. More laterally and somewhat anterior are the transverse processes. In the thoracic region, the transverse processes have a tendency to take a backward direction.

The vertebral canal which extends through the entire length of the spinal column conforms to the various spinal curvatures and to the variations in size of the spinal cord. It is triangular and large in the cervical region, somewhat small and circular in the thoracic region and then again becomes triangular in the lumbar region. The spinal column serves as an excellent protection for the spinal cord with its adjacent spinal nerves and various coverings.

PLATE 2

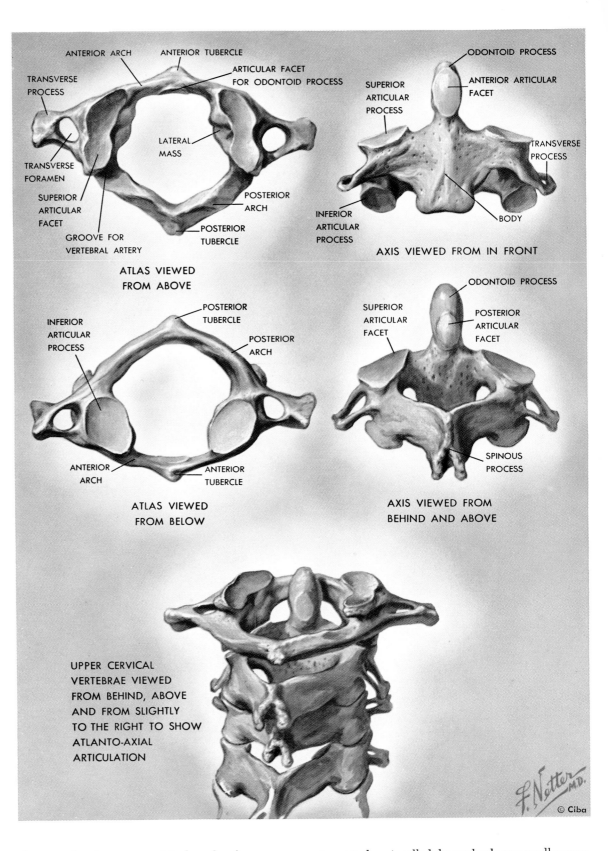

ATLAS AND AXIS

Atlas

The skull rests on the atlas, which is the first cervical vertebra. It has no body and no spinous process, but consists mainly of two lateral masses and two arches. The anterior arch is convex and carries at its midpoint a tubercle which serves as an attachment to the longus coli muscle. At the middle of the posterior surface of this arch is a smooth oval facet for articulation with the odontoid process. The posterior arch is concave backward with the posterior tubercle, a rudimentary spinous process, at the midpoint.

The two lateral masses have a superior and inferior facet. The superior facet is large, oval and concave and is shaped to form a cup for the condyles of the occipital bone. The inferior facet is circular, convex, facing downward and somewhat medially, and articulates with the axis below. Just posterior to the superior facet are small grooves through which the vertebral artery and first spinal nerve enter the skull. Lateral to each lateral mass are the transverse processes with an oval foramen through which run the vertebral artery with its accompanying vein and nerve.

Axis

The second cervical vertebra, also called the epistropheus, is most striking because of the odontoid process. This rises perpendicularly from the midportion of the upper surface of the body of the axis. A slight constriction at its base is called the neck where a small groove may be found for the attachment of the transverse atlantal ligament. On the anterior surface of the odontoid process is an oval facet for articulation with the atlas. At each side of the body of this vertebra is a superior and an inferior facet. The superior articular facet faces upward and outward articulating with the atlas, the inferior articular facet faces downward and inward and articulates with the cervical vertebrae below.

The spinous process is large, strong, and bifid, and is the meeting point of the adjacent thick laminae. The transverse processes are small and end in a single tubercle. They are perforated by a foramen through which run the vertebral artery and its accompanying vein and nerve.

22

PLATE 3

CERVICAL VERTEBRAE

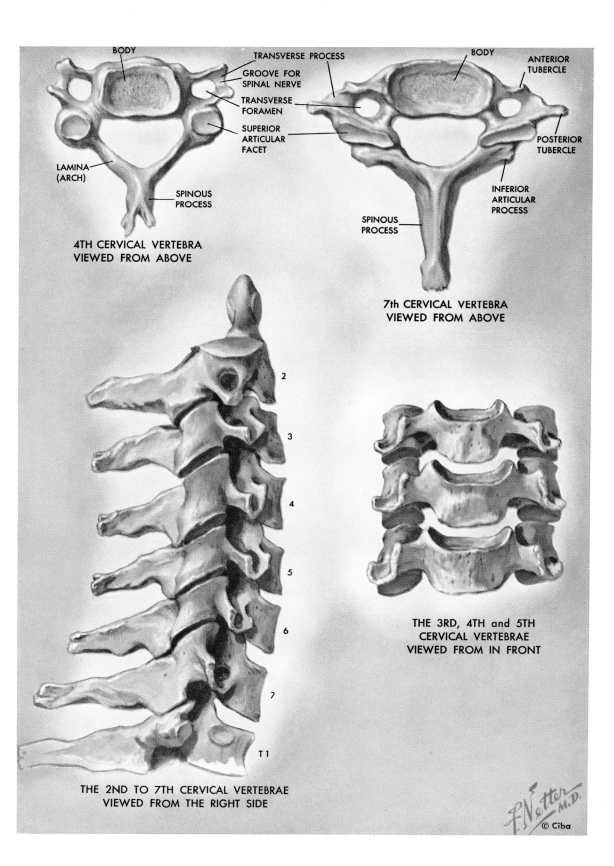

BODY
TRANSVERSE PROCESS
GROOVE FOR SPINAL NERVE
TRANSVERSE FORAMEN
SUPERIOR ARTICULAR FACET
LAMINA (ARCH)
SPINOUS PROCESS

4TH CERVICAL VERTEBRA VIEWED FROM ABOVE

BODY
ANTERIOR TUBERCLE
POSTERIOR TUBERCLE
INFERIOR ARTICULAR PROCESS
SPINOUS PROCESS

7th CERVICAL VERTEBRA VIEWED FROM ABOVE

2
3
4
5
6
7
T 1

THE 2ND TO 7TH CERVICAL VERTEBRAE VIEWED FROM THE RIGHT SIDE

THE 3RD, 4TH and 5TH CERVICAL VERTEBRAE VIEWED FROM IN FRONT

The seven cervical vertebrae have in common a foramen through their transverse processes for the vertebral artery. The first and second cervical vertebrae have already been described (Plate 2, page 22).

The seventh cervical vertebra is distinctive because of its prominent spinous process. This process runs practically in a horizontal direction and at its lowest point serves as the lowermost attachment of the ligamentum nuchae.

The other four cervical vertebrae in common show a rather smooth body broader from side to side than in an antero-posterior diameter.

The anterior surface of the body of the vertebra overlaps the upper portion of the vertebra below. The upper surface of the body of the vertebra is concave with somewhat raised edges along its margins. The lower surface of the cervical body is concave from before backward but slightly convex from side to side.

The pedicles arise from the lateral posterior aspect midway between the upper and lower margins of the vertebral bodies.

The laminae are narrow and thin and meet in the posterior midline to form short bifid spinous processes. Projecting laterally from the junction of the pedicles and laminae are the articulating facets which have a superior and an inferior surface.

The superior articulating facet is directed upward and backward and somewhat medially while the inferior facet is directed forward, downward, and laterally.

Just anterior to the facets are the transverse processes through which runs an oval foramen, a passageway for the vertebral artery, vein, and sympathetic nerves.

On the extreme outer portion of the anterior transverse process is the anterior tubercle and on the extreme posterior process is the posterior tubercle. Between these tubercles is the groove for the outgoing spinal nerve.

PLATE 4

EXTERNAL CRANIO-CERVICAL LIGAMENTS

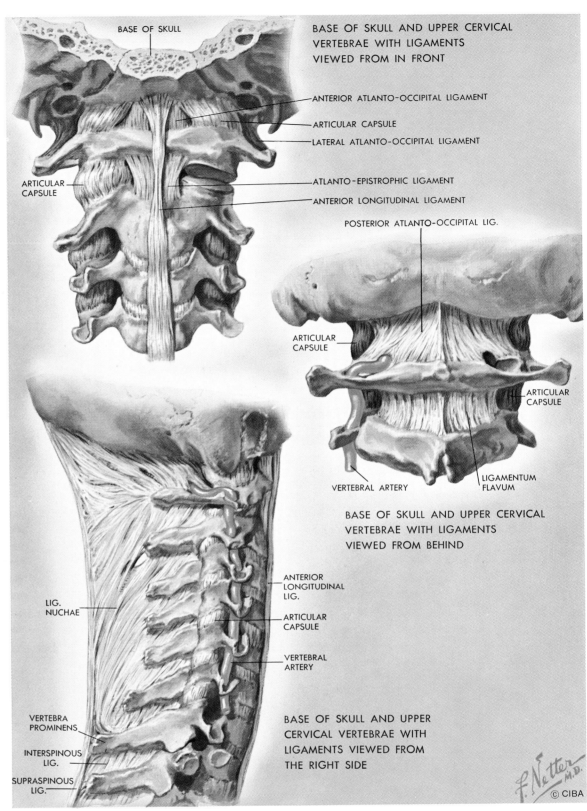

BASE OF SKULL

BASE OF SKULL AND UPPER CERVICAL VERTEBRAE WITH LIGAMENTS VIEWED FROM IN FRONT

ANTERIOR ATLANTO-OCCIPITAL LIGAMENT

ARTICULAR CAPSULE

LATERAL ATLANTO-OCCIPITAL LIGAMENT

ATLANTO-EPISTROPHIC LIGAMENT

ANTERIOR LONGITUDINAL LIGAMENT

ARTICULAR CAPSULE

POSTERIOR ATLANTO-OCCIPITAL LIG.

ARTICULAR CAPSULE

ARTICULAR CAPSULE

VERTEBRAL ARTERY

LIGAMENTUM FLAVUM

BASE OF SKULL AND UPPER CERVICAL VERTEBRAE WITH LIGAMENTS VIEWED FROM BEHIND

LIG. NUCHAE

ANTERIOR LONGITUDINAL LIG.

ARTICULAR CAPSULE

VERTEBRAL ARTERY

VERTEBRA PROMINENS

INTERSPINOUS LIG.

SUPRASPINOUS LIG.

BASE OF SKULL AND UPPER CERVICAL VERTEBRAE WITH LIGAMENTS VIEWED FROM THE RIGHT SIDE

These ligaments connect the cervical vertebrae with each other and with the cranium and are so constructed and arranged as to allow for gross and fine movements of the head and neck with freedom and security.

1. Ligamentum nuchae — is a strong, tense, fan-shaped structure stretching from the external occipital protuberance and median nuchal line down to, and in between, all the seven cervical vertebrae, giving off fibrous bands to the posterior tubercle of the atlas and the bifid spines. Joining the spinous processes of the cervical vertebrae from root to apex, it forms a septum in the midline between the muscles of the neck.

2. Anterior atlanto-occipital ligament — is a broad, dense band of fibers stretching from the anterior margin of the foramen magnum to the upper border of the anterior arch of the atlas and is continuous laterally with the articular capsule. It is reinforced at its midpoint by a rounded ligament stretching from the basilar portion of the occipital bone to the anterior

tubercle of the atlas.

3. Articular capsule — joins the posterior articular surfaces of the axis with the margins of the lateral masses of the atlas. The accessory ligament is a reinforcement of the posterior medial margin. These surround the condyles of the occipital bone and connect them with the articular processes of the atlas.

4. Lateral atlanto-occipital ligament — is a thickened portion of the articular capsule stretching from the jugular process of the occipital bone to the transverse process of the atlas.

5. Atlanto (axial)-epistrophic ligament — is a strong fibrous band extending from the anterior arch of the atlas to the front of the body of the axis. It is reinforced at its midpoint by a portion of the anterior longitudinal ligament.

6. Anterior longitudinal ligament — is a strong narrow band of fibrous tissue extending from the base of the skull down to the anterior midportion of the vertebral bodies to the sacrum. At each intervertebral space it is reinforced by fibers from the margins of the vertebral bodies and intervertebral discs.

7. Posterior atlanto-occipital ligament — is rather thin but broad and connects the margins of the foramen magnum with the upper margin of the posterior arch of the atlas. The vertebral artery and first cervical nerve pierce the lower lateral portion of this ligament to gain entry into the skull.

8. Ligamentum flavum — is also thin and broad and extends from the inner posterior margins of the vertebra above to the outer superior posterior margin of the vertebra below.

PLATE 5

INTERNAL CRANIO-CERVICAL LIGAMENTS

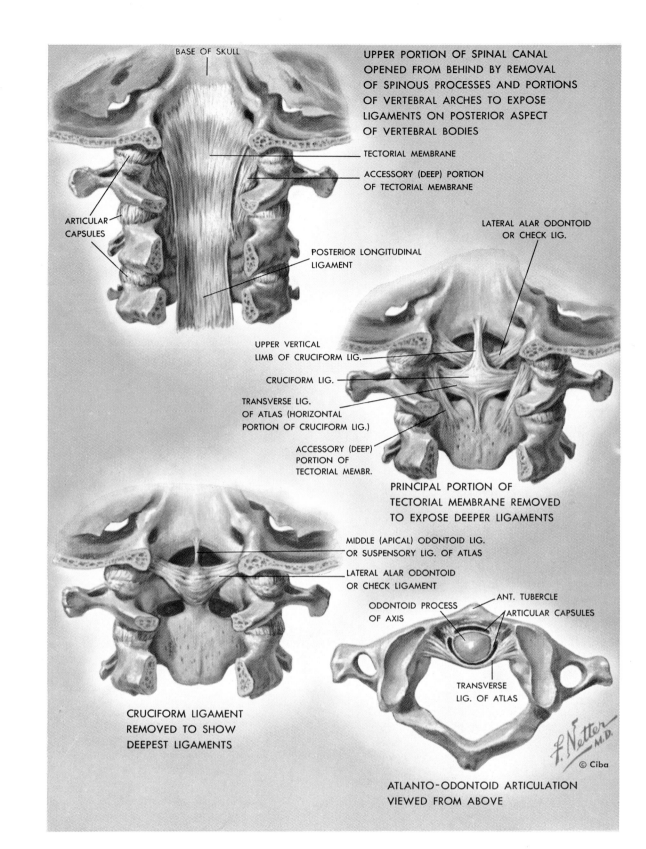

UPPER PORTION OF SPINAL CANAL OPENED FROM BEHIND BY REMOVAL OF SPINOUS PROCESSES AND PORTIONS OF VERTEBRAL ARCHES TO EXPOSE LIGAMENTS ON POSTERIOR ASPECT OF VERTEBRAL BODIES

BASE OF SKULL

TECTORIAL MEMBRANE

ACCESSORY (DEEP) PORTION OF TECTORIAL MEMBRANE

ARTICULAR CAPSULES

LATERAL ALAR ODONTOID OR CHECK LIG.

POSTERIOR LONGITUDINAL LIGAMENT

UPPER VERTICAL LIMB OF CRUCIFORM LIG.

CRUCIFORM LIG.

TRANSVERSE LIG. OF ATLAS (HORIZONTAL PORTION OF CRUCIFORM LIG.)

ACCESSORY (DEEP) PORTION OF TECTORIAL MEMBR.

PRINCIPAL PORTION OF TECTORIAL MEMBRANE REMOVED TO EXPOSE DEEPER LIGAMENTS

MIDDLE (APICAL) ODONTOID LIG. OR SUSPENSORY LIG. OF ATLAS

LATERAL ALAR ODONTOID OR CHECK LIGAMENT

ANT. TUBERCLE

ODONTOID PROCESS OF AXIS

ARTICULAR CAPSULES

CRUCIFORM LIGAMENT REMOVED TO SHOW DEEPEST LIGAMENTS

TRANSVERSE LIG. OF ATLAS

ATLANTO-ODONTOID ARTICULATION VIEWED FROM ABOVE

These ligaments also serve to permit safe and smooth movement of the head upon the neck, but in addition prevent and check trauma to the medulla oblongata and upper cervical cord.

1. Tectorial (ligament) membrane — is the upper portion of the posterior longitudinal ligament. It is fan-shaped, broad and strong and stretches from the basilar groove of the occipital bone downward over the posterior surfaces of the vertebral bodies. It covers the odontoid process, giving added strength to the transverse ligament of the atlas. This ligament has also an accessory (deep) portion with fibers more laterally placed and stretches from the lateral margins of the anterior foramen magnum to the upper postero-lateral portions of the body of the axis.

2. Posterior longitudinal ligament — is a downward continuation of the tectorial ligament forming the midportion of the posterior aspects of the vertebral bodies and receiving reinforcing fibers from the margins of the vertebral bodies and intervertebral discs.

3. Lateral alar odontoid (check) ligaments — are very strong fibrous bands which stretch from the medial aspects of the condyles of the occipital bone obliquely downward and inward to the upper lateral portions of the odontoid process. They limit rotation of the skull.

4. Cruciform ligament — has an upper vertical portion called the apical (suspensory) odontoid ligament which extends from the tip of the odontoid to midpoint of the anterior margin of the foramen magnum.

5. The transverse ligament of the atlas arises from a small tubercle on either side of the anterior arch of the atlas and stretches across and forms a sling across the posterior aspect of the odontoid holding it firmly to the facet of the mid-anterior arch. In fractures of the odontoid, this ligament usually prevents encroachment upon the cervical spinal cord and medulla.

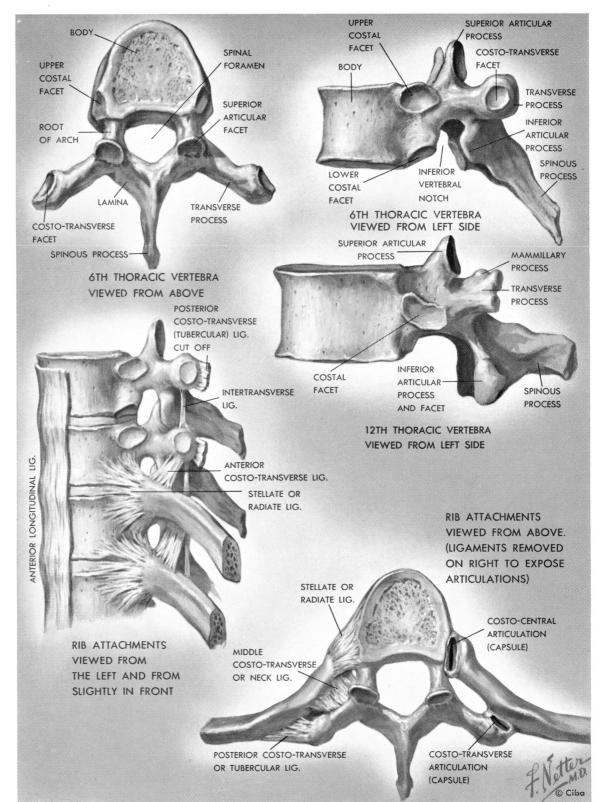

PLATE 6

THORACIC VERTEBRAE AND RIB ATTACHMENTS

The thoracic vertebrae, twelve in number, increase in size from above downward. They are distinctive in that their facets for articulation with the ribs are found on the transverse processes and vertebral bodies. The bodies of these vertebrae are thinner in front than behind and their anterior surfaces are concave and posterior surfaces are convex. In the upper thoracic vertebrae the costal facets are closer to the superior margin of the vertebral bodies and gradually are situated lower and posterior as they approach the lower thoracic cage. The pedicles of the thoracic vertebrae slant backward and upward forming a deep concavity called the inferior vertebral notch.

The upper and lower costal facets, located near the root of the pedicle, serve for articulation with the heads of the ribs. The laminae are short, broad, and fixed, with a tendency to overlap those below. At their junction with the pedicles lie the superior articular facets facing upward, backward and laterally to articulate with the corresponding inferior facets of the next higher vertebra which faces down-

ward, forward and medially.

There are several variations in articulating facets of some of the vertebrae. The articulation of the first thoracic vertebra varies in that there is an entire articular facet for the head of the first rib and a demifacet for the upper half of the head of the second rib. The eleventh thoracic vertebra varies only by having an articular facet on the pedicle and the twelfth thoracic vertebra variation consists of a convex inferior articular facet resembling the lumbar vertebra. The heads of the ribs articulate with the vertebral bodies, whereas the neck and tubercles of the ribs articulate with the facets of the transverse processes. The spinous processes are long and directed downward, at first overlapping one another, then becoming more horizontal below the eighth thoracic vertebra.

To increase the stability and motion at the various points of articulation a series of ligaments function for security. The stellate (radiate) ligament joins the anterior portion of the head of the ribs with the sides of the vertebral bodies above and below as well as with the intervertebral disc. The intertransverse ligament runs vertically joining the tips of the adjacent transverse process. The costo-transverse ligament has three bands: (1) anterior — joining the upper portion of the neck of the ribs to the lower border of the transverse process of the vertebra above, (2) middle — joining the posterior aspect of the neck of the rib to the adjacent anterior surface of the transverse process, and (3) posterior — which runs upward and backward and joins the neck of the ribs to the base of the transverse process.

PLATE 7

LUMBAR VERTEBRAE

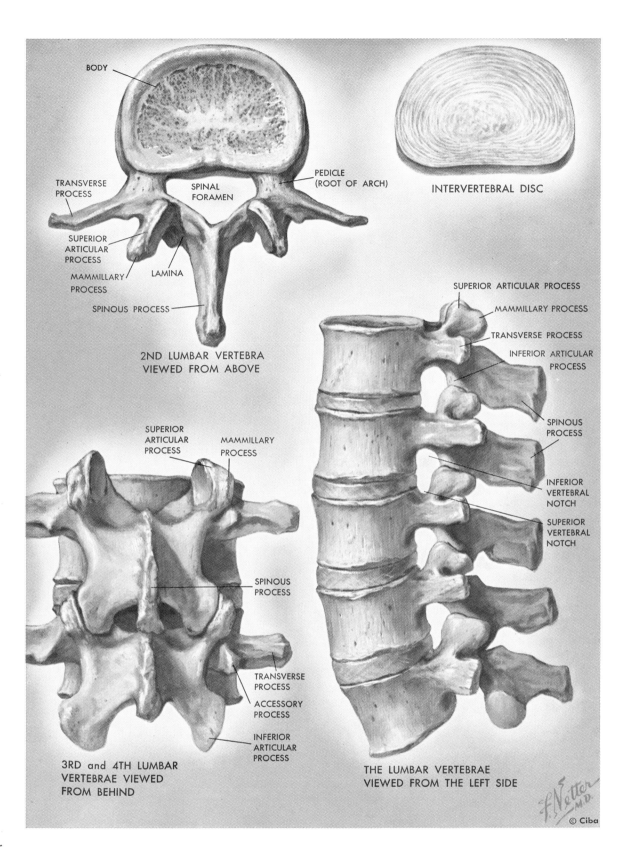

BODY

TRANSVERSE
PROCESS

SPINAL
FORAMEN

PEDICLE
(ROOT OF ARCH)

INTERVERTEBRAL DISC

SUPERIOR
ARTICULAR
PROCESS

MAMMILLARY
PROCESS

LAMINA

SPINOUS PROCESS

2ND LUMBAR VERTEBRA
VIEWED FROM ABOVE

SUPERIOR ARTICULAR PROCESS

MAMMILLARY PROCESS

TRANSVERSE PROCESS

INFERIOR ARTICULAR
PROCESS

SPINOUS
PROCESS

INFERIOR
VERTEBRAL
NOTCH

SUPERIOR
VERTEBRAL
NOTCH

SUPERIOR
ARTICULAR
PROCESS

MAMMILLARY
PROCESS

SPINOUS
PROCESS

TRANSVERSE
PROCESS

ACCESSORY
PROCESS

INFERIOR
ARTICULAR
PROCESS

3RD and 4TH LUMBAR
VERTEBRAE VIEWED
FROM BEHIND

THE LUMBAR VERTEBRAE
VIEWED FROM THE LEFT SIDE

The lumbar vertebrae, five in number, are large and massive because of their weight-bearing function and are chiefly characterized by having no foramen in their transverse processes and no articular facets on their vertebral bodies. The lumbar curve is convex anteriorly with interposing fibrocartilaginous discs for mobility.

The spinal foramen in the lumbar region is triangular in shape though smaller than in the cervical region. The body of each lumbar vertebra is narrower from before backward and wider from side to side. It is slightly taller anteriorly than posteriorly, and shows more concavity above than below. The pedicles arise from either side of the upper portion of the vertebral body. They are short, strong and proceed directly backward with grooves above and below forming the superior and inferior vertebral notches. These join to form foraminae for the exit of the spinal nerves.

Springing from the pedicles are the short, broad and powerful laminae which meet in the midline to form the spinous process. This process is thick and broad and directed backward in an almost horizontal direction.

At the base of the laminae are the articular facets. The superior articular facet is concave and directed medially and backward whereas the inferior articular facet is directed forward and laterally. The transverse processes which arise from the pedicles are comparatively slender and are situated in front of the articular processes. On the posterior superior aspect of the articular facets are slight elevations called mammillary processes. A similar elevation on the posterior aspect of the transverse process is called the accessory process.

The intervertebral disc, a fibrocartilaginous structure, acts as a cushion between the adjacent vertebral bodies. It varies in size and shape and conforms to the corresponding vertebral body. These discs are thickest in the lumbar region, increasing in size as they approach the sacrum.

The fibrocartilaginous tissue is concentrically arranged with a thick and tough outer layer called the annulus fibrosus and a soft gelatinous pulpy substance called the nucleus pulposus, the remains of the notochord. The intervertebral discs are particularly poor in blood supply.

PLATE 8

LIGAMENTS OF THE SPINAL COLUMN

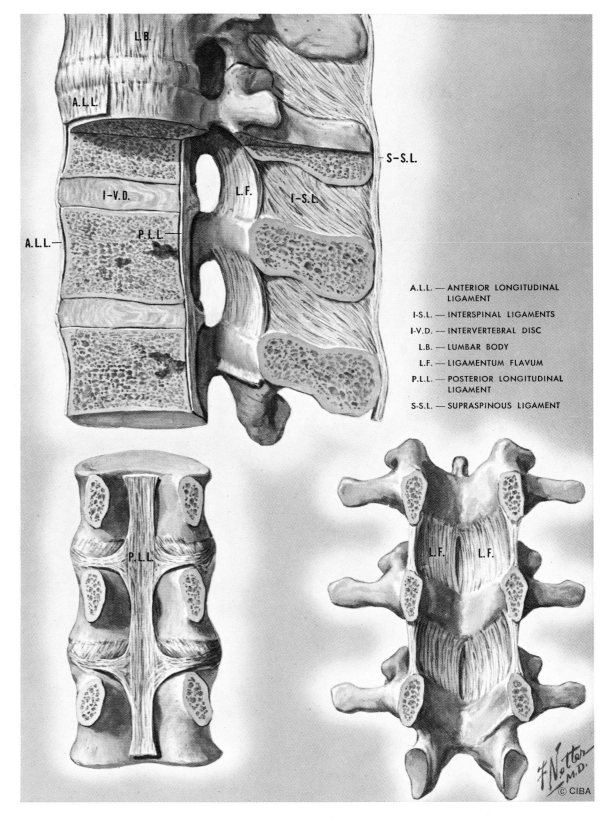

A.L.L. — ANTERIOR LONGITUDINAL LIGAMENT
I-S.L. — INTERSPINAL LIGAMENTS
I-V.D. — INTERVERTEBRAL DISC
L.B. — LUMBAR BODY
L.F. — LIGAMENTUM FLAVUM
P.L.L. — POSTERIOR LONGITUDINAL LIGAMENT
S-S.L. — SUPRASPINOUS LIGAMENT

The vertebrae are held together by a series of overlapping ligaments which not only surround the vertebral column, but aid in protecting the spinal cord. These ligaments are strong fibrous bands varying in width and strength, depending upon the function they are called upon to perform.

1. Anterior longitudinal ligament starts at the axis as a continuation of the anterior atlanto-axial ligament and extends down the entire rounded front of the bodies of the vertebrae to the sacrum intimately attached to the margins of the vertebral bodies. It is thickest in the thoracic region, less so at the cervical and lumbar levels.

2. Posterior longitudinal ligament begins on the posterior surface of the vertebral body of the axis, and extends centrally down the entire length, hugging the vertebral margins and intervertebral structures. At the margins of the vertebral bodies it fans out to reinforce these intervertebral structures. This ligament is thinnest in the cervical and lumbar regions.

3. Intervertebral fibrocartilages (discs) are interposed between the adjacent vertebral surfaces from the axis to the upper border of the sacrum. Although they vary greatly in shape, size and thickness, they conform generally to the vertebral surfaces between which they lie. They allow for great mobility in the cervical and lumbar regions, and help absorb the stress and strain transmitted to the spinal column. The discs are thicker in front, are surrounded by a thick capsule called the annulus fibrosus and are intimately attached to the hyaline cartilage of the adjacent vertebrae. Laterally, they are reinforced by the interarticular ligaments.

4. Ligamentum flavum is found to either side of the spinous process and extends laterally to the articular facets. Each is attached to the posterior margins of the lamina below and ascends obliquely to the undersurface of the lamina above. These ligaments are thinnest in the cervical region and increase in thickness as they approach the lower lumbar area.

5. Supraspinous ligament joins the tips of the spinous processes from the seventh cervical vertebra to the sacrum. It is dense and fibrous and increases in thickness and width as it approaches the lumbar region. This ligament is a continuation of the ligamentum nuchae and fuses with the interspinal ligaments.

6. Interspinal ligaments connect the adjoining spinous processes from their tips to their roots. They fuse with the supraspinous ligaments posteriorly and with the ligamentum flavum anteriorly. They are much wider and denser in the lumbar region.

PLATE 9

SACRUM AND COCCYX

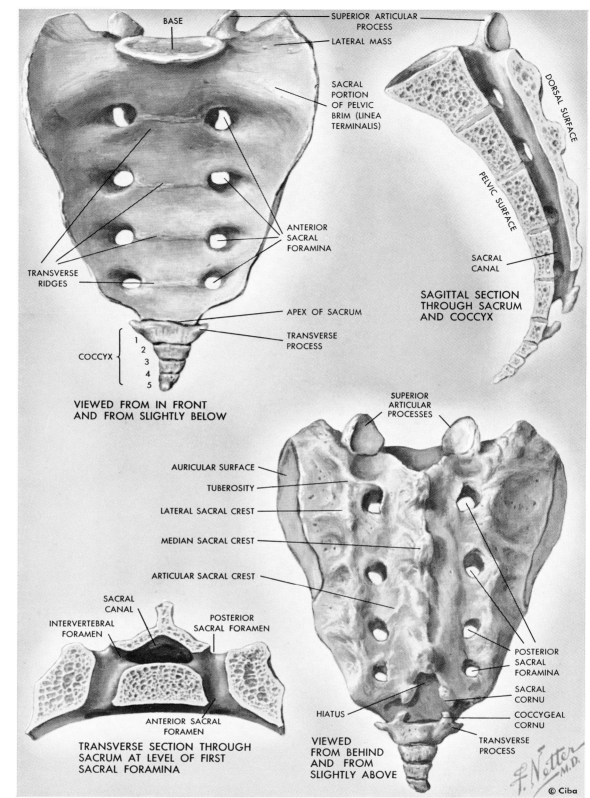

BASE

SUPERIOR ARTICULAR PROCESS

LATERAL MASS

SACRAL PORTION OF PELVIC BRIM (LINEA TERMINALIS)

DORSAL SURFACE

PELVIC SURFACE

SACRAL CANAL

SAGITTAL SECTION THROUGH SACRUM AND COCCYX

ANTERIOR SACRAL FORAMINA

TRANSVERSE RIDGES

APEX OF SACRUM

TRANSVERSE PROCESS

COCCYX 1 2 3 4 5

VIEWED FROM IN FRONT AND FROM SLIGHTLY BELOW

SUPERIOR ARTICULAR PROCESSES

AURICULAR SURFACE

TUBEROSITY

LATERAL SACRAL CREST

MEDIAN SACRAL CREST

ARTICULAR SACRAL CREST

SACRAL CANAL

INTERVERTEBRAL FORAMEN

POSTERIOR SACRAL FORAMEN

POSTERIOR SACRAL FORAMINA

SACRAL CORNU

COCCYGEAL CORNU

HIATUS

TRANSVERSE PROCESS

ANTERIOR SACRAL FORAMEN

TRANSVERSE SECTION THROUGH SACRUM AT LEVEL OF FIRST SACRAL FORAMINA

VIEWED FROM BEHIND AND FROM SLIGHTLY ABOVE

In the adult, the sacrum articulates with the fifth lumbar vertebra, the coccyx and the two hip bones. It is large, triangular and wedge-shaped and forms the posterior wall of the pelvis. Its base is oval-shaped and articulates with the inferior aspect of the body of the fifth lumbar vertebra, forming the prominent sacral vertebral angle. To either side of the sacrum are triangular areas called the alae. Just below and to either side of the base is a ridge forming the sacral portion of the pelvic brim. The lower portion of the sacrum, the apex, articulates with the coccyx.

The pelvic surface of the sacrum is concave in both dimensions, vertically and horizontally. At its middle it is grooved with four transverse ridges which mark the points of fusion of the original five vertebrae. Four anterior sacral foraminae on either side of the ridges permit passage of the anterior division of the sacral nerve and the lateral sacral arteries.

A cross-sagittal section of the sacrum demonstrates the sacral canal which encloses the lower portion of the dura and contents, the roots of the cauda equina, the filum terminale externum, fat, areolar tissue, blood vessels and fine nerve filaments.

The middle of the dorsal surface is marked by the sacral crest, the rudimentary spinous processes of the sacral vertebrae. Because the lower sacral laminae may not fuse, a hiatus may be found in the lower portion. To either side of the median sacral crest are the articular sacral crests, the remains of the fused articular processes. The lateral sacral crests represent the remains of the fused transverse processes.

The superior articular processes are large, oval, and face backward and medially. At the lowest portion the sacral cornua represent the inferior articular processes of the fifth sacral vertebra. The posterior sacral foraminae lie to either side of the median sacral crest and allow for the exit of the posterior division of the sacral nerves. The lateral sacral surface is also triangular, broadest at top, where is found an ear-shaped

articulating facet for the ilium. The sacral canal is triangular and cone-shaped as it descends toward the lower end of the sacrum.

The coccyx is made up of four rudimentary vertebrae with rudimentary body, articulating facets and transverse processes. The upper portion articulates with the sacrum and in triangular fashion diminishes in size until it reaches its lowest portion called the apex. The concave anterior surface shows three transverse grooves and the posterior convex surface shows rudimentary processes. Two remnants of articulating processes, the cornua, are found at the upper end of the coccyx. Through the hiatus runs the posterior division of the fifth sacral nerve. At the extreme lateral portions of the coccyx are the remains of the transverse processes called eminences.

PLATE 10

LIGAMENTS OF THE SACRUM AND COCCYX

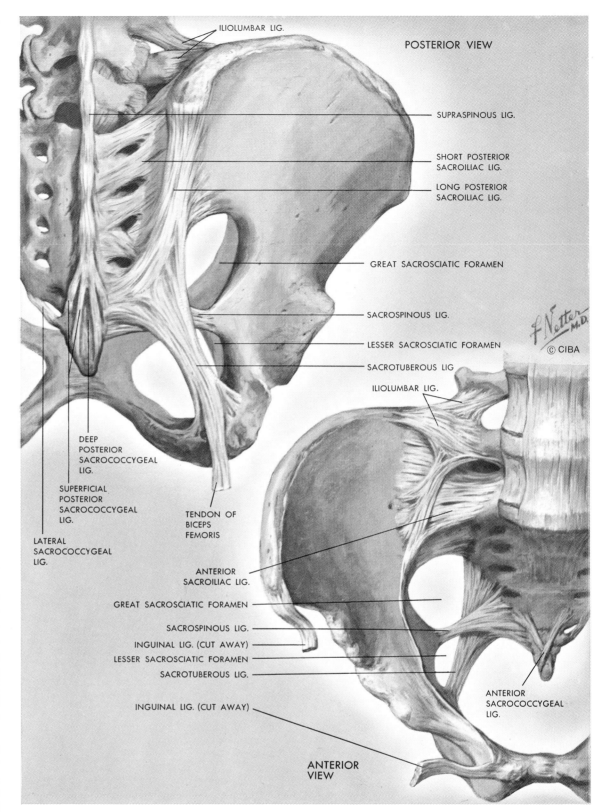

ILIOLUMBAR LIG.

POSTERIOR VIEW

SUPRASPINOUS LIG.

SHORT POSTERIOR SACROILIAC LIG.

LONG POSTERIOR SACROILIAC LIG.

GREAT SACROSCIATIC FORAMEN

SACROSPINOUS LIG.

LESSER SACROSCIATIC FORAMEN

SACROTUBEROUS LIG

ILIOLUMBAR LIG.

DEEP POSTERIOR SACROCOCCYGEAL LIG.

SUPERFICIAL POSTERIOR SACROCOCCYGEAL LIG.

LATERAL SACROCOCCYGEAL LIG.

TENDON OF BICEPS FEMORIS

ANTERIOR SACROILIAC LIG.

GREAT SACROSCIATIC FORAMEN

SACROSPINOUS LIG.

INGUINAL LIG. (CUT AWAY)

LESSER SACROSCIATIC FORAMEN

SACROTUBEROUS LIG.

INGUINAL LIG. (CUT AWAY)

ANTERIOR SACROCOCCYGEAL LIG.

ANTERIOR VIEW

The ligaments of the sacrum and coccyx are a network of fibrous bands which at points fuse and intermingle to give added strength to the wedge of the pelvis.

1. Supraspinous ligaments are dense fibrous bands joining the spinous processes of the sacrum. They fan out to become continuous with the superficial posterior sacrococcygeal ligament, which originates at the upper margin of the sacral hiatus and inserts into the posterior surface of the coccyx. Near its lower end it divides to form the deep posterior sacrococcygeal ligament.

2. Iliolumbar ligament extends as two bands from the undersurface of the transverse process of the fifth lumbar vertebra, one going to the upper portion of the iliac crest and blending with the long and short posterior sacroiliac ligaments at their iliac junction, and the other to the base of the sacrum joining the fibers of the anterior sacroiliac ligament.

3. Short posterior sacroiliac ligaments, a series of small fibrous bands radiate obliquely upward and then horizontally from the first and second transverse processes of the sacrum to the tuberosity of the ilium.

4. Long posterior sacroiliac ligaments consist of numerous fasciculi running in vertical and oblique directions from the main bonds of the sacrum to the ilium.

5. Sacrospinous ligament, triangular in shape, stretches from the lateral margin of the sacrum and coccyx to the apex of the ischial spine and crosses like a sling in front of the sacrotuberous ligament thereby forming the great sacrosciatic foramen above and the lesser sacrosciatic foramen below.

6. Sacrotuberous ligament is triangular, flat and narrow in the middle and originates from a wide margin along the fourth and fifth transverse tubercles of the sacrum and lower portion of the lateral margins of the sacrum and coccyx. It radiates obliquely downward, laterally and forward to insert into the inner margin of the ischial tuberosity. Beyond this point, the ligament continues and thickens to become the tendon of the long head of the biceps femoris.

7. The anterior portion of the iliolumbar ligament stretching from the undersurface of the transverse process of the fifth lumbar vertebra to the iliac crest and blending with the fibers of the anterior sacroiliac ligament.

8. Anterior sacroiliac ligament consists of numerous thin bands joining the anterior surface of the lateral portion of the sacrum to the margin of the auricular surface of the ilium.

9. Anterior sacrococcygeal ligament consists of irregular fibers descending like crossed slings from the lower anterior surface of the sacrum to anterior and lateral aspects of the coccyx.

10. Inguinal ligament is the reflected lower aponeurotic margin of the external oblique muscle and stretches from the anterior superior iliac spine to the pubic tubercle. In its posterolateral half it is round and cord-like, but more anteriorly it becomes wider and thinner and lies beneath the spermatic cord.

Section II

THE CENTRAL NERVOUS SYSTEM

with descriptive text by

ABRAHAM KAPLAN, M.D., F.A.C.S., D.N.S.

Clinical Professor of Neurosurgery

New York Polyclinic Medical School and Hospital

New York, N. Y.

PLATE II

DURA MATER AND MIDDLE MENINGEAL ARTERY

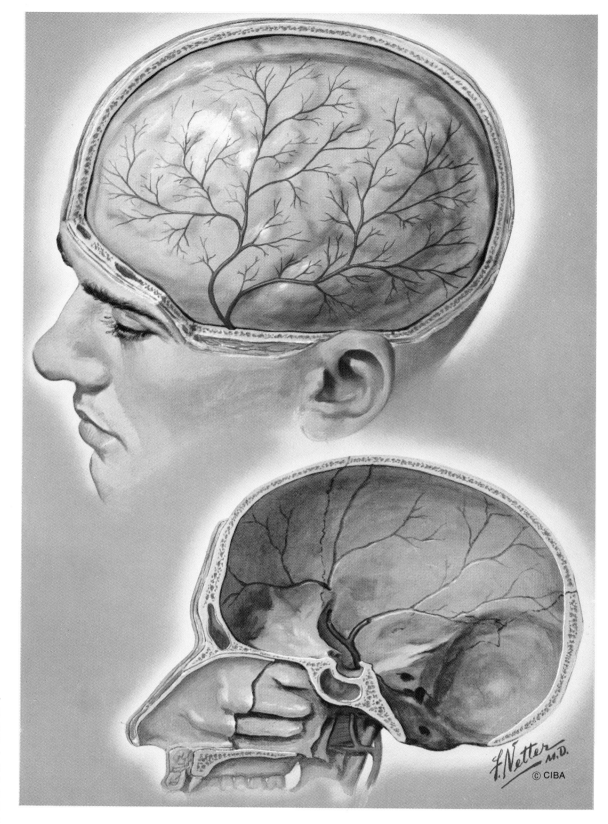

The dura mater is a shiny, tough, inelastic membrane which envelops the brain and by various folds separates the skull into adjoining compartments: (1) the falx cerebri descends vertically between the two cerebral hemispheres, is arch-shaped and attached most anteriorly to the crista galli, with its upper margin to the inner surface of the calvarium, and extends posteriorly to the internal occipital protuberance. Along the upper margin it forms a channel for the superior longitudinal sinus. The inferior margin of the falx is free, forming the channel for the inferior sagittal sinus, (2) the tentorium cerebelli is a tent-like fold which supports and separates the occipital lobes from the cerebellum. The upper convex margins, attached to the occipital bone, enclose the transverse or lateral sinus. Anteriorly it is attached to the temporal bone up to the posterior clinoid processes. Its inferior margin encloses the superior petrosal sinus, (3) the falx cerebelli is triangular and separates both cerebellar hemispheres. It is adherent superiorly to the inner margin of the occipital bone and inferiorly fuses with the dura of the

foramen magnum. Through it runs (4) the occipital sinus, stretching horizontally and joining the anterior and posterior clinoid of the sella turcica is the diaphragma sellae, separating the hypophysis from the optic chiasm and third ventricle. Through a central opening traverses the infundibulum.

At the base of the brain the dura is fused with the internal periosteum. The cranial nerves at their points of exit are enveloped by a cuff of dura. At the margin of the foramen magnum, the adherent dura becomes continuous with the spinal dura. The dura consists of two layers — the outer or endosteal layer adherent to the skull and the meningeal layer which is in close apposition to the brain.

The main blood supply, the middle meningeal artery, a branch of the internal maxillary artery, enters the skull through the foramen spinosum of the sphenoid bone. The accessory meningeal artery is

sometimes derived from the middle meningeal artery, but enters the skull through the foramen ovale, branching to the dura and to the Gasserian ganglia. The anterior meningeal artery, a branch of the ethmoidal vessels originating from the internal carotid artery, supplies the anterior fossa, the covering dura. The posterior meningeal artery, a branch of the occipital artery, enters the skull through the jugular foramen, and supplies the dura in the posterior fossa. These vessels also supply the bones through which they course, and their terminal branches anastomose with the corresponding vessels on the opposite side.

The returning veins anastomose with diploic veins, terminating in various sinuses. The dural veins communicate with the underlying cerebral veins, emissary veins, and diploe of the skull.

For the most part, the dura is insensitive except in the region of the traversing blood vessels.

PLATE 12

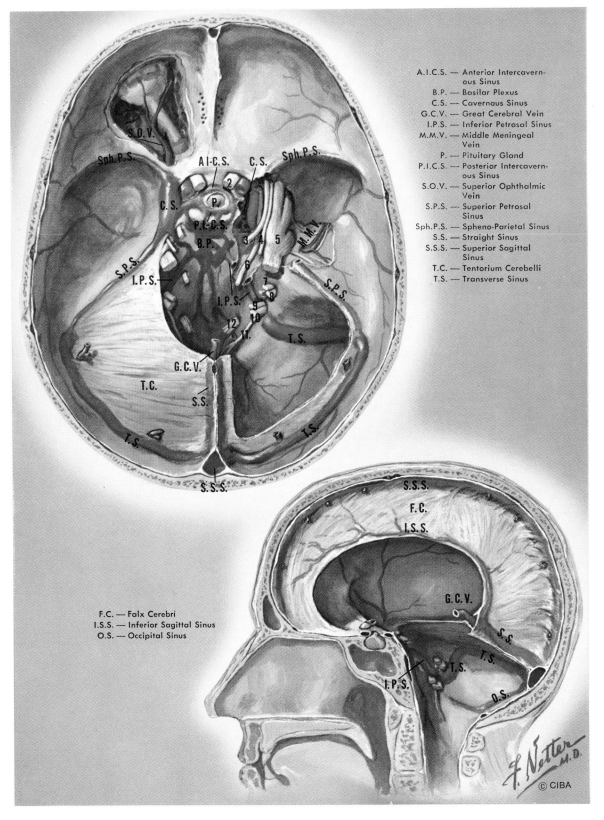

A.I.C.S. — Anterior Intercavern-
     ous Sinus
B.P. — Basilar Plexus
C.S. — Cavernous Sinus
G.C.V. — Great Cerebral Vein
I.P.S. — Inferior Petrosal Sinus
M.M.V. — Middle Meningeal
     Vein
P. — Pituitary Gland
P.I.C.S. — Posterior Intercavern-
     ous Sinus
S.O.V. — Superior Ophthalmic
     Vein
S.P.S. — Superior Petrosal
     Sinus
Sph.P.S. — Spheno-Parietal Sinus
S.S. — Straight Sinus
S.S.S. — Superior Sagittal
     Sinus
T.C. — Tentorium Cerebelli
T.S. — Transverse Sinus

F.C. — Falx Cerebri
I.S.S. — Inferior Sagittal Sinus
O.S. — Occipital Sinus

Venous Sinuses

Sinus Durae Matris

Two main groups of venous channels draining blood from the brain are encased between two dural layers.

The superior-posterior group consists of five dural sinuses:

1. Superior sagittal sinus originates at the foramen cecum with a tributary from the nasal cavity. It continues in a groove of the skull, encased within the superior margin of the falx cerebri until it approaches the occipital protuberance. There it forms the confluence of sinuses, and continues as the transverse sinus. It receives tributaries from the superior cerebral veins which, in some portions, first empty into three irregularly shaped venous spaces (venous lacuna) on either side of the sinus or into smaller lacunae or through arachnoid granulations.

2. Inferior sagittal sinus runs along the lower crescentic margin of the falx, increases in size, receiving several veins from the falx and small veins from the cerebral hemispheres. It joins the straight sinus.

3. The straight sinus runs in a dural fold at the junction of the falx cerebri and tentorium cerebelli to the occipital protuberance, where it empties into the transverse sinus receiving the great cerebral vein.

4. The two transverse sinuses are the continuation of the superior sagittal sinus (the larger) and the straight sinus (the smaller). Both curve along the groove on either side of the occipital bone, then more anteriorly in the squama of the occipital bone and mastoid parts of the parietal and temporal bone (sigmoid sinus) to end at the jugular foramen. Both receive blood from the superior petrosal

sinuses, the mastoid and condyloid emissaries, inferior cerebral and cerebellar veins (anchoring veins) and diploic veins.

5. The occipital sinus in the falx cerebelli arises by small veins from the foramen magnum, increases in size while following the cerebellar hemisphere, and empties into the confluence of sinuses.

The anterior-inferior group consists of four paired sinuses and one plexus:

1. The cavernous sinuses on both sides of the sphenoid bone are reticulated structures, beginning at the superior orbital fissure with tributaries from superior ophthalmic vein and some small cerebral veins. They empty into the superior petrosal sinus. On their most medial aspects lies the internal carotid artery. Just lateral to this artery is the abducens nerve and more laterally pass the oculomotor, trochlear, ophthalmic, and maxillary nerves.

2. Intercavernous sinuses: The anterior part passes in front, the posterior behind the hypophysis. Both join, forming the circular sinus.

3. Superior petrosal sinus connects the cavernous with the transverse sinus, runs in the margin of the tentorium cerebelli, and crosses the trigeminal nerve, receiving veins from the tympanic cavity, cerebellum and inferior cerebral parts.

4. Inferior petrosal sinus begins at the cavernous sinus, passes through the jugular foramen and ends of the internal jugular vein, receiving the internal auditory vein, veins from the medulla oblongata, pons, and cerebellum.

5. Basilar plexus lies over the basilar portion of the occipital bone, consists of interlacing venous channels, communicating with the two inferior petrosal sinuses, and drains blood from the anterior vertebral plexus.

PLATE 13

ARACHNOID
AND PIA MATER

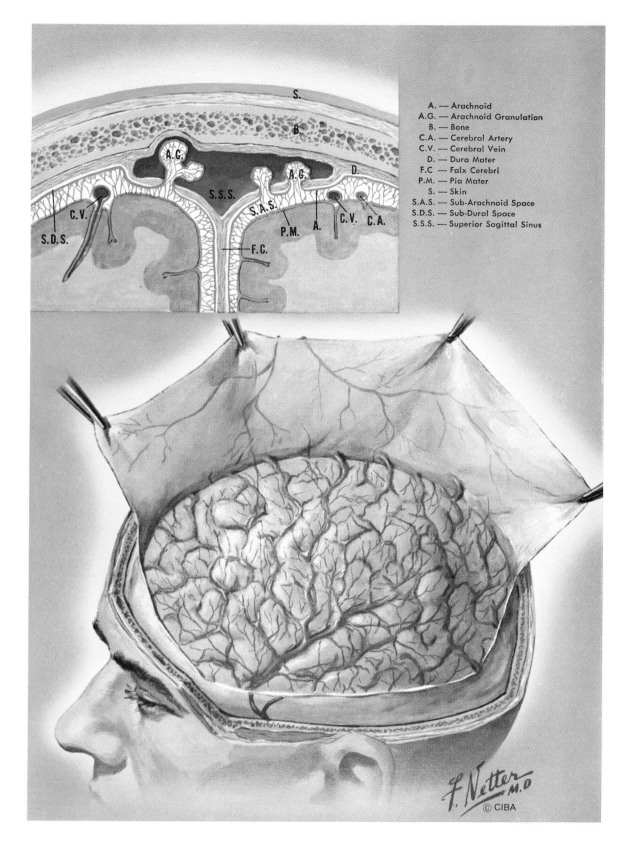

A. — Arachnoid
A.G. — Arachnoid Granulation
B. — Bone
C.A. — Cerebral Artery
C.V. — Cerebral Vein
D. — Dura Mater
F.C — Falx Cerebri
P.M. — Pia Mater
S. — Skin
S.A.S. — Sub-Arachnoid Space
S.D.S. — Sub-Dural Space
S.S.S. — Superior Sagittal Sinus

Between the dura mater and pia mater is a fine membrane, the arachnoid. It consists of two layers of fibrous and elastic tissue with low or flattened cuboidal mesothelium. It does not follow the folds and fissures of the brain, is thin and transparent over the superior surface, thicker and more opaque toward the base.

Between the layers is a spongy structure containing subarachnoid fluid, the subarachnoid space. In the grooves between the gyri the fluid is more abundant, particularly at the base of the brain. There the more freely communicating compartments form the subarachnoid cisternae: (1) the cisterna magna bridges the medulla oblongata, (2) the cisterna pontis lies on the anterior surface of the pons, (3) the cisterna interpeduncularis is located at the medial surfaces of the temporal lobes, (4) the cisterna chiasmatica surrounds the optic chiasm, (5) the cisterna fossae cerebri lateralis bridges the lateral fissure of the temporal lobes, and (6) the cisterna venae magnae cerebri occupies the space between the corpus callosum and the cerebellum.

Between the arachnoid and dura is a noncommunicating space, the subdural space. The cerebral veins traversing this space have little supporting structure and hence are most vulnerable at this point. Hemorrhage accumulating here has no pathway of escape.

Arachnoidal villi (pacchionian bodies), cluster-like projections of the dura, protrude into the superior sagittal or transverse sinus. These appear about the age of seven and increase in number and size until adult life. They push their way into the sinus, thinning out the dura and inner table of the skull. Their mesothelium serves as the pathway for the fluid into the venous system.

The pia mater, a very fine membrane rich in minute blood plexuses and mesothelial cells, is associated with the arachnoid and covers the brain intimately, following the invaginations of all sulci and conformations of the gyri.

By its various invaginations it helps form the tela choroidea, the choroid plexuses of the lateral third and fourth ventricles.

PLATE 14

BLOOD SUPPLY OF THE BRAIN

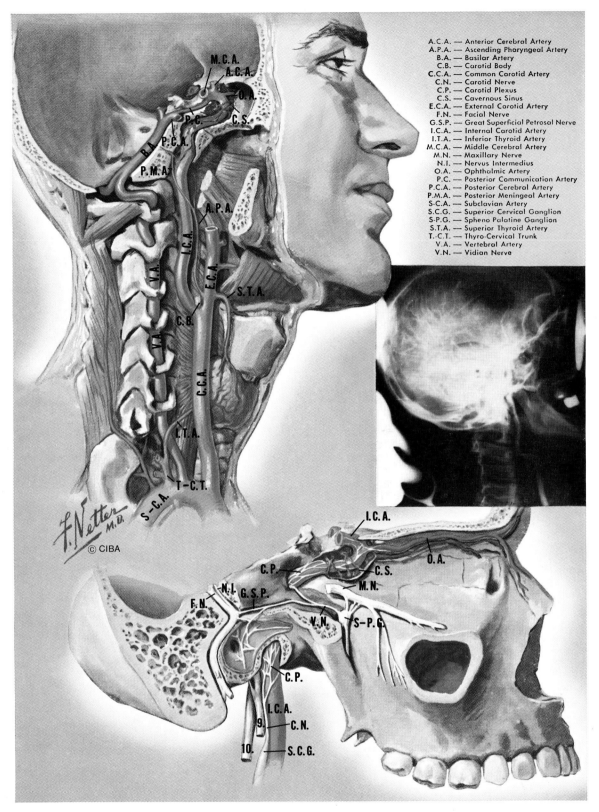

The internal carotid artery supplies the anterior portion and the vertebral artery supplies the posterior portion of the brain.

The internal carotid artery arises from the common carotid artery at the level of the thyroid cartilage, runs upward in the neck to the base of the skull without giving off any branches. At the base of the skull it lies anterior to the vagus, spinal accessory, hypoglossal, glossopharyngeal nerves, superior cervical ganglion, and internal jugular vein. Entering the carotid canal of the petrous bone, it curves forward and medially to the cochlea and tympanic cavity and is surrounded by numerous minute veins, filaments of the carotid plexus, branches of the superior cervical ganglion, and sympathetic trunk. From the middle cranial fossa, it proceeds

in the carotid groove lateral to the sphenoid bone, where it is encased between dural layers and enveloped by the cavernous sinus. At this point the artery sends off small vessels to the hypophysis, semilunar ganglion, cavernous sinus and petrosal sinus. Shortly thereafter it gives off the anterior meningeal artery. Just as the internal carotid artery emerges from the cavernous sinus, there issues the ophthalmic branch which lies medial to the anterior clinoid process, enters the orbital cavity through the optic foramen, and supplies the eyeball, ocular muscles and adjacent structures. Leaving the roof of the cavernous sinus, the internal carotid artery, again surrounded by sympathetic nerves, passes forward between the optic and the oculomotor nerves to reach the anterior perforated substance. At this point originate the following main cerebral branches:

1. Anterior cerebral artery passes forward and me-

dially across the anterior perforated substance above the optic nerve toward the longitudinal fissure. After joining its corresponding vessel by the short anterior communicating artery, the two arteries run parallel in the longitudinal fissure, curve upward and around the genu, and then backward along the superior surface of the corpus callosum to its posterior limits. In its course on the medial surface of the hemisphere it sends branches to the frontal and olfactory lobes, the rectus and internal orbital gyri, the cingular, superior frontal and central gyri, and then proceeds upward over the edge of the hemisphere at the superior and middle frontal gyri and upper portion of the anterior central gyrus. This vessel also supplies the corpus callosum, and its terminal portion sends twigs to the precuneus and adjacent lateral surface of the hemisphere, and finally ends by anastomosing with the posterior cerebral artery. *(Continued on following page)*

PLATE 15

BLOOD SUPPLY OF THE BRAIN
(continued)

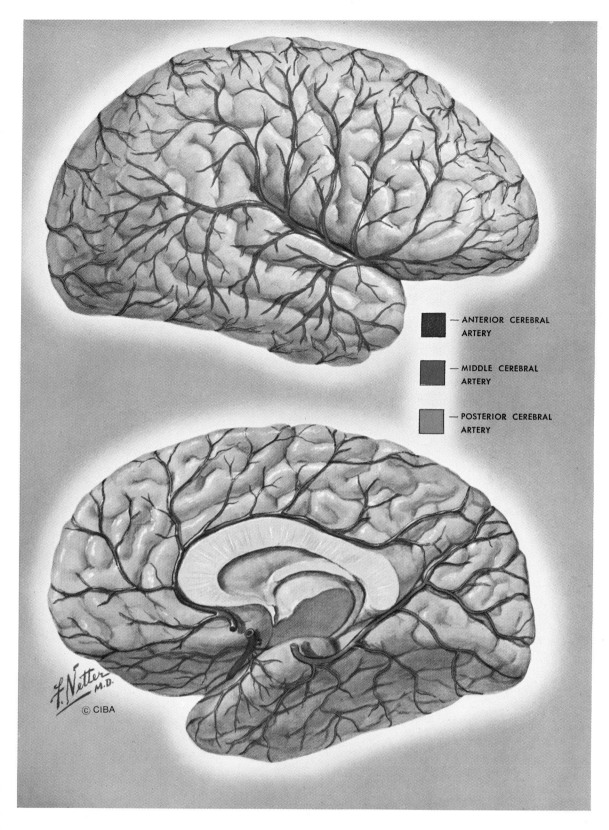

— ANTERIOR CEREBRAL ARTERY

— MIDDLE CEREBRAL ARTERY

— POSTERIOR CEREBRAL ARTERY

2. Middle cerebral artery. The largest branch of the internal carotid artery proceeds laterally in the Sylvian fissure, sending branches to the corpus striatum and internal capsule, and in its lateral portion gives off the lenticular striate artery (the artery of cerebral apoplexy) which has two main groups of finer branches, the lateral lenticular striate artery and the medial lenticular striate artery (Plate 16, page 38). It continues in its course backward and upward over the surface of the insula, and sends branches to the ventral surface of the frontal and upper surface of the temporal lobe. As it spreads over the cortex the branches supply the inferior frontal gyrus, the lateral portion of the orbital surface of the frontal lobe, the anterior central and posterior central gyrus, the lower portion of the superior parietal lobe, the supramarginal and angular gyri, the posterior portion of the superior and middle temporal gyri, and the lateral surface of the temporal lobe.

3. Posterior communicating artery arises from the internal carotid artery near the optic tract, crosses the latter anteriorly to join the posterior cerebral artery, the main branch of the basilar artery.

4. Anterior choroidal artery arises near the origin of the posterior communicating artery and passes backward and laterally between the temporal lobe and cerebral peduncle, enters the inferior horn of the lateral ventricle, and terminates in the formation of the choroid plexus.

Vertebral artery, a branch of the subclavian, ascends through the foramina of the transverse processes of the upper six cervical vertebrae, winds behind the articular process of the atlas and enters the skull through the foramen magnum. It then continues forward on the anterior surface of the medulla oblongata, and after uniting with the corresponding vessel on the opposite side at the lower border of the pons, it becomes the basilar artery.

The cranial branches of the vertebral artery are:

1. Posterior inferior cerebellar artery (the artery of thrombosis) winds around the medulla to reach the inferior surface of the cerebellum. Thrombosis of this artery results in a well-recognized clinical syndrome.

2. Posterior spinal artery arises near the side of the medulla oblongata, curves around its posterior aspect and descends downward on the dorsal surface of the spinal cord between the midline and dorsal roots.

3. Meningeal branch is formed by the union of two smaller branches near the foramen magnum, and runs between the occipital bone and the dura of the posterior fossa, sending branches also to the falx cerebelli. *(Concluded on following page)*

PLATE 16

BLOOD SUPPLY
OF THE BRAIN
(concluded)

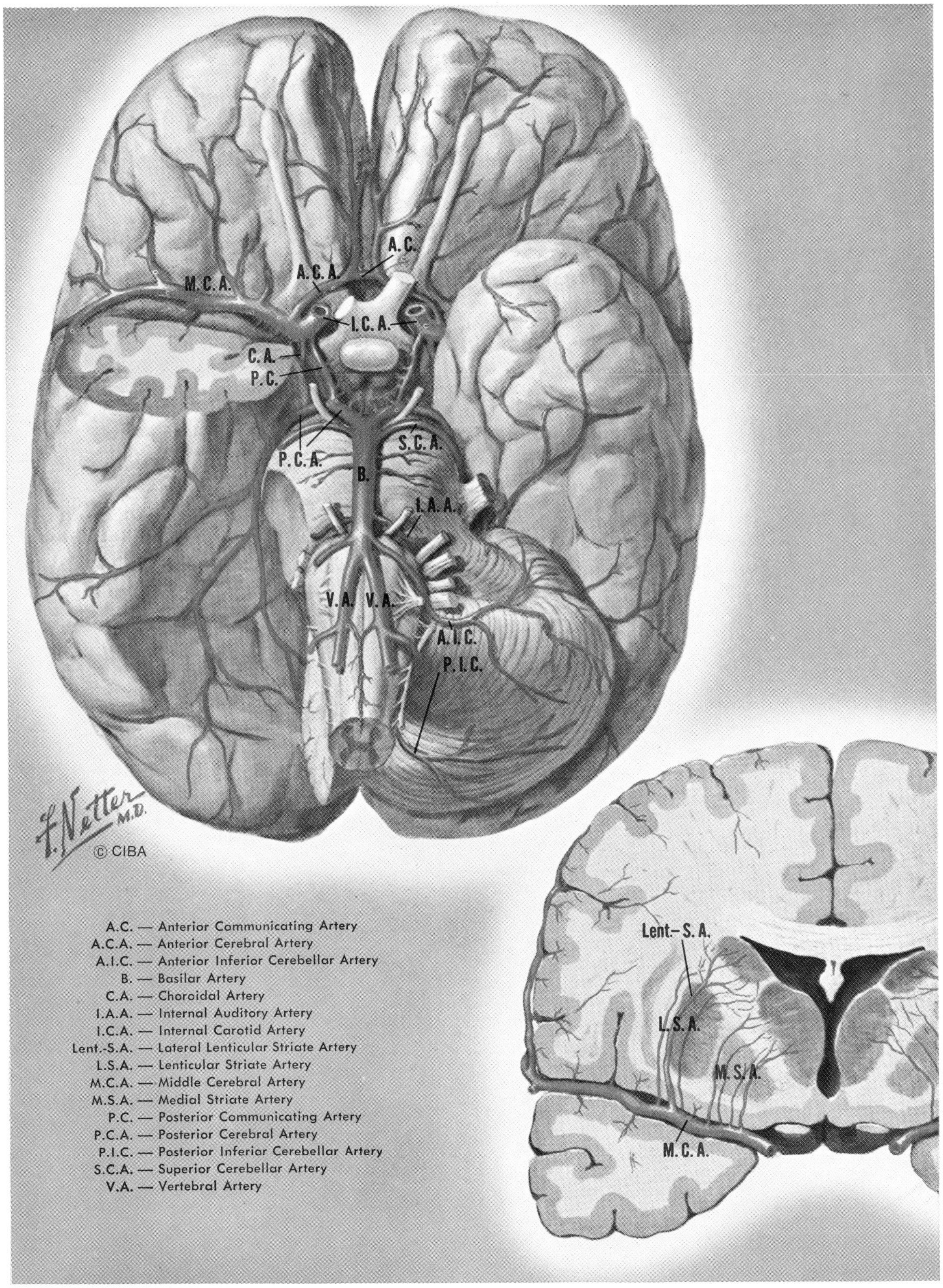

A.C. — Anterior Communicating Artery
A.C.A. — Anterior Cerebral Artery
A.I.C. — Anterior Inferior Cerebellar Artery
B. — Basilar Artery
C.A. — Choroidal Artery
I.A.A. — Internal Auditory Artery
I.C.A. — Internal Carotid Artery
Lent.-S.A. — Lateral Lenticular Striate Artery
L.S.A. — Lenticular Striate Artery
M.C.A. — Middle Cerebral Artery
M.S.A. — Medial Striate Artery
P.C. — Posterior Communicating Artery
P.C.A. — Posterior Cerebral Artery
P.I.C. — Posterior Inferior Cerebellar Artery
S.C.A. — Superior Cerebellar Artery
V.A. — Vertebral Artery

4. Anterior spinal artery arises by short branches from the medial aspect of each vertebral artery and, joining its fellow at the foramen magnum, descends in the midline on the anterior surface of the medulla oblongata, and courses downward on the anterior surface of the spinal cord.

5. Medullary arteries, several in number, are minute, and are distributed to the medulla oblongata proper.

Basilar artery, formed by the junction of the two vertebral arteries, lies in the median groove on the undersurface of the pons, from the lower to the upper margin, where it bifurcates into the two posterior cerebral arteries. From below upward it gives off the following branches:

(a) Anterior inferior cerebellar artery proceeds downward and laterally, reaching the anterior surface of the cerebellum, and anastomoses with the corresponding posterior inferior cerebellar artery.

(b) Internal auditory artery runs laterally and parallel with the acoustic nerve to its termination in the internal ear.

(c) Pontine arteries are small branches coming off laterally from the sides of the basilar artery; they supply the pons.

(d) Superior cerebellar artery arises just below the oculomotor nerve, and winds around the cerebral peduncle to reach the undersurface of the cerebellum, where its branches ramify and anastomose with the inferior cerebellar arteries. From this vessel are given off minute branches to the pineal body, anterior medullary velum and tela choroidea of the third ventricle.

(e) Posterior cerebral artery, the main terminal branch of the basilar artery, runs laterally along the curved border of the pons and, shortly after its origin, receives the posterior communicating artery, then continues in a lateral direction to wind around the cerebral peduncles, reaching the tentorial surface of the occipital lobe, where it divides, giving off branches to the temporal and occipital lobes. Its cortical branches are sent to the anterior temporal lobe, the uncus, the anterior fusiform gyrus, the fusiform and inferior temporal gyri, the gyrus lingualis, the posterior portion of the occipital cortex, the cuneus and precuneus.

Circle of Willis is a ring of blood vessels surrounding the optic chiasm and pituitary stalk. It consists of the anterior communicating artery uniting the two anterior cerebral arteries, which in turn arise from their corresponding internal carotid arteries, from which arise the posterior communicating arteries to join the corresponding posterior cerebral arteries, thereby completing a vascular cycle.

PLATE 17

LATERAL ASPECT OF THE BRAIN
Sulci and Gyri

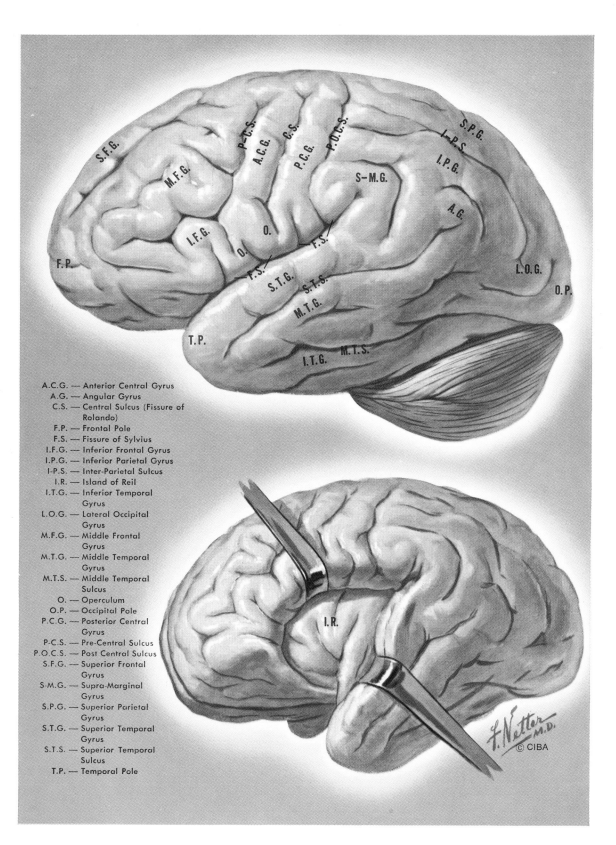

A.C.G. — Anterior Central Gyrus
A.G. — Angular Gyrus
C.S. — Central Sulcus (Fissure of Rolando)
F.P. — Frontal Pole
F.S. — Fissure of Sylvius
I.F.G. — Inferior Frontal Gyrus
I.P.G. — Inferior Parietal Gyrus
I.P.S. — Inter-Parietal Sulcus
I.R. — Island of Reil
I.T.G. — Inferior Temporal Gyrus
L.O.G. — Lateral Occipital Gyrus
M.F.G. — Middle Frontal Gyrus
M.T.G. — Middle Temporal Gyrus
M.T.S. — Middle Temporal Sulcus
O. — Operculum
O.P. — Occipital Pole
P.C.G. — Posterior Central Gyrus
P.C.S. — Pre-Central Sulcus
P.O.C.S. — Post Central Sulcus
S.F.G. — Superior Frontal Gyrus
S-M.G. — Supra-Marginal Gyrus
S.P.G. — Superior Parietal Gyrus
S.T.G. — Superior Temporal Gyrus
S.T.S. — Superior Temporal Sulcus
T.P. — Temporal Pole

Both cerebral hemispheres present inferior, medial and lateral surfaces. Only the lateral surface of the brain will be described here.

The lateral cerebral surface presents irregular grooves called sulci or fissures and elevations known as gyri or convolutions. In different individuals each hemisphere may show slight variations. The fissures divide the cerebral hemispheres into lobes.

Fissure of Sylvius (lateral cerebral fissure) separates the frontal from the temporal lobe. Of its three branches, one ascends into the inferior frontal gyrus, the second ascends at its midpoint into the same convolution, and the posterior branch extends backward, ending in the parietal lobe of the supramarginal gyrus.

Fissure of Rolando (central sulcus) arises at the upper margin (longitudinal cerebral fissure), slightly posterior to the midpoint, runs forward and downward, ending behind ascending branches of the Sylvian fissure.

Parieto-occipital fissure is about 1.5 cm. in length and is situated about 5 cm. in front of the occipital pole. Its greater part can be seen on the medial surface (see Plate 18, page 40).

Circuminsular fissure is found about the midportion of the lateral hemisphere surrounding the island of Reil.

Frontal lobe extends from the fissure of Rolando to the frontal pole and is bounded inferiorly by the fissure of Sylvius. Three frontal sulci divide the frontal lobe into superior, middle and inferior gyri. Posterior to these gyri is the anterior central sulcus (pre-central sulcus).

Parietal lobe begins at the fissure of Rolando and extends posteriorly to the parieto-occipital fissure; it is bounded below by the posterior portion of the Sylvian fissure.

The postcentral sulcus runs parallel to the fissure of Rolando. At its midpoint running horizontally is the inter-parietal sulcus, forming the posterior central gyrus, the superior parietal gyrus and the inferior parietal gyrus. The inferior parietal lobe is divided into the supramarginal gyrus which lies above the terminal curve of the Sylvian fissure, and the angular gyrus which lies above the posterior termination of the superior temporal sulcus.

Temporal lobe is bounded above by the Sylvian fissure and an imaginary line extending to the margin of the occipital lobe; inferiorly is the inferior border of the cerebral hemisphere. The superior and middle temporal sulci divide the temporal lobe into superior, middle and inferior gyri.

The island of Reil (insula) identified only when the Sylvian fissure is retracted, is divided into orbital, frontal, fronto-parietal and temporal opercula. The entire structure is called the operculum.

Occipital lobe is bounded anteriorly by the parieto-occipital fissure and from its lowest point continues to the pre-occipital notch. The lateral occipital gyrus extends horizontally from the occipital pole and forward. In this manner it divides the occipital lobe into a superior and inferior occipital gyrus.

PLATE 18

MEDIAL ASPECT
OF THE BRAIN

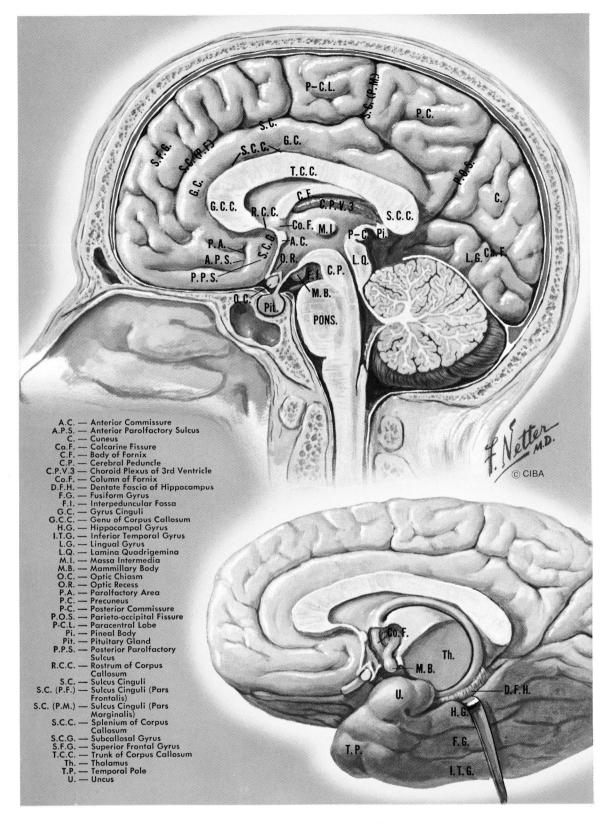

A.C. — Anterior Commissure
A.P.S. — Anterior Parolfactory Sulcus
C. — Cuneus
Ca.F. — Calcarine Fissure
C.F. — Body of Fornix
C.P. — Cerebral Peduncle
C.P.V.3 — Choroid Plexus of 3rd Ventricle
Co.F. — Column of Fornix
D.F.H. — Dentate Fascia of Hippocampus
F.G. — Fusiform Gyrus
F.I. — Interpeduncular Fossa
G.C. — Gyrus Cinguli
G.C.C. — Genu of Corpus Callosum
H.G. — Hippocampal Gyrus
I.T.G. — Inferior Temporal Gyrus
L.G. — Lingual Gyrus
L.Q. — Lamina Quadrigemina
M.I. — Massa Intermedia
M.B. — Mammillary Body
O.C. — Optic Chiasm
O.R. — Optic Recess
P.A. — Parolfactory Area
P.C. — Precuneus
P-C. — Posterior Commissure
P.O.S. — Parieto-occipital Fissure
P-C.L. — Paracentral Lobe
Pi. — Pineal Body
Pit. — Pituitary Gland
P.P.S. — Posterior Parolfactory
        Sulcus
R.C.C. — Rostrum of Corpus
        Callosum
S.C. — Sulcus Cinguli
S.C. (P.F.) — Sulcus Cinguli (Pars
        Frontalis)
S.C. (P.M.) — Sulcus Cinguli (Pars
        Marginalis)
S.C.C. — Splenium of Corpus
        Callosum
S.C.G. — Subcallosal Gyrus
S.F.G. — Superior Frontal Gyrus
T.C.C. — Trunk of Corpus Callosum
Th. — Thalamus
T.P. — Temporal Pole
U. — Uncus

The medial aspect of the frontal lobe presents the sulcus cingularis which has a frontal and marginal portion. Above and anterior to this structure lies the superior frontal gyrus and below, the gyrus cinguli. Posterior to the superior frontal gyrus is the paracentral lobule.

On the medial surface of the parietal lobe is the precuneus which is separated from the cuneus of the occipital lobe by the parieto-occipital fissure. Running more horizontally and downward is the calcarine fissure, which divides the occipital lobe into the cuneus and the lingual gyrus.

The corpus callosum joins both cerebral hemispheres, also forming the roof of the lateral ventricles. Its anterior portion (genu) arches forward and downward thinning out to form the rostrum. The midportion is called the trunk. The posterior thick portion (splenium) is bent acutely and overlies the midbrain and tela choroidea of the third ventricle. Arching anteriorly and below the splenium are two symmetrical white bands, the fornix. Its midportion is called the body and its anterior portion is called the column.

Below the fornix is the third ventricle with its choroid plexus. In the lateral walls of the third ventricle are two thalami, which are joined by a band of gray matter called the massa intermedia. In the rostral portion of the third ventricle is the anterior commissure which joins both cerebral hemispheres. This structure is closely associated with the olfactory nerve. Crossing the midline in the posterior portion of the third ventricle are sim-

ilar fibers called the posterior commissure. Posterior and superior to these fibers is a small cone-shaped mass with a stalk called the pineal body. This stalk has a small recess extending from the third ventricle, called the pineal recess.

Just above the cerebral aqueduct is the lamina quadrigemina with four elevations called colliculi, of which the two superior are larger than the two inferior ones.

Joining the pons with the cerebral hemispheres are the cerebral peduncles with a depressed area between, known as the interpeduncular fossa.

Anterior to and below the third ventricle is the optic chiasm which lies on the diaphragma sellae, and receives the fibers from each eye which cross at this point. Anterior to the optic chiasm is a diverticulum called the optic recess.

Posterior to the chiasm are two small white masses

called mammillary bodies. From the base of the third ventricle projects the infundibulum which passes through the dural roof of the pituitary fossa to join the pituitary gland. In front of the subcallosal gyrus is the parolfactory area which is separated anteriorly by the anterior parolfactory sulcus, and posteriorly by the posterior parolfactory sulcus. The olfactory bulb and tract lie on the orbital surface of the frontal lobe and divide posteriorly into two striae, one running laterally to the uncus and the other medially to the parolfactory area. Entering posteriorly from the uncus is the hippocampal gyrus which is continuous posteriorly with the cingular gyrus and inferiorly with the lingual gyrus. Extending above the hippocampal gyrus is a narrow band called the fascia dentata hippocampi. When these structures are visualized from the undersurface of the temporal lobe, the fusiform gyrus and the inferior temporal gyrus can readily be identified.

PLATE 19

BASAL GANGLIA

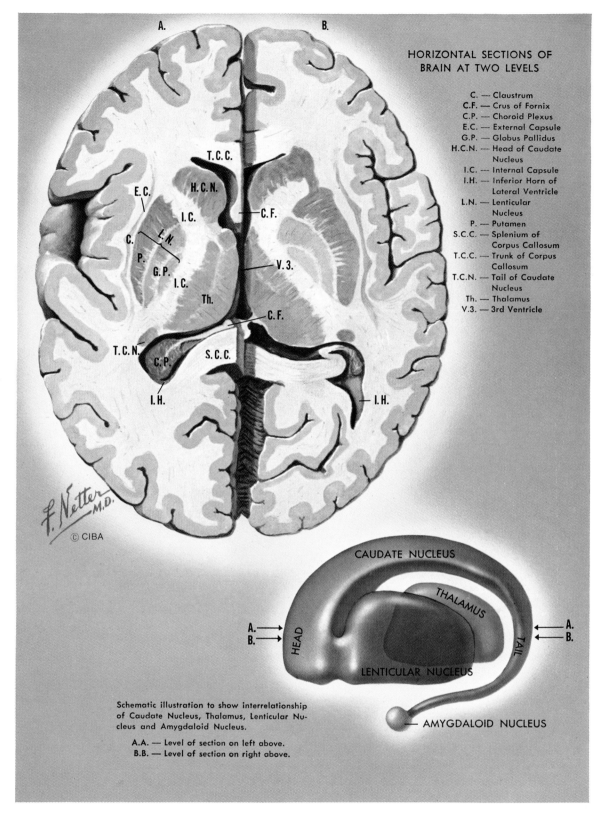

HORIZONTAL SECTIONS OF
BRAIN AT TWO LEVELS

C. — Claustrum
C.F. — Crus of Fornix
C.P. — Choroid Plexus
E.C. — External Capsule
G.P. — Globus Pallidus
H.C.N. — Head of Caudate
Nucleus
I.C. — Internal Capsule
I.H. — Inferior Horn of
Lateral Ventricle
L.N. — Lenticular
Nucleus
P. — Putamen
S.C.C. — Splenium of
Corpus Callosum
T.C.C. — Trunk of Corpus
Callosum
T.C.N. — Tail of Caudate
Nucleus
Th. — Thalamus
V.3. — 3rd Ventricle

Schematic illustration to show interrelationship
of Caudate Nucleus, Thalamus, Lenticular Nucleus and Amygdaloid Nucleus.

A.A. — Level of section on left above.
B.B. — Level of section on right above.

A. Corpus striatum:

1. The caudate nucleus is a mass of gray matter; its anterior portion is the head, extending into the anterior margin of the lateral ventricle, where it is also continuous with the anterior end of the lenticular nucleus. As the caudate nucleus extends posteriorly it becomes narrow and slender, lies lateral to the thalamus, and then continues downward into the roof of the inferior cornu, ending in the putamen as the amygdaloid nucleus.

2. The lenticular nucleus, shaped like a biconvex lens, lies between the insula and the caudate nucleus and thalamus, but is separated from the insula by the claustrum. Ventrally it rests on the inferior horn of the lateral ventricle and anterior perforated substance. The most lateral portion of the lenticular nucleus is the putamen and the two medial portions are called the globus pallidus.

3. The internal capsule, between the caudate and lenticular nuclei, containing fibers connecting them, is "V"-shaped, having its apex directed medially. The rostral portion, called the anterior limb, contains fibers going from the thalamus to the frontal lobe, fibers from the cerebral cortex forming a portion of the corpus striatum, and fibers from the frontal lobe to the cerebral peduncle and pontine nuclei. Through the midportion of the internal capsule traverse the motor fibers from the cerebral cortex toward the base of the cerebral peduncle. The posterior limb of the internal capsule extends lat-

erally between the lenticular nucleus and the thalamus. Through the anterior two-thirds of the posterior limb run the fibers from the motor area of the cerebral cortex which pass through the middle three-fifths of the base of the cerebral peduncle, then forming the pyramid of the medulla oblongata. Passing through the posterior third are sensory fibers from the thalamus, fibers from the optic radiation in the lower visual center, acoustic fibers from the lateral lemniscus and temporal lobe, and finally fibers from the occipital and temporal lobes to the pontine nuclei.

These fibers radiating from the cortex form a fan-shaped structure called the corona radiata.

B. Amygdaloid nucleus, the tail end of the caudate nucleus, is located in the roof of the terminal portion of the inferior ventricle.

C. Thalamic radiation consists of four main parts: (1) the frontal group, called the anterior thalamic

radiation, arises from the anterior portion of the thalamus, and is directed to the cortex of the frontal lobe, (2) the parietal group starts from the lateral surface of the thalamus, and connects the posterior frontal lobe with the parietal cortex. Some fibers terminating in the posterior portion of the frontal lobe mediate cutaneous sensations, muscle and joint sensibility, (3) the occipital group, containing no visual fibers, arises from the posterior portion of the thalamus, passes through the pulvinar and along the lateral ventricle, (4) the ventral group originates on the ventral surface of the thalamus, passes laterally under the cover of the lenticular nucleus, and finally ends in the cortex of the temporal lobe and insula.

D. Claustrum lies between the external capsule and the insula. It is made up of a thin layer of gray substance having a wavy course, corresponding to the sulci and gyri of the insula.

PLATE 20

CRANIAL NERVES

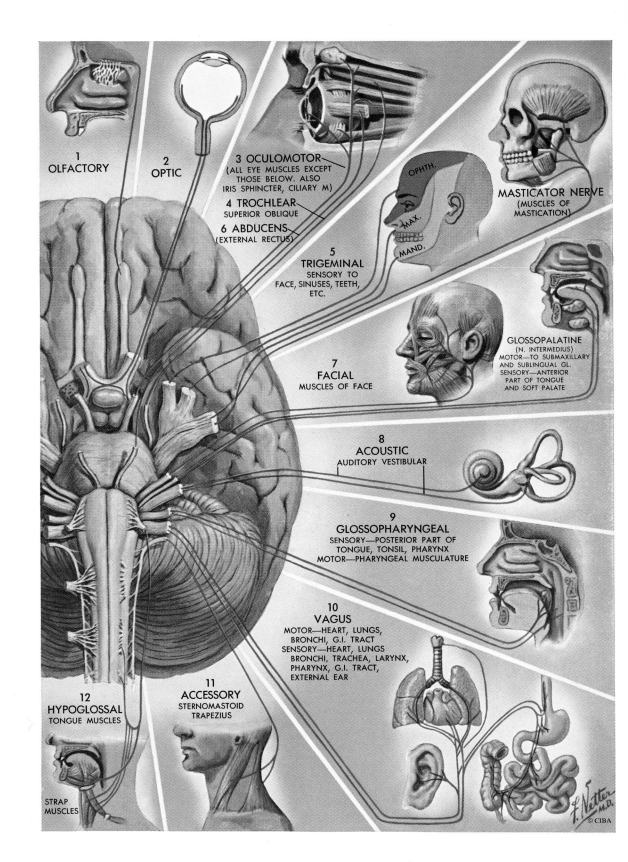

Within the illustration:

1 OLFACTORY

2 OPTIC

3 OCULOMOTOR
(ALL EYE MUSCLES EXCEPT THOSE BELOW. ALSO IRIS SPHINCTER, CILIARY M)

4 TROCHLEAR
SUPERIOR OBLIQUE

6 ABDUCENS
(EXTERNAL RECTUS)

5 TRIGEMINAL
SENSORY TO FACE, SINUSES, TEETH, ETC.

OPHTH.
MAX.
MAND.

MASTICATOR NERVE
(MUSCLES OF MASTICATION)

7 FACIAL
MUSCLES OF FACE

GLOSSOPALATINE
(N. INTERMEDIUS)
MOTOR—TO SUBMAXILLARY AND SUBLINGUAL GL. SENSORY—ANTERIOR PART OF TONGUE AND SOFT PALATE

8 ACOUSTIC
AUDITORY VESTIBULAR

9 GLOSSOPHARYNGEAL
SENSORY—POSTERIOR PART OF TONGUE, TONSIL, PHARYNX
MOTOR—PHARYNGEAL MUSCULATURE

10 VAGUS
MOTOR—HEART, LUNGS, BRONCHI, G.I. TRACT
SENSORY—HEART, LUNGS, BRONCHI, TRACHEA, LARYNX, PHARYNX, G.I. TRACT, EXTERNAL EAR

11 ACCESSORY
STERNOMASTOID TRAPEZIUS

12 HYPOGLOSSAL
TONGUE MUSCLES

STRAP MUSCLES

F. Netter M.D.
©CIBA

CRANIAL NERVES	ORIGIN AND COURSE	TERMINATION AND FUNCTION
1. OLFACTORY:	Olfactory cells in nasal mucosa. Through cribriform plate to the olfactory bulb, then backward and along the olfactory nerve below the frontal lobe dividing into two branches.	Medial branch ending in subcallosal gyrus and parolfactory area; lateral branch in uncus and hippocampal gyrus. Smell.
2. OPTIC:	Ganglion cells of the retina. Optic nerve through the optic foramen to the optic chiasm; a point of decussation. Mixed fibers from the corresponding portions of the retina pass back along the optic tract to the lateral geniculate body.	The second neuron goes from the geniculate body to the cortical visual center in the cuneus. Vision.
3. OCULOMOTOR:	Floor of the aquaeductus cerebri. Emerging near the midline at the upper pons from where it proceeds lateral to the posterior clinoid, in the lateral wall of the cavernous sinus, then through the superior orbital fissure into the orbit.	Motor to all the ocular muscles except the lateral rectus and superior oblique, also parasympathetic fibers to the sphincter of the pupil and to the ciliary muscle.

4. TROCHLEAR:	Floor of the aquaeductus cerebri. Emerging at junction of upper pons and cerebral peduncle, proceeds laterally to posterior clinoid, in lateral wall of the cavernous sinus, crosses the oculomotor nerve before entering the orbit through superior orbital fissure.	Innervates the superior oblique muscle, which rotates eyeball outward and downward.
5. TRIGEMINAL: *Sensory* Division	Floor of the fourth ventricle. Emerging at the lateral portion of the pons, passes over the petrous apex forming the Gasserian ganglion where it divides into three branches. 1. *Ophthalmic* branch from the upper portion of the ganglion enters superior orbital fissure. 2. *Maxillary* branch from midportion of the ganglion to foramen rotundum, through inferior orbital fissure and infra-orbital groove to infra-orbital foramen. 3. *Mandibular* branch from lowest portion of the ganglion leaving skull through foramen ovale uniting with motor division at its exit.	*Ophthalmic* branch: Sensation to cornea, ciliary body, iris, lacrimal gland, conjunctiva, nasal mucous membrane, eyelid, eyebrow, forehead and nose. *Maxillary:* Sensation to skin of cheek, lower lid, side of nose and upper jaw, teeth, mucosa of mouth, sphenopalatine-pterygoid regions, and maxillary sinus. *Anterior:* Muscles of mastication, mucosa of lower mouth and skin. *Posterior:* Skin of external ear, ear canal, temporal area, parotid gland, mandibular joint, lower jaw and teeth, mucosa of mouth, gums, sublingual glands, and anterior two-thirds of tongue.
Motor Division	From pons beneath the Gasserian ganglion leaving through foramen ovale where it unites with mandibular nerve forming two branches.	
6. ABDUCENS:	Near midline of the furrow at lower portion of the pons. Passes through an aperture of the petrous apex, then through lateral portion of cavernous sinus entering orbit by superior orbital fissure.	Rotates the eyeball outward by supplying the two heads of the lateral rectus muscle.
7. FACIAL: *Motor* Division	Lower portion of pons in recess between inferior peduncle and olive. Passes through internal acoustic meatus along facial canal and makes its exit at stylomastoid foramen. Running forward through parotid gland, it divides into many branches.	Motor supply of facial muscles, scalp, auricle, buccinator, platysma, stapedius, stylohyoid, posterior belly of digastric.
Sensory Division "intermedius"	Geniculate ganglion in facial canal. Branches run by way of chorda tympani to periphery. Centrally it proceeds through acoustic meatus entering brain between inferior peduncle and olive.	Taste in anterior two-thirds of tongue. Sensation to soft palate. Innervation of salivary glands.
8. ACOUSTIC: *Cochlear* Division	Spiral ganglion of cochlea; peripheral fibers to the organ of Corti; central fibers go to the internal auditory meatus and enter the inferior peduncle.	Hearing. Terminates in the ventral and dorsal cochlear nuclei.
Vestibular Division	Bipolar cells in the vestibular ganglion. Superior, inferior and posterior branches end in the utricle, superior and lateral semicircular canals, the saccule and in the ampule of posterior semicircular canal respectively.	Maintenance of equilibrium; terminates in the medial, lateral, superior and spinal vestibular nuclei and in cerebellum.
9. GLOSSOPHARYNGEAL:	Passes from medulla oblongata laterally to the jugular foramen, through the petrous temporal bone, making its exit between internal carotid artery and internal jugular vein.	Taste in posterior third of tongue. Sensation to fauces, tonsils, pharynx, and soft palate. Motor for pharynx and stylopharyngeus muscle. Impulses to parotid gland.
10. VAGUS:	Arises in the groove between inferior peduncle and olive, passes through the jugular foramen where it is joined by the cranial portion of the spinal accessory nerve and continues down the neck and thorax into the abdomen.	*Sensory* fibers to skin in back of auricle, posterior portion of external acoustic meatus, pharynx, larynx, thoracic and abdominal viscera. *Motor* fibers to pharynx, base of tongue, larynx, and to autonomic ganglia innervating thoracic and abdominal viscera.
11. SPINAL ACCESSORY:	*Cranial portion:* Derives from four to five rootlets at side of medulla, runs laterally below vagus at jugular foramen where it is joined by *spinal portion* which arises from motor cells in the anterior gray column as low as the fifth cervical segment. Ascends between posterior root and dentate ligaments; enters skull through foramen magnum, and leaves through the jugular foramen.	*Cranial portion:* Motor to pharynx, upper larynx, uvula and palate. Sends fibers to the recurrent laryngeal and cardiac nerves. *Spinal portion:* Motor to upper portion of sternomastoid and trapezius muscles. Sends branches to C2, 3 and 4 nerves.
12. HYPOGLOSSAL:	Rootlets emerge between olive and medullar pyramid, unite while entering hypoglossal canal in occipital bone. Leaving canal, the nerve turns downward, passes between internal carotid artery and jugular vein, loops around occipital artery, crosses digastric muscle, giving off a descending ramus to form the ansa hypoglossi.	Motor to strap muscles of neck and tongue — stylohyoid, mylohyoid, inferior belly of omohyoid, sternothyroid, styloglossus, hyoglossus, genioglossus, geniohyoid and intrinsic muscles of tongue.

PLATE 21

CEREBROSPINAL FLUID CIRCULATION

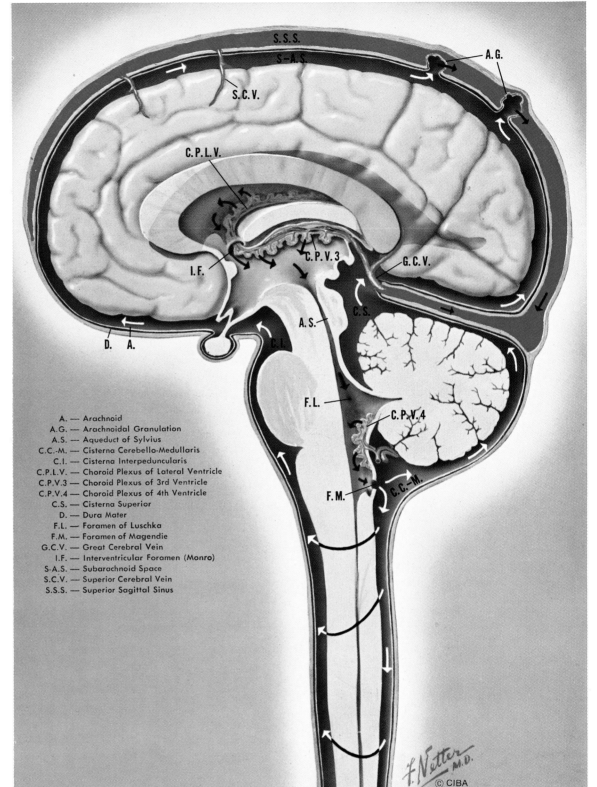

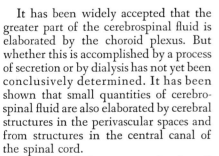

A. — Arachnoid
A.G. — Arachnoidal Granulation
A.S. — Aqueduct of Sylvius
C.C.-M. — Cisterna Cerebello-Medullaris
C.I. — Cisterna Interpeduncularis
C.P.L.V. — Choroid Plexus of Lateral Ventricle
C.P.V.3 — Choroid Plexus of 3rd Ventricle
C.P.V.4 — Choroid Plexus of 4th Ventricle
C.S. — Cisterna Superior
D. — Dura Mater
F.L. — Foramen of Luschka
F.M. — Foramen of Magendie
G.C.V. — Great Cerebral Vein
I.F. — Interventricular Foramen (Monro)
S-A.S. — Subarachnoid Space
S.C.V. — Superior Cerebral Vein
S.S.S. — Superior Sagittal Sinus

It has been widely accepted that the greater part of the cerebrospinal fluid is elaborated by the choroid plexus. But whether this is accomplished by a process of secretion or by dialysis has not yet been conclusively determined. It has been shown that small quantities of cerebrospinal fluid are also elaborated by cerebral structures in the perivascular spaces and from structures in the central canal of the spinal cord.

The choroid plexuses are tufts of small capillary vessels (like a glomerulus) of the tela choroidea which are fringe-shaped and which are covered by a very fine layer of ependymal cells. These are located in the various ventricles. A choroid plexus is found in each lateral ventricle, the third ventricle and the fourth ventricle. In the lateral ventricles they extend from the interventricular foramen along the dependent portion of the medial wall of the ventricle posteriorly to the inferior horn. Another pair of choroid plexuses project downward on either side of the roof of the third ventricle into

its lumen. The choroid plexus of the fourth ventricle is fairly large and may be found in the lower portion of the latter's roof. It is "T"-shaped with the vertical portion in the midline.

The major portion of the cerebrospinal fluid, elaborated by the choroid plexuses, passes into the lateral ventricles. Then it flows through the interventricular foramen (Monro) into the third ventricle and by way of the aqueduct of Sylvius into the fourth ventricle. A small quantity of fluid reaches the fourth ventricle through the central canal of the spinal cord. From the fourth ventricle the spinal fluid escapes into the subarachnoid space by one of three exits: (1) through the foramen of Magendie in the roof of the fourth ventricle, thereby entering the cisterna magna or the cisterna cerebello-medullaris, or (2) through either foramina of Luschka (situated at the extreme lateral portions of the fourth ventricle), thereby emptying

into the cisterna pontis, or (3) from the cisterna magna the cerebrospinal fluid may be directed over the cerebellar hemispheres to the cisterna superior. From the cisterna pontis the flow of the cerebrospinal fluid is forward to the cisterna interpeduncularis and cisterna chiamatis. From these cisternae the fluid sweeps upward over the surface of both lateral hemispheres, anteriorly, upward between the two hemispheres along the longitudinal fissure, over the corpus callosum, along the Sylvian fissure and over the temporal lobes.

The fluid finally reaches the arachnoidal villi where, by a process of osmosis, it is emptied into the great venous dural sinuses, particularly the superior sagittal sinus. Small quantities of fluid may also be absorbed along the perineural and perivascular spaces. The total quantity of cerebral fluid in the ventricular and subarachnoid spaces varies usually between 125 and 150 cc.

PLATE 22

FOURTH VENTRICLE AND MEDULLA OBLONGATA

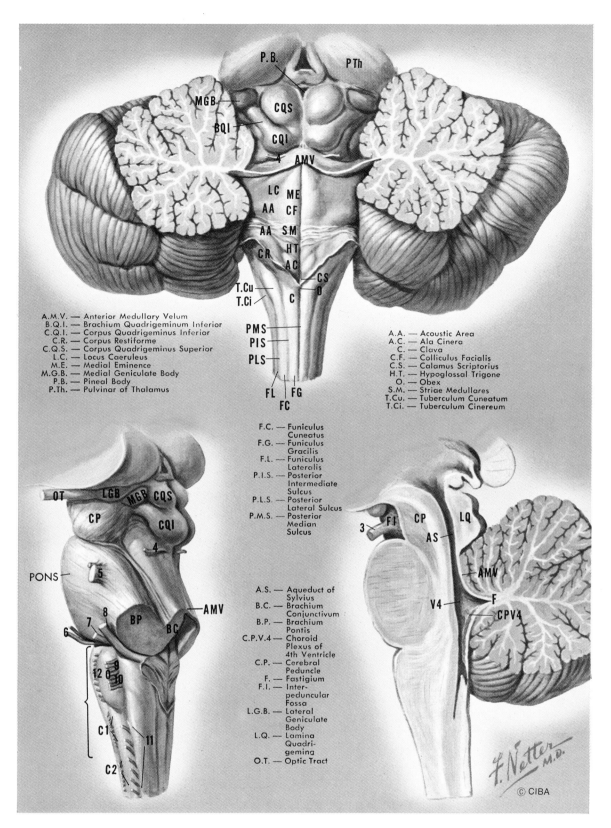

A.M.V. — Anterior Medullary Velum
B.Q.I. — Brachium Quadrigeminum Inferior
C.Q.I. — Corpus Quadrigeminus Inferior
C.R. — Corpus Restiforme
C.Q.S. — Corpus Quadrigeminus Superior
L.C. — Locus Caeruleus
M.E. — Medial Eminence
M.G.B. — Medial Geniculate Body
P.B. — Pineal Body
P.Th. — Pulvinar of Thalamus

A.A. — Acoustic Area
A.C. — Ala Cinera
C. — Clava
C.F. — Colliculus Facialis
C.S. — Calamus Scriptorius
H.T. — Hypoglossal Trigone
O. — Obex
S.M. — Striae Medullares
T.Cu. — Tuberculum Cuneatum
T.Ci. — Tuberculum Cinereum

F.C. — Funiculus Cuneatus
F.G. — Funiculus Gracilis
F.L. — Funiculus Lateralis
P.I.S. — Posterior Intermediate Sulcus
P.L.S. — Posterior Lateral Sulcus
P.M.S. — Posterior Median Sulcus

A.S. — Aqueduct of Sylvius
B.C. — Brachium Conjunctivum
B.P. — Brachium Pontis
C.P.V.4 — Choroid Plexus of 4th Ventricle
C.P. — Cerebral Peduncle
F. — Fastigium
F.I. — Interpeduncular Fossa
L.G.B. — Lateral Geniculate Body
L.Q. — Lamina Quadrigemina
O.T. — Optic Tract

The fourth ventricle is a rhomboid-shaped cavity lying on the posterior aspect of the pons, continuous with the aqueduct of Sylvius above and with the medulla oblongata below. Lateral to the lower portion of the third ventricle is the pulvinar of the thalamus. Just above the beginning of the aqueduct of Sylvius is the pineal body while below this structure is the quadrigeminal plate, consisting of the corpus quadrigeminus superior and inferior. Fibers from the inferior colliculi proceed laterally, forming the brachium quadrigeminum inferior, and end in the median geniculate body. Laterally the fourth ventricle is bounded by the two brachia conjunctiva which are joined by a thin layer called the anterior medullary velum. Below is a small groove known as the locus caeruleus.

In the midline of the floor of the fourth ventricle is the sulcus limitans. To either side at its midpoint is the medial eminence which includes the facial colliculus and trigone of the hypoglossal nerve. More laterally is an elevated structure called the area acoustica. At the lateral inferior border of the fourth ventricle is the corpus restiforme which joins the spinal cord and the medulla oblongata with the cerebellum. Crossing transversely the lower portion of the fourth ventricle are several fine strands, the striae medullares, below which are two symmetrical triangular areas called the hypoglossal trigone. Beneath these are the nuclei of the hypoglossal nerves. Just below is a similar triangular area, the ala cinera, marking the nucleus of the vagus

nerve. The lowermost tip of the fourth ventricle, shaped like a penpoint, is called calamus scriptorius; its terminal triangular lamina is called the obex.

The roof of the fourth ventricle is triangular. Its anterior portion is the fastigium (nucleus fastigii), and underneath its posterior portion lies the choroid plexus. Below and lateral to the floor of the fourth ventricle are the tuberculum cuneatum and, more medially, the clava.

The medulla oblongata is pyramidal and rests upon the basilar portion of the occipital bone. It extends from the lowermost portion of the pons to about the first pair of cervical nerves where it becomes the spinal cord. Its upper portion in part forms the floor of the fourth ventricle, but its lower portion is covered by the cerebellum.

The posterior median sulcus is a continuation of a similar narrow groove of the spinal cord which

becomes shallower as it proceeds upward, ending in the expansion of the fourth ventricle. The posterior intermediate sulcus runs parallel and ends in the same manner.

From the anterior lateral sulcus emerge the root filaments of the hypoglossal nerve, and from the groove of the posterior lateral sulcus emerge the rootlets of the glossopharyngeal, vagus, and spinal accessory nerves. At the lower limits of these sulci are the fasciculus gracilis and the fasciculus cuneatus. Both of these fasciculi diverge as they approach the lower end of the fourth ventricle, and end in elevations (fasciculus gracilis) forming the clava, the fasciculus cuneatus forming the cuneate tubercle. These fasciculi constitute the posterior sensory fibers ending in nuclei, gracilis, and cuneatus. Funiculus lateralis is an almost invisible groove corresponding to the line of origin of the dorsal roots.

PLATE 23

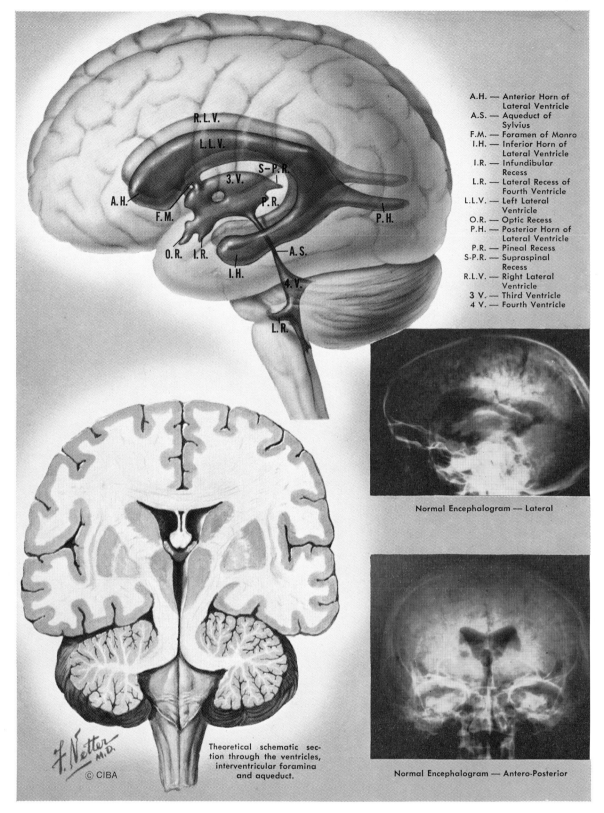

A.H. — Anterior Horn of Lateral Ventricle
A.S. — Aqueduct of Sylvius
F.M. — Foramen of Monro
I.H. — Inferior Horn of Lateral Ventricle
I.R. — Infundibular Recess
L.R. — Lateral Recess of Fourth Ventricle
L.L.V. — Left Lateral Ventricle
O.R. — Optic Recess
P.H. — Posterior Horn of Lateral Ventricle
P.R. — Pineal Recess
S-P.R. — Suprapineal Recess
R.L.V. — Right Lateral Ventricle
3 V. — Third Ventricle
4 V. — Fourth Ventricle

Normal Encephalogram — Lateral

Theoretical schematic section through the ventricles, interventricular foramina and aqueduct.

Normal Encephalogram — Antero-Posterior

VENTRICLES OF THE BRAIN

Within the substance of the brain are four ventricles — two lateral ventricles, a third and a fourth ventricle. These communicate with each other, and with the subarachnoid space. The choroid plexus within each ventricle elaborates the cerebrospinal fluid which flows from the lateral ventricles through the interventricular foramina (Monro) into the third ventricle, then through the cerebral aqueduct (Sylvius) into the fourth ventricle, and from there escapes into the subarachnoid space.

Lateral ventricles are situated in the lower medial portion of each cerebral hemisphere. They are separated by a thin layer called septum pellucidum. Each lateral ventricle consists of a body and three cornua (horns). The body which extends from the foramen of Monro to the splenium, is triangular in cross section with its apex pointing medially and downward. The anterior horn passes laterally forward and then slightly downward into the frontal lobe with its apex curving around the anterior portion of the caudate nucleus. The posterior horn extends laterally and backward into the occipital lobe. The inferior horn curves around the posterior end of the thalamus, passes backward, then laterally downward and forward within the temporal lobe.

The choroid plexus of the lateral ventricle stretches along the medial aspect of the floor of the ventricle and extends from the foramen of Monro to the end of the inferior horn. Through the foramen of Monro it also joins the plexus of the opposite side.

The third ventricle is a thin, centrally placed cleft below the body of the lateral ventricles and lies between the two thalami. It communicates anteriorly with the lateral ventricles through the foramen of Monro and with the fourth ventricle through the cerebral aqueduct (Sylvius). Anteriorly it has a funnel-shaped prolongation — the infundibulum — and just above the optic chiasm there is another angular prolongation — the optic recess. At the upper margin of the posterior boundary of the third ventricle is a diverticulum called the suprapineal recess. The massa intermedia crosses horizontally from one lateral wall of the third ventricle to the other at about midportion. The choroid plexus lies on either side of the roof of this ventricular cavity close to the interventricular foramina.

The cerebral aqueduct (Sylvius) is a thin tubular channel between the third and fourth ventricles.

The fourth ventricle is rhomboid-shaped. Its floor has four angles, the superior angle being continuous with the cerebral aqueduct, the inferior with the central canal of the medulla oblongata. Its lateral angles extend to the brachia and inferior peduncles. The roof of the fourth ventricle is triangular in shape and above it lie the vermis and cerebellum. Within the apex of the fourth ventricle is found the "T"-shaped choroid plexus with its vertical portion in the midline. In the roof of the fourth ventricle is the foramen of Magendie, through which cerebrospinal fluid escapes into the cisterna magna. At the lateral margins of the fourth ventricle are the two foramina of Luschka emptying into the lateral recess.

When the fluid in the ventricles or subarachnoid space is replaced by oxygen or air, x-ray films of the skull will show the size, shape and position of these spaces. This procedure is known as encephalography.

PLATE 24

CRANIAL NERVE NUCLEI

The cranial nerve nuclei consist of nerve cells, and their fibers arrange themselves according to functional units. Motor and sensory nuclei are diagrammatically represented on opposite sides.

Motor Nuclei

1. Edinger-Westphal nucleus. Its fibers, which run to the oculomotor nerve and thence to the ciliary ganglion, innervate the intrinsic eye muscles.

2. Oculomotor nucleus has a median and a lateral group of cells. Their fibers supply all the extrinsic eye muscles except the lateral rectus and superior oblique.

3. Trochlear nucleus. After coursing caudally to enter the anterior medullary velum, its fibers then decussate to make their exit to supply the superior oblique muscle.

4. Motor nucleus of trigeminal nerve. Its fibers run laterally with the mandibular nerve to innervate the muscles of mastication.

5. Abducens nucleus. Fibers from this nucleus are directed ventrally to supply the lateral rectus muscle.

6. Motor nucleus of facial nerve. Its fibers run dorsomedially, hook around the abducens nucleus and then proceed ventrolaterally, emerging at the lower end of the pons to innervate the voluntary facial muscles.

7. Superior salivatory nucleus sends fibers through the chorda tympani to the submaxillary ganglion to supply the submaxillary and sublingual glands.

8. Inferior salivatory nucleus sends fibers to the otic ganglion to supply the parotid gland.

9. Hypoglossal nucleus sends fibers downward and laterally to the lower border of the pyramid to supply the tongue.

10. Dorsal motor nucleus of vagus sends fibers through the medulla oblongata to the vagus and spinal accessory nerves which end in vagal sympathetic plexuses in the chest and abdomen.

11. Nucleus ambiguus sends fibers through the glossopharyngeal, vagus and spinal accessory nerves to supply the pharynx and larynx.

12. Nucleus of spinal accessory. Its

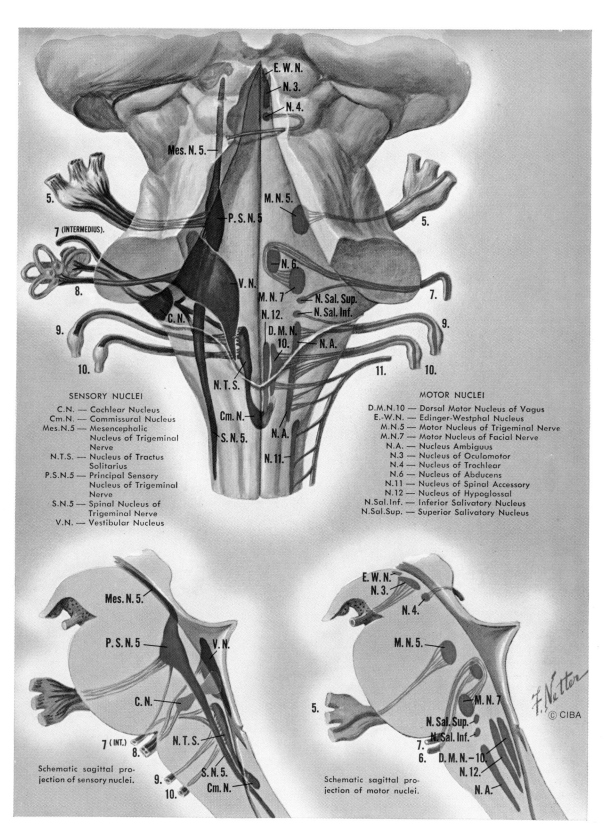

SENSORY NUCLEI

C.N. — Cochlear Nucleus
Cm.N. — Commissural Nucleus
Mes.N.5 — Mesencephalic Nucleus of Trigeminal Nerve
N.T.S. — Nucleus of Tractus Solitarius
P.S.N.5 — Principal Sensory Nucleus of Trigeminal Nerve
S.N.5 — Spinal Nucleus of Trigeminal Nerve
V.N. — Vestibular Nucleus

MOTOR NUCLEI

D.M.N.10 — Dorsal Motor Nucleus of Vagus
E.-W.N. — Edinger-Westphal Nucleus
M.N.5 — Motor Nucleus of Trigeminal Nerve
M.N.7 — Motor Nucleus of Facial Nerve
N.A. — Nucleus Ambiguus
N.3 — Nucleus of Oculomotor
N.4 — Nucleus of Trochlear
N.6 — Nucleus of Abducens
N.11 — Nucleus of Spinal Accessory
N.12 — Nucleus of Hypoglossal
N.Sal.Inf. — Inferior Salivatory Nucleus
N.Sal.Sup. — Superior Salivatory Nucleus

Schematic sagittal projection of sensory nuclei.

Schematic sagittal projection of motor nuclei.

fibers form rootlets which join bulbar rootlets of the spinal accessory nerve to innervate the trapezius and sternomastoid muscles.

Sensory Nuclei

1. Mesencephalic nucleus of trigeminal nerve. Fibers from extrinsic eye muscles and muscles of mastication end in this nucleus from which arises the mesencephalic root of this nerve.

2. Principal sensory nucleus of trigeminal nerve. Fibers carrying impulses of pain, temperature and touch from the head and face reach the pons and divide into short ascending fibers which end in this nucleus and long descending branches which terminate in the spinal nucleus of trigeminal nerve.

3. Spinal nucleus of trigeminal nerve. Its fibers mediate pain and temperature exclusively and become continuous with the substantia gelatinosa Rolandi.

4. Vestibular nucleus. Fibers from the vestibular bipolar ganglion cells terminate in this nucleus. Its short ascending fibers end in the lateral (Deiters') nucleus; the longer descending fibers terminate in a large principal nucleus, a descending spinal nucleus, a superior nucleus (Bechterew) and the cerebellum.

5. Cochlear nucleus. Central fibers arising from bipolar cells in the spiral ganglion of the cochlea terminate in this nucleus. From its ventral portion fibers cross through the lateral lemniscus to the inferior colliculus. From its dorsal portion fibers pass through the medial geniculate body to the inferior colliculus, ending in the auditory area of the cerebral cortex.

6. Nucleus of tractus solitarius receives visceral afferent fibers from the facial, glossopharyngeal and vagus nerves.

7. Commissural nucleus joins the nucleus of the tractus solitarius.

PLATE 25

Thalamus

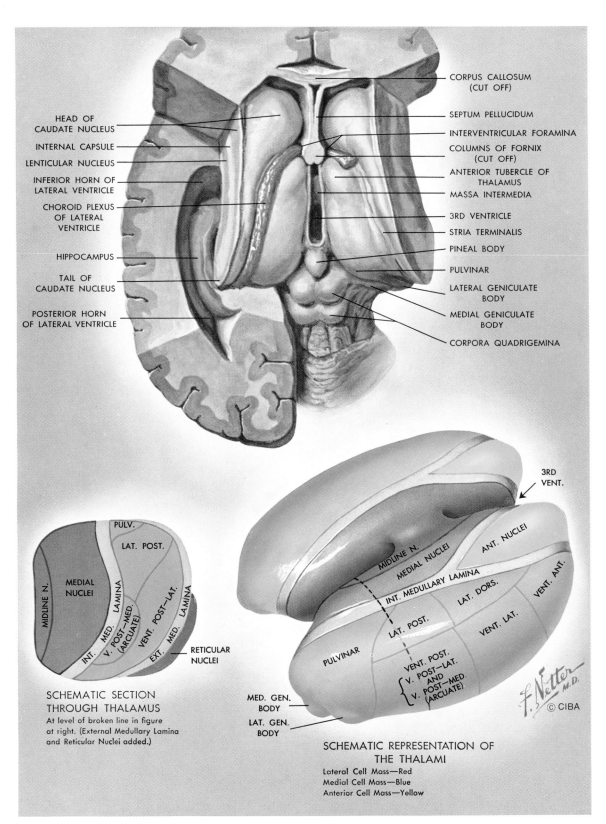

HEAD OF CAUDATE NUCLEUS
INTERNAL CAPSULE
LENTICULAR NUCLEUS
INFERIOR HORN OF LATERAL VENTRICLE
CHOROID PLEXUS OF LATERAL VENTRICLE
HIPPOCAMPUS
TAIL OF CAUDATE NUCLEUS
POSTERIOR HORN OF LATERAL VENTRICLE

CORPUS CALLOSUM (CUT OFF)
SEPTUM PELLUCIDUM
INTERVENTRICULAR FORAMINA
COLUMNS OF FORNIX (CUT OFF)
ANTERIOR TUBERCLE OF THALAMUS
MASSA INTERMEDIA
3RD VENTRICLE
STRIA TERMINALIS
PINEAL BODY
PULVINAR
LATERAL GENICULATE BODY
MEDIAL GENICULATE BODY
CORPORA QUADRIGEMINA

PULV.
LAT. POST.
MEDIAL NUCLEI
MIDLINE N.
INT. MED. LAMINA
V. POST.-MED. (ARCUATE)
VENT. POST.-LAT.
EXT. MED. LAMINA
RETICULAR NUCLEI

SCHEMATIC SECTION THROUGH THALAMUS
At level of broken line in figure at right. (External Medullary Lamina and Reticular Nuclei added.)

3RD VENT.
MIDLINE N.
MEDIAL NUCLEI
ANT. NUCLEI
INT. MEDULLARY LAMINA
LAT. DORS.
VENT. ANT.
LAT. POST.
VENT. LAT.
PULVINAR
VENT. POST.
V. POST.-LAT. AND V. POST.-MED. (ARCUATE)
MED. GEN. BODY
LAT. GEN. BODY

SCHEMATIC REPRESENTATION OF THE THALAMI
Lateral Cell Mass—Red
Medial Cell Mass—Blue
Anterior Cell Mass—Yellow

The thalamus is a mass of ganglionic nuclei which are end stations for ascending tracts of the tegmen and fibers from the optic tract. These nuclei also serve as points of origin of cells and fibers radiating to almost every portion of the cortex (thalamocortical radiation). Similarly from various parts of the cerebral cortex come streams of fibers to the thalamus (corticothalamic radiation).

The thalami (optic), two ovoid masses, are situated on either side of the third ventricle. Each is about four cm. long and made up mainly of gray substance with a covering layer of white substance and ependymal cells. They each have an anterior and posterior pole as well as superior, inferior, medial and lateral surfaces. The smaller anterior pole lies just posterior to the foramen of Monro. On its dorsal surface is an elevation — the anterior tubercle. The posterior, somewhat wider and more rounded, pole overlies the superior colliculus. Its prominent, slightly angulated bulge is called the pulvinar.

The superior surface, in its medial portion a part of the floor of the lateral ventricle, is convex and separated laterally from the caudate nucleus by the stria terminalis and its overlying vein. Its posterior medial margin is covered by choroid plexus from the third ventricle. Fibers representing ascending tegmental paths, medial lemniscus, spinothalamic tract and brachium conjunctivum enter the thalamus through the inferior surface.

The medial surface forms part of the lateral wall of the third ventricle and is connected by the massa intermedia to the opposite thalamus.

The lateral surface lies adjacent to the occipital portion of the internal capsule by which it is separated from the lenticular nucleus of the corpus striatum. Fibers from this area radiate to the internal capsule to reach the cerebral cortex (thalamic radiation).

The thalamic gray matter is divided by a vertical septum of white matter, the "internal medullary lamina." As this lamina passes forward it bifurcates to partly surround the anterior pole. This portion, the "anterior tubercle," is somewhat raised. It contains several cell groups, the anterior nuclei.

Medial to the internal medullary lamina lie the medial nuclei and still more medially, close to the wall of the third ventricle the midline nuclei. The latter extend into the massa intermedia.

Lateral to the internal medullary lamina is the lateral nuclear mass of the thalamus. This is again subdivided into ventral nuclei and dorsal or lateral nuclei. The ventral nuclei are the ventral anterior, the ventral lateral and the ventral posterior. The latter is again subdivided (see cross section) into the ventral posterolateral and the ventral posteromedial, or the "arcuate" or "semilunar" nucleus.

Posterior to the lateral nuclear mass lie the posterior nuclei of the thalamus consisting of the "pulvinar" and the medial and lateral geniculate bodies.

On the lateral surface of the lateral nuclear mass is a layer of myelinated fibers known as the external medullary lamina and just outside this are the reticular nuclei (see cross section).

An attempt has been made here only to present and classify the principal nuclei. The afferent and efferent connections of the various nuclei are described in a subsequent plate.

PLATE 26

Spinal Cord in Situ

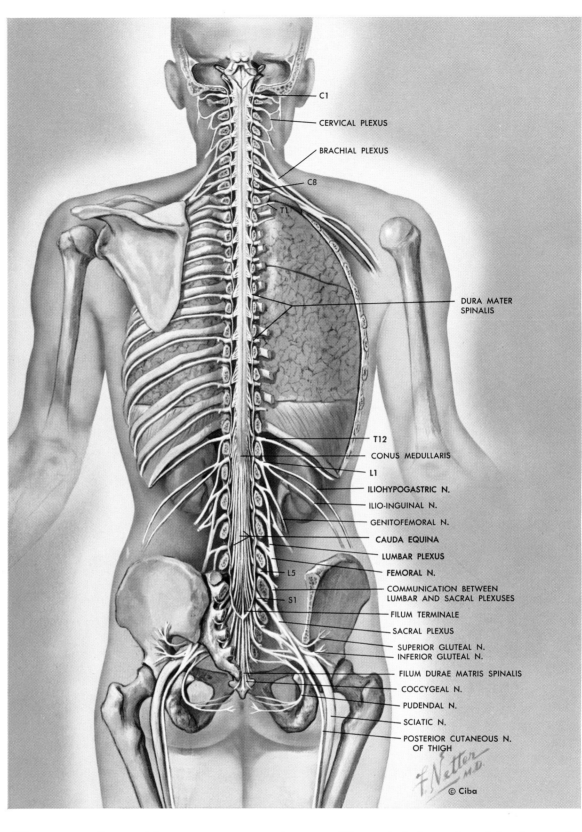

Labels on figure:
C1
CERVICAL PLEXUS
BRACHIAL PLEXUS
C8
T1
DURA MATER SPINALIS
T12
CONUS MEDULLARIS
L1
ILIOHYPOGASTRIC N.
ILIO-INGUINAL N.
GENITOFEMORAL N.
CAUDA EQUINA
LUMBAR PLEXUS
FEMORAL N.
L5
COMMUNICATION BETWEEN LUMBAR AND SACRAL PLEXUSES
S1
FILUM TERMINALE
SACRAL PLEXUS
SUPERIOR GLUTEAL N.
INFERIOR GLUTEAL N.
FILUM DURAE MATRIS SPINALIS
COCCYGEAL N.
PUDENDAL N.
SCIATIC N.
POSTERIOR CUTANEOUS N. OF THIGH

F. Netter M.D.
© Ciba

The spinal cord, a direct downward continuation of the medulla oblongata, starts at the upper border of the atlas and ends at the lower border of the first lumbar vertebra as the conus medullaris. Though cylindrical, it is slightly flattened in its anteroposterior diameter. Corresponding to the large nerves supplying the upper and lower limbs we find a cervical enlargement from cervical 3 to thoracic 2, and a lumbar enlargement from thoracic 9 to 12. From the lowermost end of the spinal cord — the conus medullaris — extends a delicate median prolongation, the filum terminale interna, which ends with the dural sac at the second sacral vertebra. Its extradural prolongation — filum terminale externa — ends at the coccyx.

The spinal cord is enveloped by the dura, arachnoid and pia mater. External to the dura is the epidural space filled by a thin layer of fat, areolar tissue and veins. The arachnoid and subarachnoid spaces are filled with fluid which cushions the spinal cord. The pia mater intimately surrounding the spinal cord also has lateral extensions to the inner dural surface.

These are equally spaced between nerve roots and are known as dentate ligaments.

In fetal life the spinal cord fills the entire length of the vertebral canal and the spinal nerves run in a horizontal direction. As the vertebral column elongates with growth, the spinal cord is drawn upward and the roots therefore assume an increasingly oblique and downward direction toward their foramina of exit, forming at its lowest portion the cauda equina.

The spinal nerves emerge from the spinal cord in pairs, eight in the cervical region, twelve in the thoracic region, five in the sacral region, one pair of coccygeal nerves, and five lumbars, making a total of 31 pairs of spinal nerves. These also correspond to varying segments of neuromeres of the spinal cord.

Each spinal nerve has an anterior and posterior root, the latter showing an oval enlargement called the ganglion. These nerve roots join to form plexuses:

1. The cervical plexus, formed by the anterior divisions of the upper four cervical nerves.

2. The brachial plexus, which is formed by the anterior divisions of C5, 6, 7, 8, and first thoracic nerves.

3. The lumbar plexus, formed by the anterior division of lumbar 1, 2, 3, and greater part of lumbar 4.

4. The sacral plexus, formed by the roots of lumbar 4 and 5, and sacral 1, 2, and 3 nerves.

In addition to the twelve pairs of intercostal nerves, some of the most significant nerves are the iliohypogastric nerve arising from the first lumbar root; the ilio-inguinal nerve arising also from the first and second lumbar roots; the femoral nerve arising from the second, third and fourth lumbar roots; the sciatic nerve which is the main nerve of the sacral plexus; and the coccygeal nerve which also receives filaments from the fourth and fifth sacral nerves.

PLATE 27

EXIT OF SPINAL NERVES

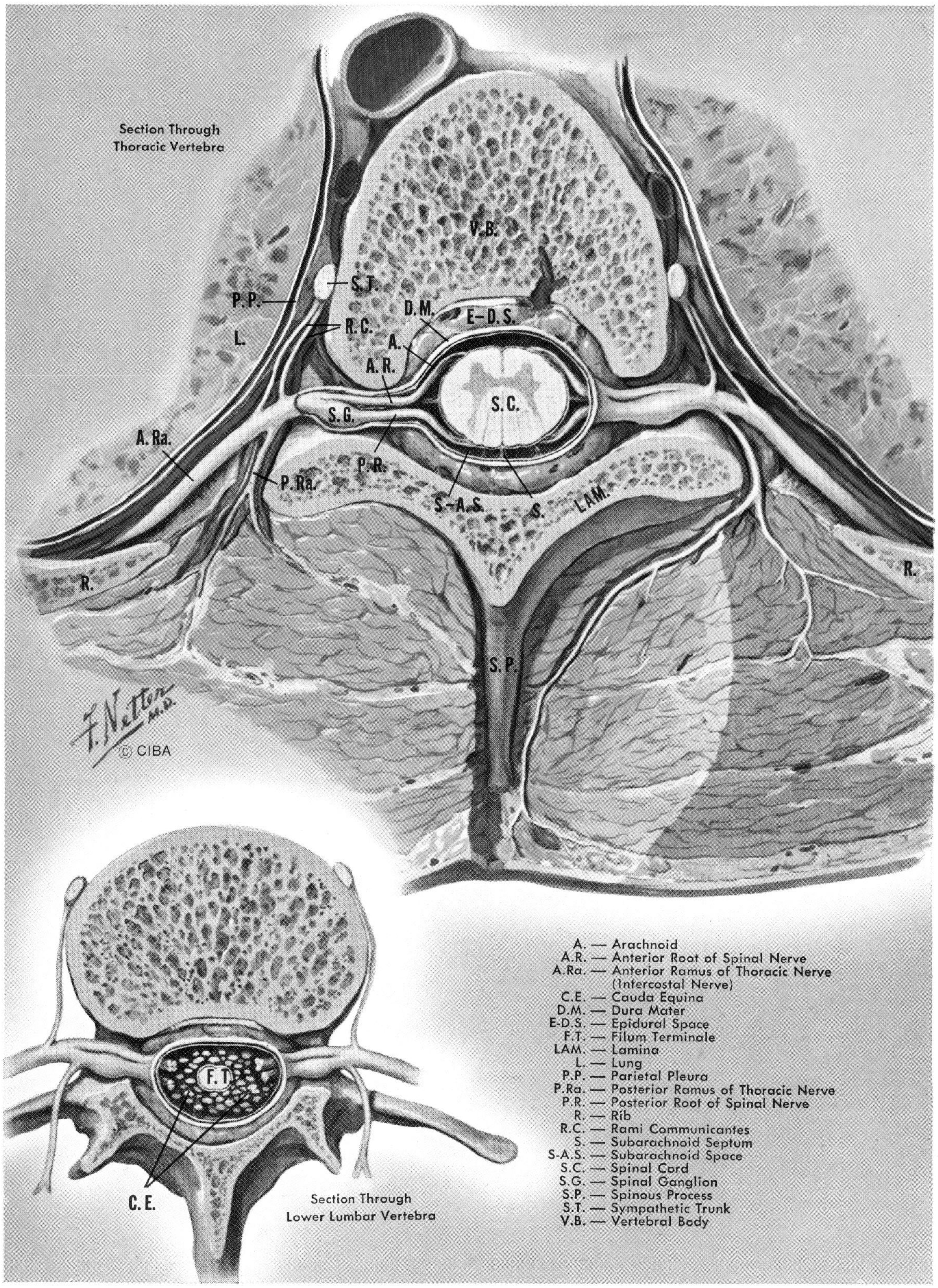

Section Through
Thoracic Vertebra

F. Netter
© CIBA

Section Through
Lower Lumbar Vertebra

A. — Arachnoid
A.R. — Anterior Root of Spinal Nerve
A.Ra. — Anterior Ramus of Thoracic Nerve
(Intercostal Nerve)
C.E. — Cauda Equina
D.M. — Dura Mater
E-D.S. — Epidural Space
F.T. — Filum Terminale
LAM. — Lamina
L. — Lung
P.P. — Parietal Pleura
P.Ra. — Posterior Ramus of Thoracic Nerve
P.R. — Posterior Root of Spinal Nerve
R. — Rib
R.C. — Rami Communicantes
S. — Subarachnoid Septum
S-A.S. — Subarachnoid Space
S.C. — Spinal Cord
S.G. — Spinal Ganglion
S.P. — Spinous Process
S.T. — Sympathetic Trunk
V.B. — Vertebral Body

As the anterior root of the spinal cord emerges from the anterior and lateral gray columns, it traverses the surrounding membranes of pia, arachnoid and dura. The posterior root, which is attached to the posterolateral portion of the spinal cord, originates from two bundles of fibers in the spinal ganglion. Both anterior and posterior roots pierce the dura separately as they make their exit through their respective intervertebral foramina. As a rule, the posterior root is thicker and larger than the anterior root. They are enclosed in a common dural sheath just beyond the spinal ganglion where they become the spinal nerve and are surrounded by epineurium.

The spinal ganglia, which lie at the outer portion of the intervertebral foramina, are oval-shaped and vary in size corresponding to their nerve roots.

The spinal nerves lie horizontally in the cervical region but below these segments the spinal nerves assume an increasingly oblique and downward direction as they approach the lumbar region where they are almost vertical, forming the cauda equina. At the lower thoracic level there is a difference of two vertebral segments between the origin of the spinal nerve and the level of exit.

From each sympathetic trunk ganglion, which lies on the posterolateral surface of the vertebral body, a branch (gray ramus communicans) joins the adjacent spinal nerve.

Efferent, preganglionic sympathetic fibers (white ramus communicans), which originate in the lateral columns, pass along with the anterior root to the corresponding sympathetic ganglion or along its trunk to sympathetic plexuses.

Shortly after emerging from the intervertebral foramen each spinal nerve gives off a meningeal branch which turns back through the same foramen to supply the spinal cord membranes, blood vessels, intervertebral ligaments and joint surfaces.

The spinal nerve then divides into two branches, each with fibers from both roots:

1. Anterior division supplies the anterior and lateral portions of the trunk and limbs. In the thoracic region it spans the space between the pleura and intercostal membranes, runs below the lower rib margin and supplies the intercostal muscles and adjacent skin. In the cervical and lumbar regions the anterior divisions form plexuses.

2. Posterior division is directed backward shortly beyond the formation of the spinal nerve. Its medial branch supplies the multifides, longissimus, semispinalis and trapezius, then proceeds along the spinous process, and supplies the skin. Its lateral branch traverses the longissimus and supplies the intercostal muscle and adjacent skin.

In the lumbar region the medial branches of the posterior division hug the articular processes of the vertebrae and end in the multifides, and the lateral branches supply the group of sacrospinalis muscles, adjacent fascia and skin.

PLATE 28

SECTIONS THROUGH THE SPINAL CORD

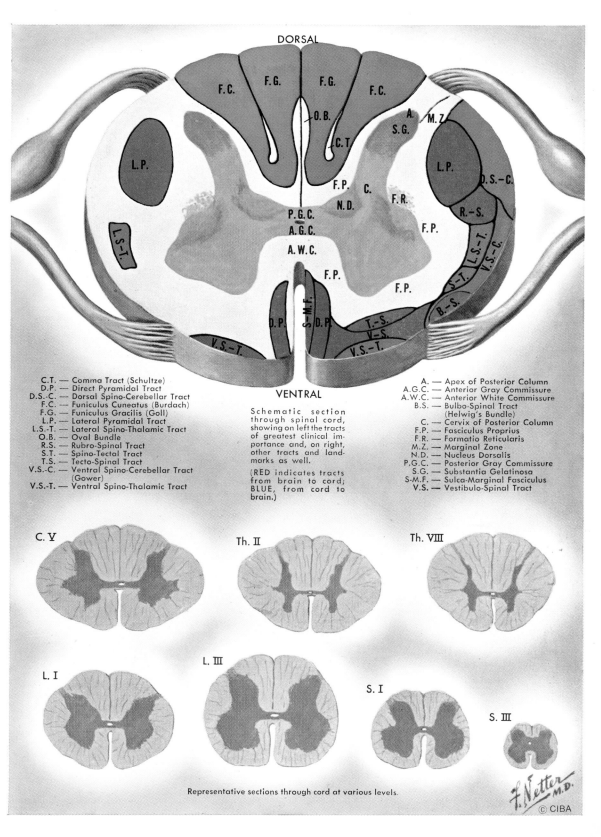

DORSAL

VENTRAL

Schematic section through spinal cord, showing on left the tracts of greatest clinical importance and, on right, other tracts and landmarks as well.

(RED indicates tracts from brain to cord; BLUE, from cord to brain.)

C.T. — Comma Tract (Schultze)
D.P. — Direct Pyramidal Tract
D.S.-C. — Dorsal Spino-Cerebellar Tract
F.C. — Funiculus Cuneatus (Burdach)
F.G. — Funiculus Gracilis (Goll)
L.P. — Lateral Pyramidal Tract
L.S.-T. — Lateral Spino-Thalamic Tract
O.B. — Oval Bundle
R.S. — Rubro-Spinal Tract
S.T. — Spino-Tectal Tract
T.S. — Tecto-Spinal Tract
V.S.-C. — Ventral Spino-Cerebellar Tract (Gower)
V.S.-T. — Ventral Spino-Thalamic Tract

A. — Apex of Posterior Column
A.G.C. — Anterior Gray Commissure
A.W.C. — Anterior White Commissure
B.S. — Bulbo-Spinal Tract (Helwig's Bundle)
C. — Cervix of Posterior Column
F.P. — Fasciculus Proprius
F.R. — Formatio Reticularis
M.Z. — Marginal Zone
N.D. — Nucleus Dorsalis
P.G.C. — Posterior Gray Commissure
S.G. — Substantia Gelatinosa
S-M.F. — Sulca-Marginal Fasciculus
V.S. — Vestibulo-Spinal Tract

C. V   Th. II   Th. VIII   L. I   L. III   S. I   S. III

Representative sections through cord at various levels.

F. Netter, M.D.
© CIBA

Cross sections of the spinal cord at various levels show considerable variation in size and shape. The proportion of gray to white matter also varies and is much greater in the cervical and lumbar regions and greatest in the conus medullaris. The anterior and posterior gray columns in the thoracic region are equally thin, but in the cervical region the anterior gray columns are larger; in the lumbar region and below, both gray columns are about equally wide and in much greater proportion to the white matter.

Through the entire length of the spinal cord runs the central canal, which is lined with ciliated ependymal cells. Superiorly it opens into the fourth ventricle, and inferiorly extends into the filum terminale. The horizontal gray matter which joins the gray columns surrounds the central canal and is divided by it into anterior and posterior gray commissures.

Through the spinal cord run fibers carrying impulses to and from various portions of the brain. These fibers group themselves into tracts. Only those of known clinical importance will be described.

Funiculus gracilis (Goll) and funiculus cuneatus (Burdach) carry muscle and joint sensations and lie between the posterior median and posterolateral sulcus. In the cervical and thoracic regions these tracts are separated by a septum at the lower portion of which is found the comma tract (Schultze).

Lateral spinothalamic tract mediates pain and temperature sensation. It arises in the posterior column, crosses to the opposite side in the anterior commissure and ascends in the lateral funiculus to the thalamus.

Ventral spinothalamic tract transmits impulses of touch. It also arises in the posterior column, crosses in the anterior commissure to the opposite side and ascends in the anterior funiculus to the thalamus.

Dorsal spinocerebellar tract transmits impulses from leg muscles and trunk between the sixth cervical and second lumbar segments. It is located on the lateral surface ventral to the posterior lateral sulcus, and ascends to the cerebellum via the restiform body.

Ventral spinocerebellar tract (Gower) carries impulses to the cerebellum via medulla, pons and anterior medullary velum. It lies at the periphery on the ventrolateral aspect of the cord.

Spinotectal tract arises from cells in the posterior gray column, crosses over and ascends in the lateral funiculus, and ends in the corpora quadrigemina.

Rubrospinal tract carries impulses for cerebellar reflexes. It arises in the red nucleus, crosses over and descends near the center of the lateral funiculus.

Lateral pyramidal tract carries impulses to the primary motor neuron. It arises from large cells in the precentral gyrus and, after decussation in the medulla, enters the lateral funiculus lying between the dorsal spinocerebellar tract and lateral funiculus.

Direct pyramidal tract is small; it arises from cells in the central motor area, passes down the same side close to the anterior median fissure, then crosses in the anterior commissure to the opposite side and at various levels ends by synapses with the anterior horn cells.

Tectospinal tract mediates optic and auditory reflexes. It arises in the superior colliculi, crosses and then descends in the anterior funiculus to end in the motor cells of the anterior column.

PLATE 29

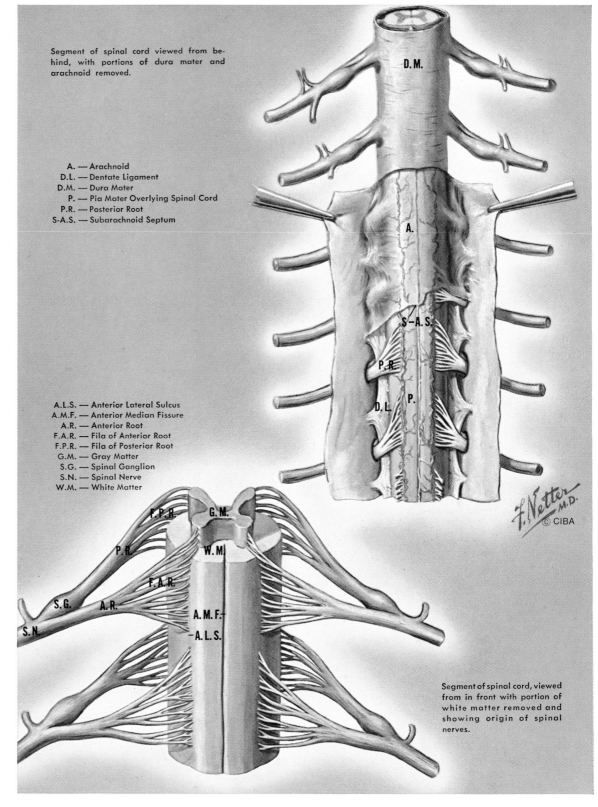

Segment of spinal cord viewed from behind, with portions of dura mater and arachnoid removed.

A. — Arachnoid
D.L. — Dentate Ligament
D.M. — Dura Mater
P. — Pia Mater Overlying Spinal Cord
P.R. — Posterior Root
S-A.S. — Subarachnoid Septum

A.L.S. — Anterior Lateral Sulcus
A.M.F. — Anterior Median Fissure
A.R. — Anterior Root
F.A.R. — Fila of Anterior Root
F.P.R. — Fila of Posterior Root
G.M. — Gray Matter
S.G. — Spinal Ganglion
S.N. — Spinal Nerve
W.M. — White Matter

Segment of spinal cord, viewed from in front with portion of white matter removed and showing origin of spinal nerves.

SPINAL MEMBRANES AND NERVE ROOTS

The spinal cord is enveloped by membranes which are a direct continuation of those surrounding the brain.

Dura mater extends direct from the cranial dura, beginning at the foramen magnum and continuing as far down as the second sacral vertebra. This membrane adheres anteriorly to the posterior longitudinal ligament and corresponds in shape to the enlargements of the spinal cord. The dura also invests the spinal nerves as they leave the lateral margins of the spinal cord to their points of exit.

The subdural space is a potential space containing a minute quantity of fluid and is found between the arachnoid and the dura.

Arachnoid and subarachnoid consist of a delicate meshwork of mesothelial cells with spaces filled with cerebrospinal fluid. These membranes also envelop the spinal nerves to their intervertebral foramina.

Pia mater is a delicate fibrous layer which intimately invests the spinal cord. At its lateral margins the pia forms denser pointed prolongations to the inner dural surface. These are spaced equally between the nerve roots, and also separate the anterior from the posterior spinal roots.

Although there are no visible demarcations, the spinal cord is said to be made up of segments of varying lengths. These segments correspond approximately to the attachments of a pair of spinal nerves. The widest segments are in the midthoracic region.

On cross section of the spinal cord one can see the white matter on the periphery, which is made up of medullated nerve fibers held together by neuroglia. In the central portion of the spinal cord we find the gray matter which has the form of the letter "H." This consists of numerous nerve cells and nonmedullated nerve fibers, held together by neuroglia.

The spinal nerves consist of an anterior spinal root and posterior spinal root with its ganglion. These are attached to the corresponding gray matter of the spinal cord.

The anterior root arises from nerve cells in the anterior and lateral columns of the gray matter, and as the fibers pass through the white matter they become medullated. They leave the spinal cord in two or three irregular rows (fila) to efferent pathways.

The posterior root arises from the medial afferent fibers of the spinal ganglion and reaches the posterolateral sulcus in the form of six or eight fasciculi (fila).

The spinal ganglia are enveloped by the continuation of the dural sheath and contain irregularly spherical cells. These cells give off a unipolar coiled axon which divides into a medial and lateral portion. The former is directed toward the spinal cord and becomes the posterior root, while the latter is directed peripherally to sensory end organs of muscles, joints, skin and viscera.

The anterior median fissure, lined by an overlapping fold of pia, dips into the greater part of the anterior portion of the spinal cord.

The anterior lateral sulcus is a fine depression about midway between the anterior median fissure and the lateral margin of the spinal canal and marks the exit of the fila of the anterior roots.

PLATE 30

ARTERIES OF THE SPINAL CORD

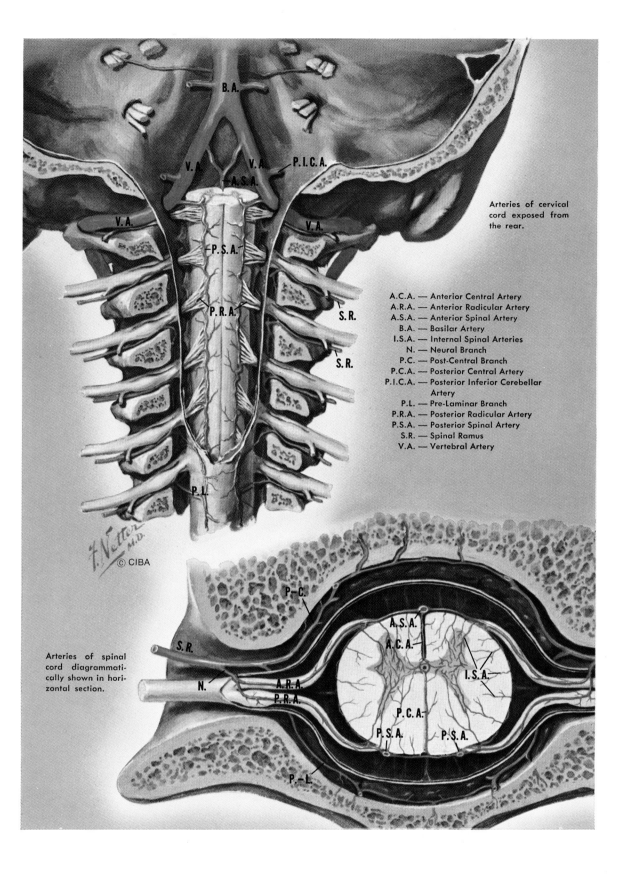

Arteries of cervical cord exposed from the rear.

A.C.A. — Anterior Central Artery
A.R.A. — Anterior Radicular Artery
A.S.A. — Anterior Spinal Artery
B.A. — Basilar Artery
I.S.A. — Internal Spinal Arteries
N. — Neural Branch
P.C. — Post-Central Branch
P.C.A. — Posterior Central Artery
P.I.C.A. — Posterior Inferior Cerebellar Artery
P.L. — Pre-Laminar Branch
P.R.A. — Posterior Radicular Artery
P.S.A. — Posterior Spinal Artery
S.R. — Spinal Ramus
V.A. — Vertebral Artery

Arteries of spinal cord diagrammatically shown in horizontal section.

The spinal cord derives its blood supply from the vertebral artery and from a series of spinal rami which enter the intervertebral foramina at successive levels.

The posterior spinal artery is a branch of the vertebral artery which begins near the lateral margin of the medulla oblongata and descends on the dorsolateral surface of the spinal cord posterior to the spinal roots. In its downward course to the cauda equina the posterior spinal artery receives a succession of small arterial branches which enter the spinal canal through the intervertebral foramina. These vessels and their branches anastomose freely around the posterior roots and with the corresponding vessels on the opposite side, dipping also into the substance of the spinal cord, and in the midline form the posterior central artery.

The anterior spinal artery is formed by the union of two branches from the terminal portion of the vertebral artery at the level of the foramen magnum. The artery descends as a single trunk on the anterior aspect of the spinal cord to the conus medullaris, then continues along the cauda equina and ends as a fine arteriole accompanying the filum terminale. At successive levels it, too, is reinforced by spinal branches entering through the intervertebral foramina. Along its course small twigs from this artery enter the substance of the spinal cord and in the anterior median fissure these form the anterior central artery.

The spinal branches arise at various levels from the sacral, iliolumbar, intercostal, inferior thyroid and vertebral arteries which enter the spinal canal through the intervertebral foramina. Each spinal branch divides into two rami: (1) a peripheral ramus which after entering the spinal canal divides into an ascending and descending branch and then anastomoses with the one above and below to form two lateral chains on the posterior surfaces of the vertebral bodies near the junction of the pedicles, and (2) a central ramus which supplies the spinal cord and its membranes by dividing into anterior and posterior arteries which anastomose with the anterior and posterior arteries of the spinal cord.

PLATE 31

VENOUS DRAINAGE OF SPINAL CORD AND VERTEBRAL COLUMN

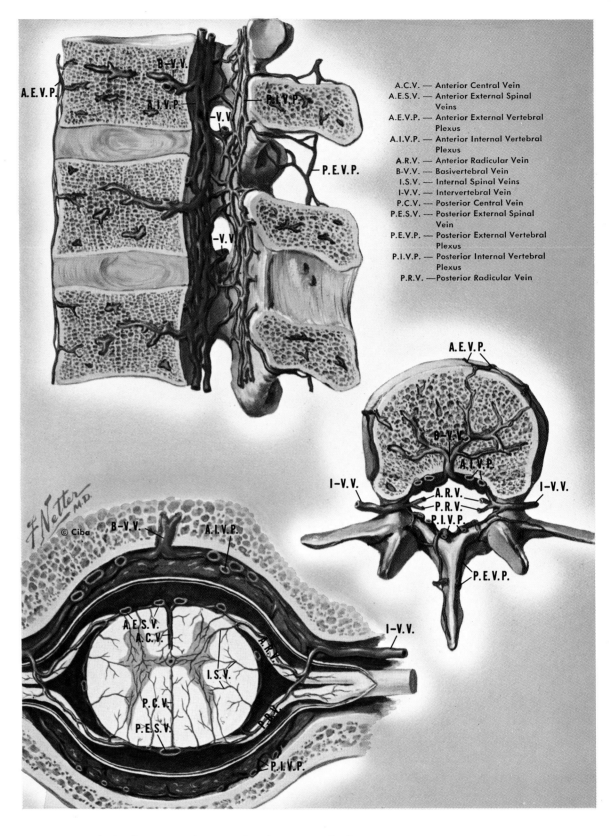

A.C.V. — Anterior Central Vein
A.E.S.V. — Anterior External Spinal Veins
A.E.V.P. — Anterior External Vertebral Plexus
A.I.V.P. — Anterior Internal Vertebral Plexus
A.R.V. — Anterior Radicular Vein
B-V.V. — Basivertebral Vein
I.S.V. — Internal Spinal Veins
I-V.V. — Intervertebral Vein
P.C.V. — Posterior Central Vein
P.E.S.V. — Posterior External Spinal Vein
P.E.V.P. — Posterior External Vertebral Plexus
P.I.V.P. — Posterior Internal Vertebral Plexus
P.R.V. — Posterior Radicular Vein

Outside and inside the vertebral canal, running along the entire length, is a series of venous plexuses which freely anastomose with each other and end in intervertebral veins.

Two groups of venous plexuses are found on the outside of the vertebral canal: (1) the anterior group lies in front of the vertebral bodies. This group receives some venous tributaries from vertebral bodies and communicates with the basivertebral and intervertebral veins, and (2) the posterior group which forms a network of venous plexuses spreading over the spinous processes, laminae, facets and adjacent deep musculature. In the cervical region these veins com-

municate with the deep cervical, occipital and cerebral veins.

The venous plexuses on the inside of the vertebral canal lie between the dura and inner vertebral surfaces. These veins receive tributaries from the adjacent bony structures and the spinal cord. Although they form a close network, running vertically within the spinal canal, they may be subdivided into (1) a pair of anterior internal venous plexuses which lie on either side of the posterior longitudinal ligament and into which basivertebral veins empty, and (2) a single posterior internal venous plexus which lies anterior to, and on either side of, the vertebral arches and ligamentum flavum, and anastomoses with the posterior external veins.

These plexuses form almost a series of venous rings at the level of each vertebra, found most strikingly at

the foramen magnum.

Tunneling the bony structure of each vertebral body is the basivertebral vein which has a small valve-like opening as it joins the anterior internal venous plexus.

The intervertebral veins leave the spinal cord through the intervertebral foramina in company with the spinal nerves. They also have a valve-like mechanism as they join the intercostal, lumbar and sacral veins.

The veins of the spinal cord are minute and delicate. They emerge from the anterior median fissure as the anterior central vein, and from the posterior sulcus as the posterior central vein. There are also two lateral longitudinal veins on either side of the spinal cord, and they all empty into the intervertebral veins. However, those near the foramen magnum empty into the inferior petrosal sinus or cerebellar veins.

PLATE 32

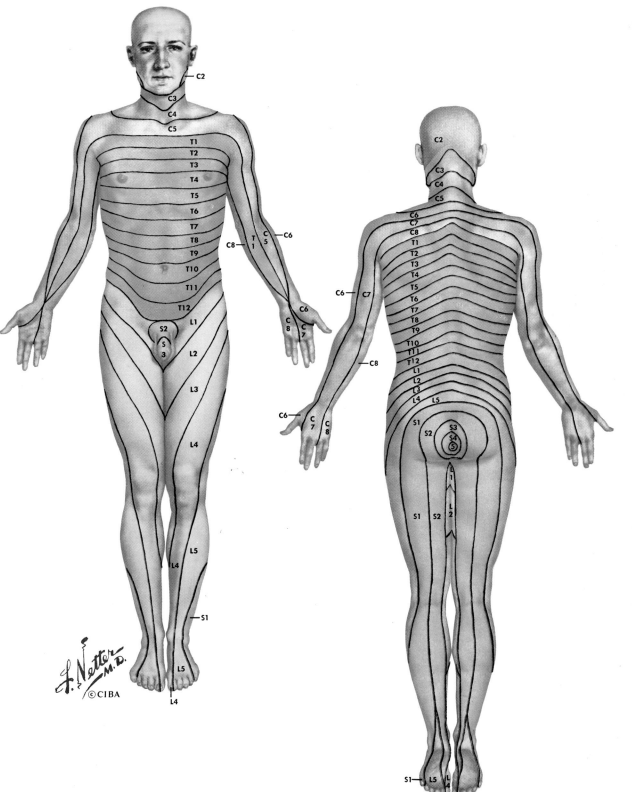

DERMAL SEGMENTATION

Sensations from the outside world are carried to the consciousness by the spinal and some cranial nerves to the brain. They travel over the posterior roots; their further detailed course is for the moment not of interest. All the cell bodies are situated in ganglia outside of the central nervous system proper; they have a peripheral branch going to the sense organ and a central branch going to the spinal cord or the brain.

We include here the fibers carrying hot and cold, pain and touch. Vibration sense and position sense are probably complicated sensations involving several of the primitive sensations, including the proprioceptive sensations, which in the spinal cord go also into the ganglia, but in the head region end in the mesencephalic nucleus of the trigeminal nerve.

In the head, sensations are mediated by the trigeminus, and in a small region behind the external auditory meatus by the facial and the vagus nerves. In the body, the various spinal nerves take over. These are by and large arranged metamerically, that is to say, one segment lies behind the other in an orderly sequence. But these sequences are interrupted in the arm and the leg regions where several segments have been carried out to the periphery of the limb and are, therefore, no more represented near the axis of the body. Hence, on the ventral side of the body, C5 borders on T1, and L1 on S2.

Two other important points should be realized: The segmentations given in almost all diagrams are based on pain, but the borders for the reception of pain are not the same as those for the reception of, say, touch, which generally involves a somewhat narrower sphere. The second point is that the different nerves overlap to some extent, so that frequently no more than a hypesthesia develops after one root has been cut.

If one is familiar with the cutaneous distribution of various nerve roots, it is possible to localize the site and level of any pathologic disturbance.

A chart outlining the exact sensory dermal segments serves as a good reference, but it is valuable to remember some surface landmarks which will serve as a general guide to localization:

1. The clavicular region is supplied by cervical 5 sensory root.
2. The deltoid region is supplied by cervical 5 and 6 sensory roots.
3. The nipple area is supplied by thoracic 4 sensory root.
4. The umbilicus is supplied by thoracic 10 sensory root.
5. The groin region is supplied by thoracic 12 sensory root.
6. The lateral aspect of the arm is supplied by cervical 5, 6 and 7 sensory roots.
7. The inner aspect of the arm is supplied by cervical 8 and thoracic 1 sensory roots.
8. The inner and anterior surfaces of the thigh are supplied from above down by lumbar 1, 2, 3 and 4 sensory roots.
9. The outer and posterior surfaces of the thigh are supplied by lumbar 5 and sacral 1 and 2 sensory roots.
10. The perineum is supplied by sacral 2, 3, 4 and 5 sensory roots.
11. The hand is supplied from the radial to the ulnar borders by cervical 6, 7 and 8 sensory roots. Cervical 6 supplies the thumb, cervical 7 the middle of the hand, including the index and middle fingers, and cervical 8 the ulnar border, including the ring and little fingers.
12. The foot is supplied from its lateral to its medial surface by sacral 1, lumbar 5 and lumbar 4 sensory roots.

NOTE: Some discrepancies exist in the definition of the dermal segments as published by different authors, but the chart produced here is based essentially on the work of Dr. J. Jay Keegan, University of Nebraska College of Medicine. We herewith express our appreciation for his contributions and personal communication.

Keegan, J. J.: *J. Neurosurg.* 4:115, 1947
Keegan, J. J.: *J. Bone Jt. Surg.* 26:238, 1944
Eaton, L. M.: *Surg. Clin. N. Amer.* 26:810, 1946

Section III

FUNCTIONAL NEURO-ANATOMY

with descriptive text by

GERHARDT VON BONIN, M.D.

Professor of Anatomy, University of Illinois College of Medicine
Chicago, Illinois

PLATE 33

POSTCENTRAL GYRUS

INTERNAL CAPSULE

POSTEROLATERAL VENTRAL NUCLEUS OF THE THALAMUS

MESENCEPHALON

F.E. — Free Nerve Endings
H. — Nerve Endings on Hair Follicle
M. — Meissner's Corpuscle
M.S. — Muscle Spindle
V.P. — Vater-Pacini Corpuscle

NUCLEUS GRACILIS

NUCLEUS CUNEATUS

MEDIAL LEMNISCUS

LOWER MEDULLA

MEDIUM MYELINATED FIBERS (TOUCH)

UNMYELINATED FIBERS (PAIN, HOT AND COLD)

FUNICULUS CUNEATUS

FUNICULUS GRACILIS

LATERAL SPINO-THALAMIC TRACT

VENTRAL SPINO-THALAMIC TRACT

CERVICAL CORD

HEAVILY MYELINATED FIBERS (PROPRIOCEPTION)

SUBSTANTIA GELATINOSA

SOMESTHETIC SYSTEM
Body

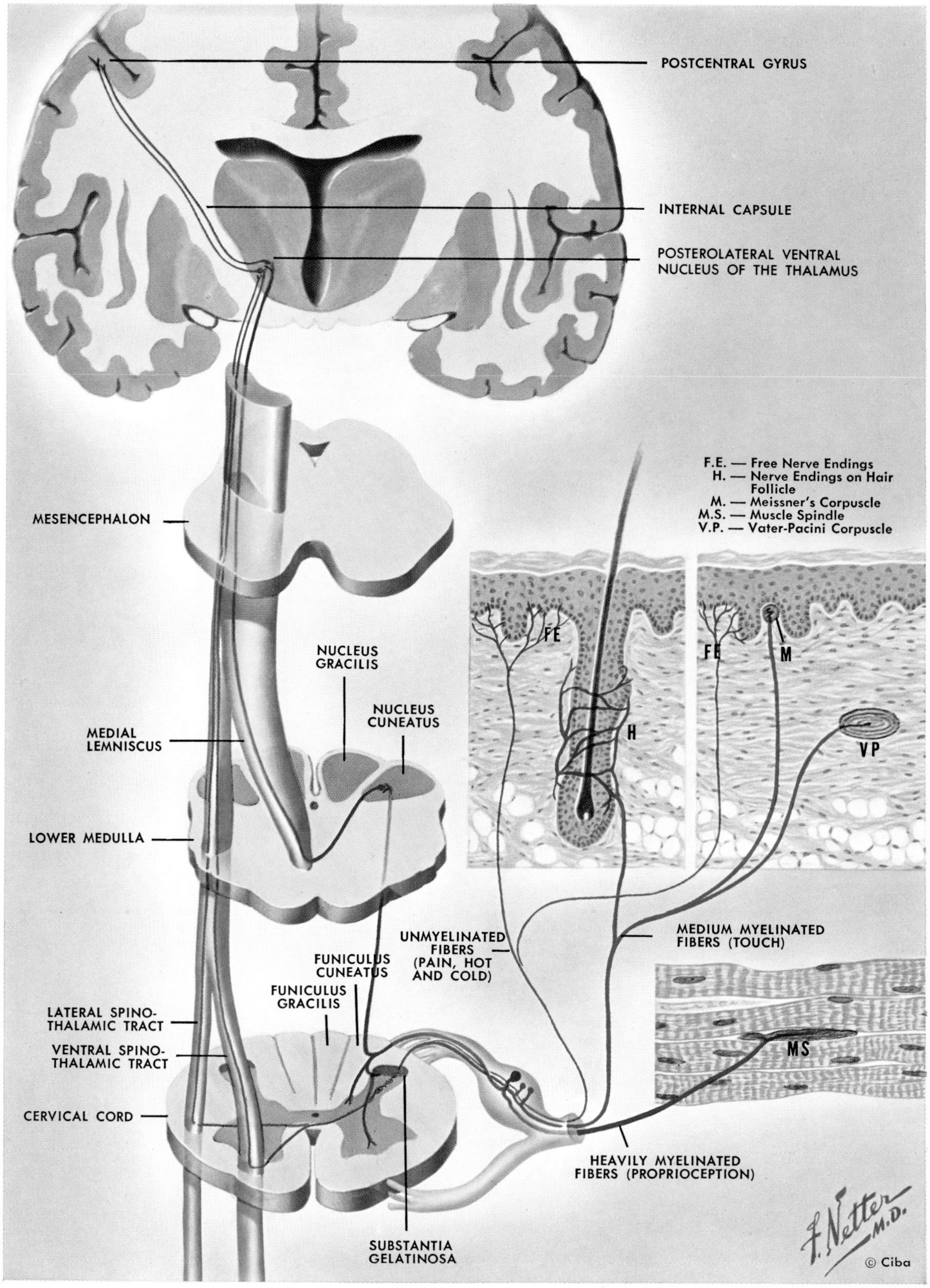

Somesthetic messages are either exteroceptive (from the skin) or proprioceptive (from muscles, tendons and joints). In the thick skin on the palmar surface of hand and fingers and the plantar surface of foot and toes (right half of skin picture), free nerve endings (FE), Meissner's corpuscles (M), and bodies of Vater-Pacini (VP) are found. In the thin skin covering the rest of the body (left half of skin picture), Meissner's corpuscles are rare, but hairshafts (H) receive a liberal supply of sensory nerves. Proprioceptive end-organs are muscle or tendon spindles of which only the former are shown (MS). They react to stretch. The nerve fibers bringing proprioceptive messages to the spinal cord are heavily myelinated, "touch fibers" are medium myelinated, "pain fibers" are unmyelinated.

In the posterior root heavy and medium myelinated fibers form a medial moiety. They enter the posterior funiculus. Proprioceptive fibers give off collaterals to Clarke's column, to the anterior horn, and to the posterior horn entering it from its ventral side (the last two are shown as one fiber in the figure). Exteroceptive fibers ascend in the posterior funiculus, lying lateral to corresponding fibers coming from lower levels. The fibers shown in illustration (cervical level, arm) course through the cuneate funiculus (or fasciculus), to end in the cuneate nucleus, shown in the section of the lower medulla. The messages from the leg pour into the nucleus gracilis. The axons of the cells composing these two nuclei cross over and ascend through the brain stem as the medial lemniscus ending in the posterolateral ventral nucleus of the thalamus.

Thin and unmyelinated fibers, the lateral moiety of the posterior root, enter the marginal zone of Lissauer, and then impinge upon the posteromarginal cells and/or the gelatinous substance of Rolando. These cell masses influence in turn the nucleus proprius of the posterior horn. The cells in the nucleus proprius send their axons into the opposite lateral or ventral spinothalamic tract. The branched axon shown in the illustration is merely a convenient symbol. The lateral spinothalamic tract carries pain and temperature; the ventral spinothalamic tract carries touch. The spinothalamic tracts unite on the dorsal and then on the lateral side of the medial lemniscus. They, too, end in the ventrolateral nucleus of the thalamus, occipitad to the medial lemniscus. Somesthetic impulses are relayed along the axons of the thalamic neurons to the cerebral cortex just behind the Rolandic sulcus.

REFERENCES

Association for Research in Nervous and Mental Diseases, Pain: Proceeding of the Association, Dec. 18 and 19, 1942. Vol. XXIII. Baltimore, Williams and Wilkins, 1943
Lloyd, D. P. C.: Physiol. Rev. 24: 1-17, 1944

PLATE 34

SOMESTHETIC SYSTEM
Head

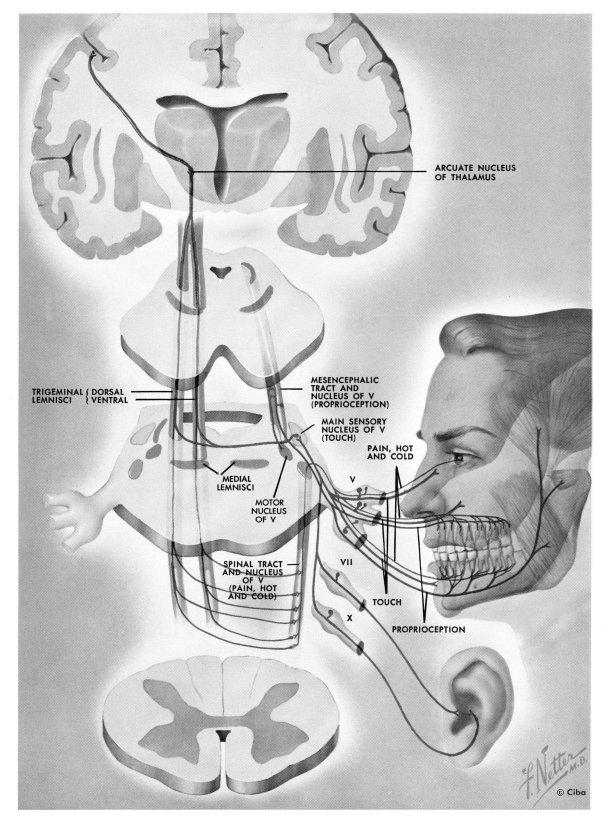

The face is supplied with sensory nerves by the trigeminus (V), the facial (VII) and the vagus (X) nerves. The trigeminus and cervical nerves overlap. Roughly, only that part of the face which is not bearded in the male is exclusively innervated by the trigeminus. The ophthalmic and the maxillary divisions of this nerve are purely sensory, the mandibular division contains also motor fibers to the muscles of mastication. Just as in the rest of the body, dichotomy of lemniscus and spinothalamic system is present — touch is conducted over myelinated fibers to the main sensory nucleus in the pons, while pain is conducted over unmyelinated fibers to the spinal nucleus of the trigeminus. This nucleus extends from the pons down to the uppermost cervical levels of the cord where it merges into the gelatinous substance of Rolando. For a short space below the pons the spinal tract of the trigeminus lies directly at the surface of the brain stem; else-

where it is covered by the dorsal spinocerebellar tract (Sjöqvist). Many fibers turn ventral without bifurcating into the spinal tract, others bifurcate and thus supply both nuclei (Gerard).

The facial (VII) sends sensory fibers (nervus intermedius) to a small patch in the anterior wall of the external auditory meatus, while the vagus (X) sends sensory branches to a small patch on the posterior wall of that meatus. The central processes of these sensory neurons feed into the main and spinal trigeminal nuclei respectively (Brodal).

The neurons in the main sensory nucleus and in the spinal nucleus send their axons to the opposite side where they ascend in either of two bundles known as the dorsal and ventral trigeminal lemnisci. They end in the arcuate nucleus of the thalamus, just

medial to the ventrolateral nucleus (Plate 33, page 58). The thalamic cells send their axons to the face, field of the somesthetic area in the postcentral gyrus.

Proprioceptive impulses, evoked by stretching the muscles of mastication or by pressure on the teeth (Corbin and Harrison), reach the mesencephalic root. These fibers are the only sensory fibers of the somesthetic system which do not arise within ganglia but from cell bodies within the central nervous system.

The further course of impulses arriving at the mesencephalic nucleus is not known.

REFERENCES

Brodal, A.: *Arch. Neurol. & Psychiat.* 57: 292-306, 1947
Corbin, K. B., and Harrison, F.: *J. Neurophysiol.* 3: 423-435, 1940
Gerard, M. W.: *Arch. Neurol. & Psychiat.* 9: 306-338, 1923
Sjöqvist, Olaf: *Zentralbl. f. Neurochir.* 2: 274-281, 1937

PLATE 35

TASTE

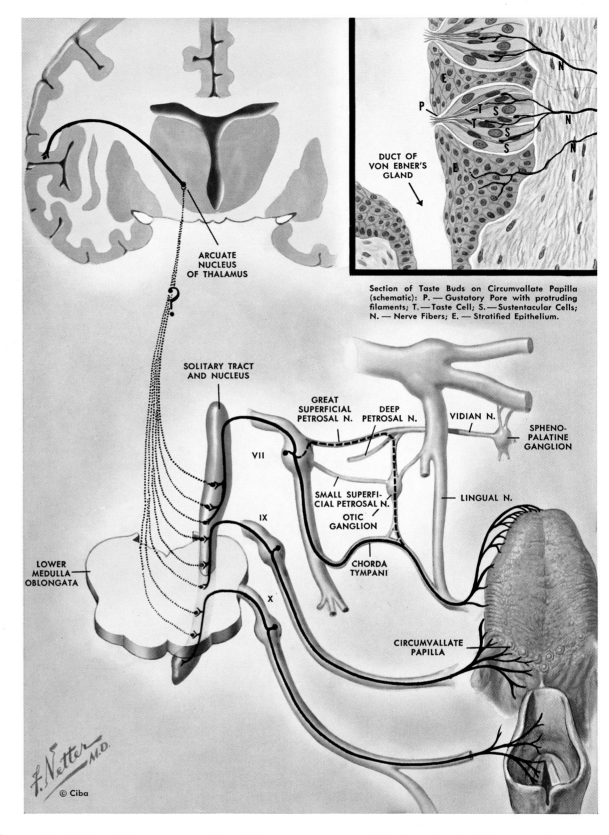

ARCUATE NUCLEUS OF THALAMUS

SOLITARY TRACT AND NUCLEUS

GREAT SUPERFICIAL PETROSAL N.

DEEP PETROSAL N.

VIDIAN N.

SPHENO-PALATINE GANGLION

VII

SMALL SUPERFI-CIAL PETROSAL N.

OTIC GANGLION

LINGUAL N.

IX

LOWER MEDULLA OBLONGATA

X

CHORDA TYMPANI

CIRCUMVALLATE PAPILLA

DUCT OF VON EBNER'S GLAND

Section of Taste Buds on Circumvallate Papilla (schematic): P. — Gustatory Pore with protruding filaments; T. —Taste Cell; S.—Sustentacular Cells; N. — Nerve Fibers; E. — Stratified Epithelium.

F. Netter M.D.
© Ciba

Tastebuds are found (lower right-hand corner of illustration) on the tip of the tongue, on the banks of the moats surrounding the circumvallate papillae at the back of the tongue, and on the pharynx, epiglottis and larynx. The circumvallate papillae contain the densest population of tastebuds.

Each bud contains sensory cells (T), with filaments protruding from the pore (P) and sustentacular cells (S), (upper right-hand corner of illustration). Into the surrounding moats empty von Ebner's glands whose watery secretion is considered to flush the moat and to prepare the surface of the tastebuds for new stimuli.

Four basic qualities, sweet, sour, salty and bitter, are generally distinguished and each tastebud responds to only one of these qualities. But all tastebuds look alike. The total number of tastebuds decreases with old age. Most tastebuds are innervated by the glossopharyngeus (IX). The facial (VII) innervates the tip of the tongue and the vagus (X) sends branches to epiglottis and larynx.

The peripheral pathway of the taste fibers in the facial nerve is tortuous. The cell body in the geniculate ganglion usually sends its peripheral fiber by way of the chorda tympani through the petrotympanic fissure to the lingual nerve of the mandibular branch of the trigeminus (V). However, the cell body may occasionally send its fiber by way of the great superficial petrosal and past the otic ganglion to the lingual

nerve and, finally, to the tip of the tongue. Sometimes extirpation of the gasserian ganglion causes loss of taste at the tip of the tongue (Schwartz and Weddell).

In the brain stem, taste fibers from VII, IX and X stream into the solitary nucleus. The connections between this nucleus and cerebral cortex are obscure. In all likelihood, axons of the cells in the solitary nucleus cross and ascend, in connection with those of the trigeminal lemniscus (Plate 34, page 59), to the arcuate nucleus of the thalamus. This nucleus appears to relay messages concerned with taste to the infraparietal plane or the medial side of the parietal operculum (Ruch and Patton).

REFERENCES

Ruch, T. C., and Patton, H. D.: *Fed. Proc.* 5: 89-90, 1946
Schwartz, H. G., and Weddell, G.: *Brain* 61: 99-115, 1938

PLATE 36

CONTROL
OF RESPIRATION

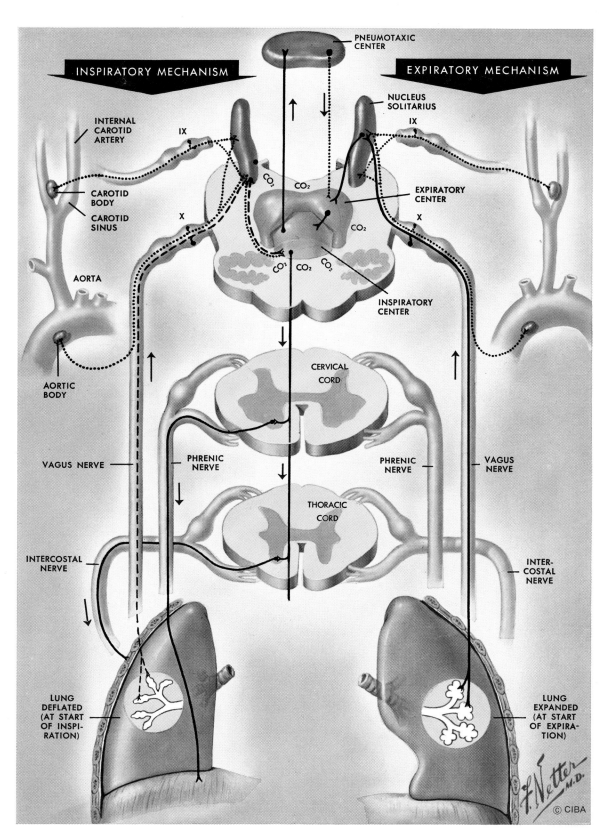

Though the solitary nucleus is concerned with taste, control of respiration appears to be its primary function, for it is present even in animals which have no tastebuds, such as birds.

At least three stimuli are effective in respiratory control and are indicated in the illustration: (1) CO_2, bathing the respiratory center directly (and acting, perhaps, by influencing the actual reaction of the blood), (2) the chemical composition of the circulating blood, acting on the chemoreceptors in the carotid and aortic bodies, and (3) the degree to which the lung is distended.

The motor neurons to the phrenic nerve (in C_4 and C_5), to the intercostal muscles (in the thoracic segments, particularly the upper half) and presumably those to the auxiliary muscles of respiration are under the control of an expiratory and an inspiratory center in the medulla oblongata, approximately at the level of the inferior olive. These centers are in the "reticular substance" and appear to be a part of the inhibitory and the facilitatory

centers recently described by Magoun and Rhines. These two respiratory centers, in their turn, receive afferent fibers from the pneumotaxic center near the hypothalamus and from the solitary nucleus. The latter is under the influence of the messages sent by the chemoreceptors of the carotid body over the glossopharyngeus (IX) and vagus (X) and by the stretch receptors in the lung sent over the vagus. When the lung is collapsed (expiration, left half), impulses traveling from stretch receptors over the vagus to the solitary nucleus have a low frequency. They are picked up by the inferior portion of the solitary nucleus and are relayed, probably via the reticulospinal tract and motor neurons in the spinal cord, to the inspiratory center which then causes the diaphragm and external intercostal muscles to contract. Expansion of

the lung in inspiration (right half) stimulates the stretch receptors, and impulses are sent along the vagus at high frequency. They are now picked up by a more superior portion of the solitary nucleus which relays impulses to the expiratory center; the latter inhibits the inspiratory muscles and may, in exceptional circumstances, also stimulate the expiratory muscles.

This mechanism (Wyss) appears sufficient in itself to insure the play of alternate inspiration and expiration. Chemoreceptors and CO_2 provide additional security, perhaps by changing the threshold of response of the neurons composing the respiratory centers.

REFERENCES

Magoun, H. W., and Rhines, R.: *Spasticity*. Springfield, Ill., Charles C Thomas, 1948

Wyss, O. A. M.: *J. Neurophysiol.* 10: 315-320, 1947

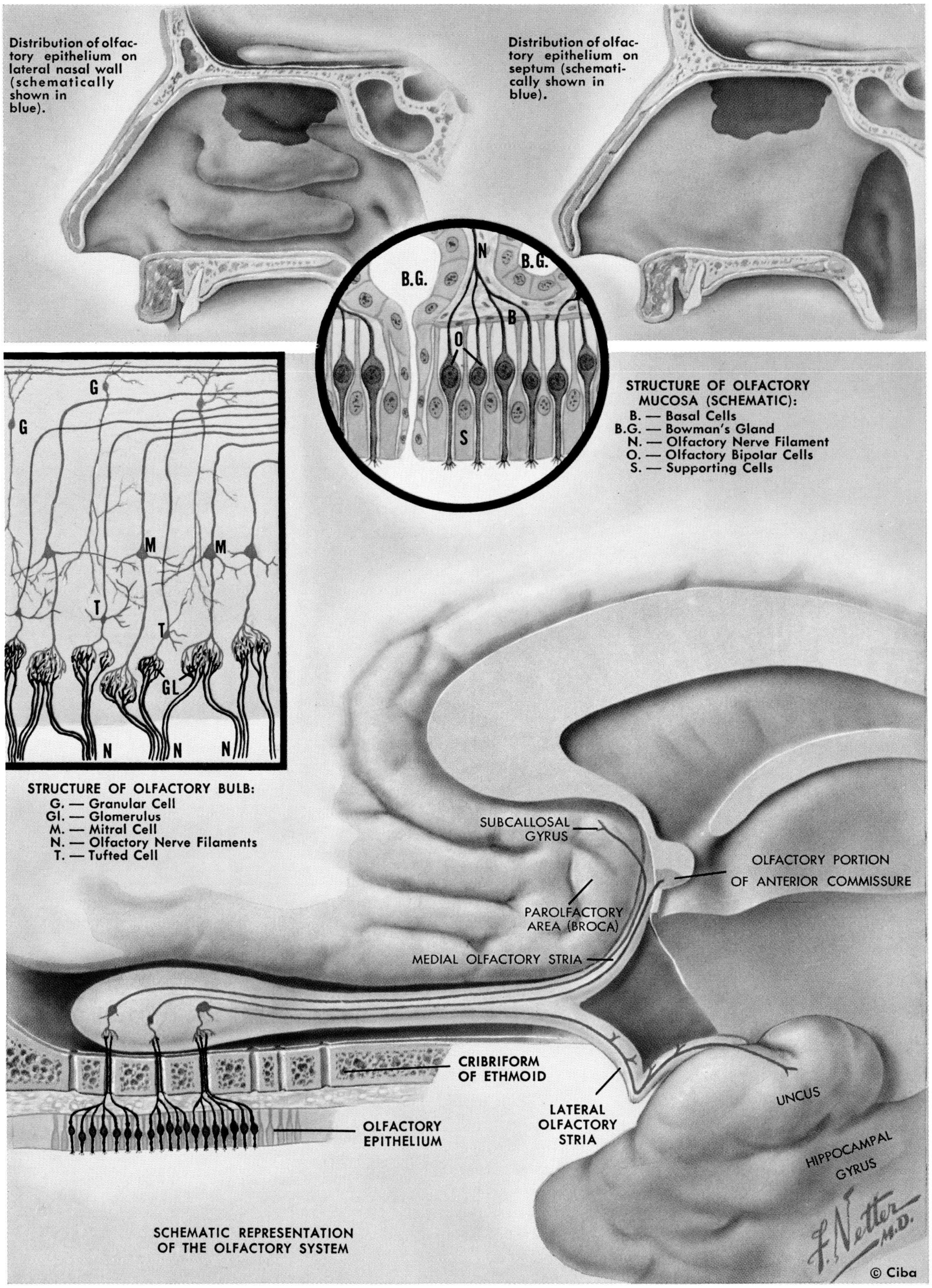

PLATE 37

Distribution of olfactory epithelium on lateral nasal wall (schematically shown in blue).

Distribution of olfactory epithelium on septum (schematically shown in blue).

STRUCTURE OF OLFACTORY MUCOSA (SCHEMATIC):
B. — Basal Cells
B.G. — Bowman's Gland
N. — Olfactory Nerve Filament
O. — Olfactory Bipolar Cells
S. — Supporting Cells

Olfactory System

STRUCTURE OF OLFACTORY BULB:
G. — Granular Cell
Gl. — Glomerulus
M. — Mitral Cell
N. — Olfactory Nerve Filaments
T. — Tufted Cell

SUBCALLOSAL GYRUS

OLFACTORY PORTION OF ANTERIOR COMMISSURE

PAROLFACTORY AREA (BROCA)

MEDIAL OLFACTORY STRIA

CRIBRIFORM OF ETHMOID

LATERAL OLFACTORY STRIA

UNCUS

OLFACTORY EPITHELIUM

HIPPOCAMPAL GYRUS

SCHEMATIC REPRESENTATION OF THE OLFACTORY SYSTEM

Olfactory stimuli are received by the olfactory cells which are found in a small patch extending over both the lateral and medial walls and the roof of the upper nasal meatus (upper section of illustration). Within this olfactory mucosa, often described as being of a yellow-brownish color in life (the blue color in plate is purely symbolical), olfactory cells are embedded between sustentacular cells.

An olfactory cell is thin, bulging out where the nucleus is situated, and bears "hairs" at its free end. Toward its base it tapers into a long thread. These threads make up the olfactory filaments which pierce the cribriform plate and enter the olfactory bulb (lowest figure of plate).

The olfactory cells are the only sensory cells in the human body which conduct impulses. In the olfactory bulb, the fila form an extremely complicated plexus. Each sensory cell sends signals to many glomeruli, dense balls composed of fila olfactoria and of dendrites from the mitral and the "tufted" cells of the olfactory bulb.

Some degree of spatial localization in the projection of different areas of the olfactory epithelium onto different regions of the bulb has been shown (Clark). The projection is somewhat diffuse but with regard to some areas rather precise. Both mitral and tufted cells send their axons into the olfactory tract, but they also send signals to a "feed-back" mechanism represented by the granular cells which send their axons back to the mitral and tufted cells. Whether this reinforces or inhibits subsequent messages is not known.

The fibers of the olfactory tract are definitely known to course through the lateral olfactory striae toward the uncus. The fibers gradually become exhausted on their way; the last fibers reach the amygdaloid nucleus, but no olfactory impulse can be traced, electrically or anatomically, to the entorhinal area or any part of the hippocampus.

The medial olfactory stria contains fibers coursing through the olfactory portion of the anterior commissure to the opposite olfactory bulb. In man, the number of these fibers is very small. Whether fibers end in the parolfactory area and the subcallosal gyrus has become doubtful in the light of recent evidence.

According to modern investigations, much of the "rhinencephalon" of classical anatomy, in particular the hippocampus (cornu ammonis), is not involved in the function of smell, but is built into yet unknown circuits (Brodal).

REFERENCES
Brodal, A.: Brain 70: 179-222, 1947
Clark, W. E. LeGros: The Projection of the Olfactory Epithelium on the Olfactory Bulb in the Rabbit. J. Neur., Neurosurg. & Psychiat. 14: 1-10, 1951
Meyer, M., and Allison, A. C.: An Experimental Investigation of the Connections of the Olfactory Tracts in the Monkey. J. Neur., Neurosurg. & Psychiat. 12: 274-286, 1949

PLATE 38

OPTIC SYSTEM

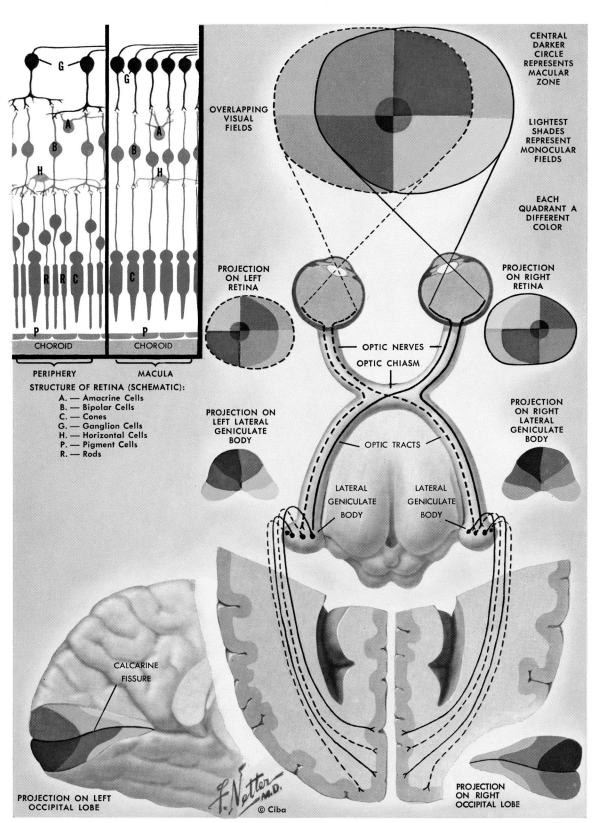

STRUCTURE OF RETINA (SCHEMATIC):
A. — Amacrine Cells
B. — Bipolar Cells
C. — Cones
G. — Ganglion Cells
H. — Horizontal Cells
P. — Pigment Cells
R. — Rods

The human retina (and that of most primates) has a macula lutea which contains only cones, while the peripheral field chiefly contains rods. Rods contain visual purple and have a very low threshold (a few quanta excite them, Hecht), with a minimum at a spectral frequency of 544 mμ. Cones do not contain visual purple, have a much higher threshold, with a minimum at 590 mμ (Purkinje shift), and are responsible for photopic vision. Different cones respond to different wavelengths of light. Cones responding to red, green, and blue (moderators) have been found (Granit).

Both rods (R) and cones (C) have short central processes which conduct excitation to a dendrite of a bipolar cell (B, upper left diagram). These in their turn transmit messages to the ganglion cells whose axons form the optic nerve, chiasm and tract and end in the lateral geniculate body of the diencephalon (right side of plate). Amacrine cells (A) and horizontal cells (H) may constitute a regulatory "feed-back mechanism." In the macula, cones, bipolar and ganglion cells are present in equal numbers. In the periphery, many rods and cones impinge upon one bipolar cell, and many bipolar cells on one ganglion cell (Polyak). There are altogether about 125,000,000 rods and cones but only about 1,250,000 fibers in the optic nerve or tract.

The cells of the lateral geniculate body are arranged in six laminae, two ventral, large-celled ones and four dorsal, small-celled ones. The semidecussation in the optic chiasm contains fibers from both eyes, but from corresponding (right or left) halves of each retina to each geniculate body. Fibers from each eye end by splitting into three rami in alternate layers. The two lowest layers relay optic impulses in part at least to the anterior quadrigeminal body on the roof of the midbrain (not shown in plate). The four dorsal laminae contain cells which send their axons into the optic radiation of Gratiolet which runs lateral to the posterior horn of the ventricle (lower right of plate) and ends in the striate area of the cerebral cortex. This area, easy to identify in fresh brain by the stripe of Gennari or of Vicq d'Azyr, covers both walls of the posterior calcarine fissure and the adjacent parts of the occipital pole. Retina and striate areas correspond "point-to-point" (Marshall and Talbot). Each hemisphere is directed toward the opposite side, i.e., toward that side of the body which it governs, the upper lip of the calcarina is directed downward, the lower lip upward (corresponding to the location of leg and face in the somesthetic area). The macula lutea is presented in a rather large area at the occipital pole, the temporal demilune in the most anterior portion of the striate area. Peripheral parts of the retina are projected to a comparatively small part of the striate area.

REFERENCES
Chacko, L. W.: The Laminar Pattern of the Lateral Geniculate Body in the Primates. J. Neur., Neurosurg. & Psychiat. 11: 211-224, 1948
Granit, R.: Sensory Mechanisms of the Retina. . . . Oxford University Press, 1947
Hecht, S.: Amer. Sci. 32: 159-177, 1944
Marshall, W. H., and Talbot, S. A.: Biological Symposia 7: 117-164, 1942
Polyak, S. L.: The Retina. Chicago, Ill., Univ. of Chicago Press, 1941

PLATE 39

ACOUSTIC SYSTEM

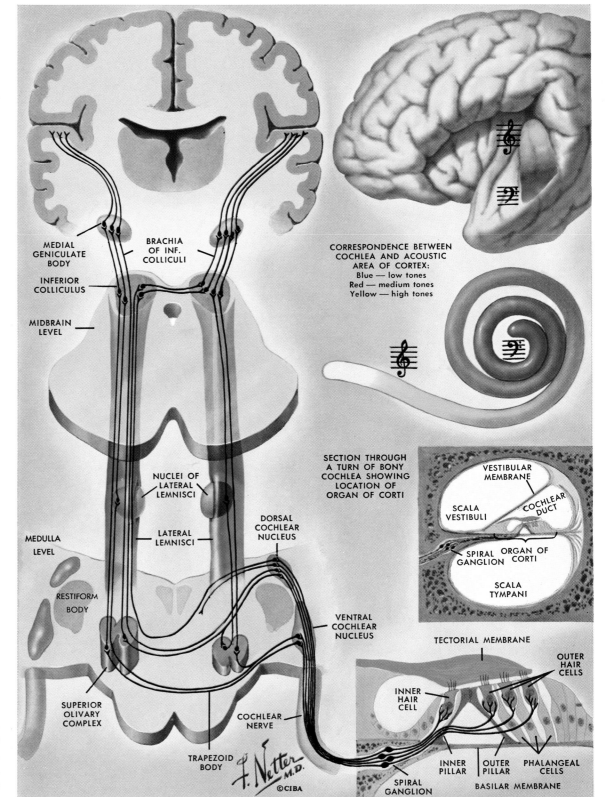

Acoustic stimuli, *i.e.*, longitudinal vibrations of air or other ponderable media, impinge upon Corti's organ (lower right of plate) after having passed through the middle ear and through the scala vestibuli and scala tympani.

In Corti's organ, hair cells, embedded within a scaffold of phalangeal and pillar cells, are rubbed against the tectorial membrane.

In the cochlea, low tones are picked up near the tip (helicotrema), high tones near the oval window. The basilar membrane is shorter near the oval window than near the tip.

Excitations of the hair cells are picked up by the cochlear nerve (VIII) whose (bipolar) ganglion cells are embedded in the petrous bone. The fibers enter the brain stem at the lateral side of the pons, lateral to the restiform body and immediately split up to enter the dorsal and **ventral** cochlear nuclei (Lorente de No).

The acoustic pathways to the cortex are complex. The further cell stations are: the superior olive, the nucleus of the lateral lemniscus, the inferior colliculus on the roof of the midbrain and the medial geniculate body.

Between cochlear nuclei and medial geniculate body are at least two neurons. The synapse may be located in any of the three cell masses mentioned. Many but not all fibers decussate. Of these decussations, the most ventral one at the level of the superior olive is the strongest; it is known as the trapezoid body. The pathway between superior olive and inferior colliculus is a compact bundle of fibers known as the lateral lemniscus.

From the medial geniculate body, the acoustic radiation emerges to end on Heschl's gyrus on the supratemporal plane (upper left and right of plate).

There is a point-to-point correspondence between cochlea and the acoustic area of the cortex. This was first worked out in the cat where low tones are transmitted to the frontal, high tones to the occipital end of the acoustic area (Howell). In man and primates, the twist by which the temporal lobe develops ontogenetically has brought about an almost complete reversal of the location of high and low tones.

REFERENCES

Ades, H. W., and Felder, R. E.: *J. Neurophysiol.* 8: 463-470, 1945
Bailey, P., von Bonin, G., Carol, H. W., and McCulloch, W. S.: *J. Neurophysiol.* 6: 121-128, 1943
Barnes, W. T., Magoun, H. W., and Ranson, S. W.: *J. Comp. Neurol.* 79: 129-152, 1943
Lorente de No, R.: *Laryngoscope* 43: 327-380, 1933
Stevens, S. S., and Davis, H.: *Hearing, Its Psychology and Physiology.* New York City, J. Wiley & Sons, 1938

PLATE 40

SPINAL EFFECTOR MECHANISM

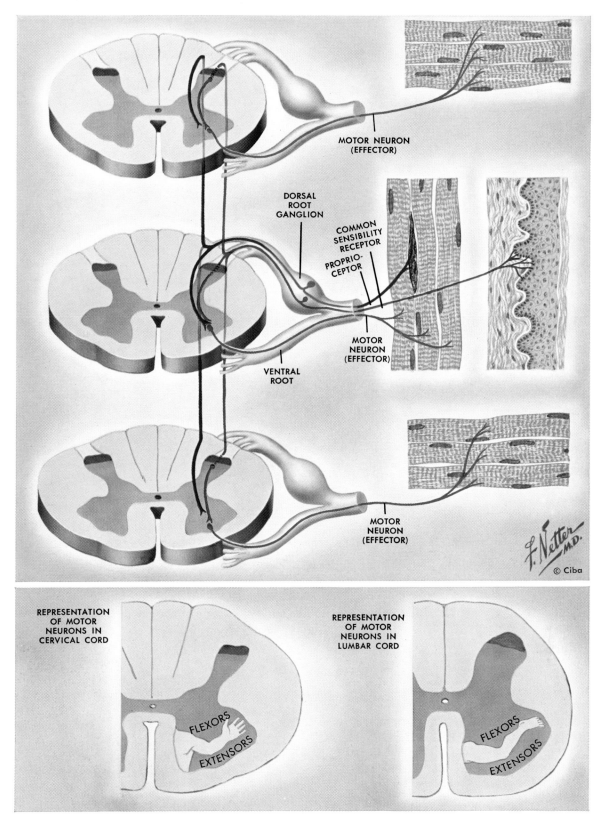

MOTOR NEURON
(EFFECTOR)

DORSAL
ROOT
GANGLION

COMMON
SENSIBILITY
RECEPTOR

PROPRIO-
CEPTOR

MOTOR
NEURON
(EFFECTOR)

VENTRAL
ROOT

MOTOR
NEURON
(EFFECTOR)

F. Netter M.D.

© Ciba

REPRESENTATION
OF MOTOR
NEURONS IN
CERVICAL CORD

FLEXORS

EXTENSORS

REPRESENTATION
OF MOTOR
NEURONS IN
LUMBAR CORD

FLEXORS

EXTENSORS

With this plate the motor apparatus is introduced. The detailed analysis of it is discussed in Plate 43, page 68, and Plate 44, page 69. All controls of movements, from the cerebral cortex to the proprioceptors, play directly or indirectly on the motor neurons in the anterior column of the spinal cord — which, therefore, was called by Sherrington the "final common pathway." Each cell in the anterior horn innervates several muscle fibers known as the "motor unit." The number varies in mammals from about 4 in the ocular and laryngeal muscles to more than 100 in some muscles of the leg. No data on man exist. The cells in the anterior horn are arranged in ill-defined groups. The medial ones innervate the muscles of the trunk, the lateral groups, only present in the cervical and lumbar enlargement, innervate the extremities, cells innervating the flexors being more dorsal than those innervating the extensors (lowest figures in plate).

The motor neurons can be influenced by both proprioceptive and exteroceptive ("common sensibility," see illustration) fibers (Lloyd). The former, streaming in through the medial moiety of the posterior root (Plate 33, page 58), send a branch directly to the motor neuron at the level

of their entrance. They also have ascending and descending collaterals ending by numerous branches in the adjacent levels. The direct branch extends well into the anterior column, and makes contact with cells innervating extensors. The branches reaching the anterior horn at higher and lower levels do not extend quite as far ventrad and end in the neighborhood of the flexor neurons. The net result is that proprioceptive impulses will cause contraction of extensors and relaxation of flexors (kneejerk, Achilles tendon reflex, etc.). Exteroceptive, particularly painful impulses (labeled "common sensibility" in the middle panel) pass through the "filter" of the posterior column. The cells of the nucleus proprius of the posterior horn send collaterals into the ventral column, where they influence preponderantly the flexor group. This is the

structural basis for the "flexor reflex."

In life these sensory stimuli are not as massive as those evoked by the reflex hammer (or the pin) of the physician. They serve to adjust a delicate balance of muscular tension rather than to evoke brisk and meaningless jerks. To stress this point the term "feed-back mechanism," of which the governor of the steam engine is a simple example, has recently been introduced.

It is partly by changing the "gain" of these simple reflexes or feed-back mechanisms that the higher centers control the motor neurons in the spinal cord.

REFERENCES

Lloyd, D. P. C.: *Physiol. Rev.* 24, 1-17, 1944
Sherrington, C. S.: *The Integrative Action of the Nervous System.* London, Constable & Co. Ltd., 1906, 412 pp.

PLATE 41

VESTIBULAR CONTROLS

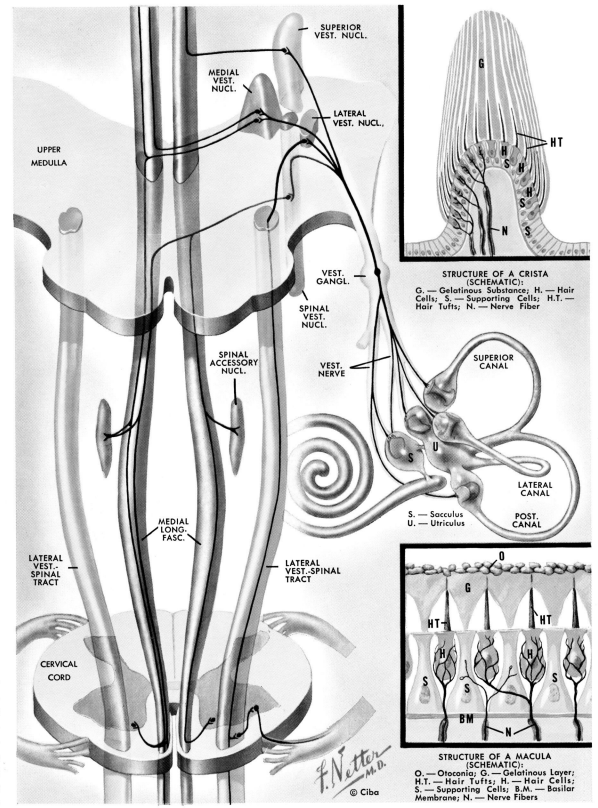

STRUCTURE OF A CRISTA
(SCHEMATIC):
G. — Gelatinous Substance; H. — Hair
Cells; S. — Supporting Cells; H.T. —
Hair Tufts; N. — Nerve Fiber

S. — Sacculus
U. — Utriculus

STRUCTURE OF A MACULA
(SCHEMATIC):
O. — Otoconia; G. — Gelatinous Layer;
H.T. — Hair Tufts; H. — Hair Cells;
S. — Supporting Cells; B.M. — Basilar
Membrane; N. — Nerve Fibers

Vestibular sensations are almost exclusively used for control of the muscles. There are two kinds of receptors in the vestibular labyrinth: Cristae in the semicircular canals and maculae in the sacculus (S) and utriculus (U), (middle right of plate). The former (upper right) are hair cells (H) on the cristae of the three ampullae. These hair cells are between supporting cells (S) and bear on their free end long tufts of hair (HT), embedded in a gelatinous substance (G). The endolymph flowing past the crista when the head is moved (because the fluid has inertia) provides the adequate stimulus which is picked up by the nerve fibers of the vestibular nerve (Scarpa's ganglion). The sacculus and utriculus each bear the latter, viz., the maculae acusticae (lower right). That in the sacculus is folded so that its two halves are roughly at right angles to both surfaces of the saccular macula. Each macula consists of supporting cells (S) which provide lodgings for hair cells (H) bearing hair tufts (HT). The tufts are embedded in a

gelatinous mass (G), but this forms a much thinner layer than on the cristae ampullae, and contains moreover on its free surface otoconia, small grains of "ear-dust," consisting mostly of calcium carbonate.

The vestibular nerve, which carries the messages from these receptors, enters the brain stem next to the acoustic nerve (Plate 39, page 64) but veers medially to the restiform body, to end soon either in one of the four vestibular nuclei (the spinal, lateral, medial or superior), or in the cerebellum (beyond scope of picture).

The cells of the vestibular nuclei send their axons either to the cerebellum or to one of two tracts: the medial longitudinal bundle or the lateral vestibulospinal tract. Superior, medial and spinal nuclei supply fibers to both medial longitudinal fasciculi. The lat-

eral nucleus sends its axons into the lateral vestibulospinal tract (some of its cells send their axons back to the vestibular labyrinth — not shown in plate). The medial longitudinal fasciculus (Plate 42, page 67) contains additional fibers emanating from other cell masses. It conveys messages to the nuclei of the eye muscles, to the cells innervating the muscles moving head and neck, i.e., spinal accessory nucleus, and, at least in lower mammals, to the cells innervating the muscles of the trunk (cervical cord, lower left). It cannot be traced beyond the cervical levels in man. The lateral vestibulospinal tract enters the cord in the anterior fasciculus and ends on the motor neurons of the muscles of the limbs. Powerful in lower mammals, it is a very small and perhaps insignificant bundle in man.

PLATE 42

CONTROL OF
EYE MOVEMENTS

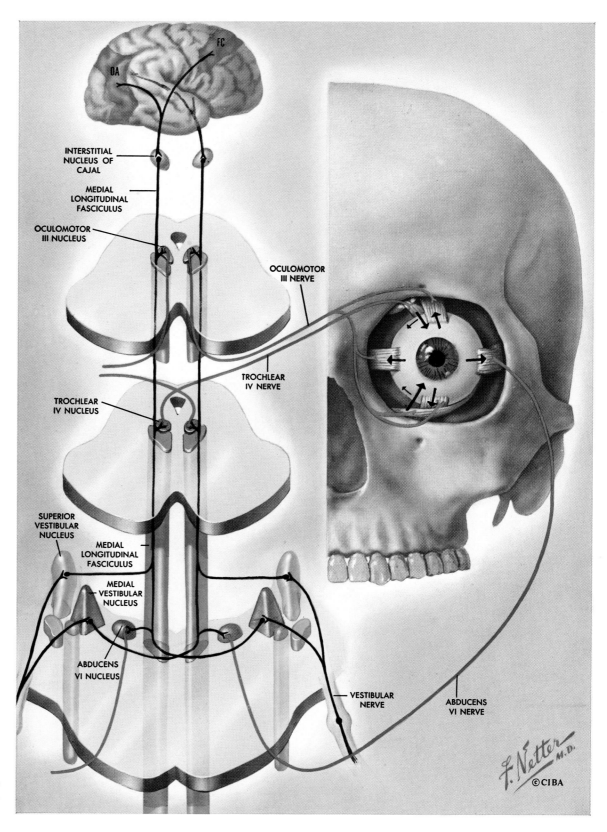

The oculomotor nerve (III) sends fibers to the superior, internal and inferior recti and to the inferior oblique muscle; the trochlear nerve (IV) innervates the superior oblique muscle; and the abducens nerve (VI) innervates the external rectus. These muscles are shown on the right of the plate, the arrows symbolize their action. The nuclei of all three nerves are closely adjacent to the medial longitudinal fasciculus. Plate 41, page 66, and the lower left side of Plate 42, above, illustrate that fibers from the vestibular nuclei enter this bundle thus allowing the vestibular organ to influence eye movements (nystagmus). But the medial longitudinal bundle contains also fibers which are axons of cells situated in gray masses at the rostral level of the midbrain. The exact location is doubtful;

the plate depicts the interstitial nucleus of Cajal for which better arguments have been presented than for the nucleus of Darkshevitch in the central gray near the aqueduct of Sylvius. Fibers emerging from the superior corpora quadrigemina (not shown in plate) and from the cortex and going to the nucleus of Cajal constitute the pathways for the cortical control of ocular movements. The fibers from the cerebral cortex come from the occipital and from the frontal eyefields. The former corresponds roughly to Brodmann's area 19, Economo's OA, the latter corresponds to Brodmann's 8, Economo's FC — zones which will be described later. Direct connections from area FC to the oculomotor nucleus have recently been demonstrated (Ward and Reed).

Whether eye muscles are supplied with propriocep-

tive fibers is still doubtful. Proprioceptive end-organs, *i.e.,* muscle spindles, have been found in some mammalian genera, but not in primates. In any event, it should be remembered that man and primates are among the few mammals which can change the direction of their gaze by isolated movements of their eyes. Hence, it is more important for man to compensate by eye movements for the changing position of his head or for the change in space of the object of attention than to keep the relative positions of eyes and head constant.

REFERENCES

Crosby, E. C., and Henderson, J. W.: The Mammalian Midbrain and Isthmus Regions. *J. Comp. Neur.* 88: 53-92, 1948

Ward, A. A., Jr., and Reed, H. L.: *J. Neurophysiol.* 9: 329-336, 1946

PLATE 43

PYRAMIDAL SYSTEM

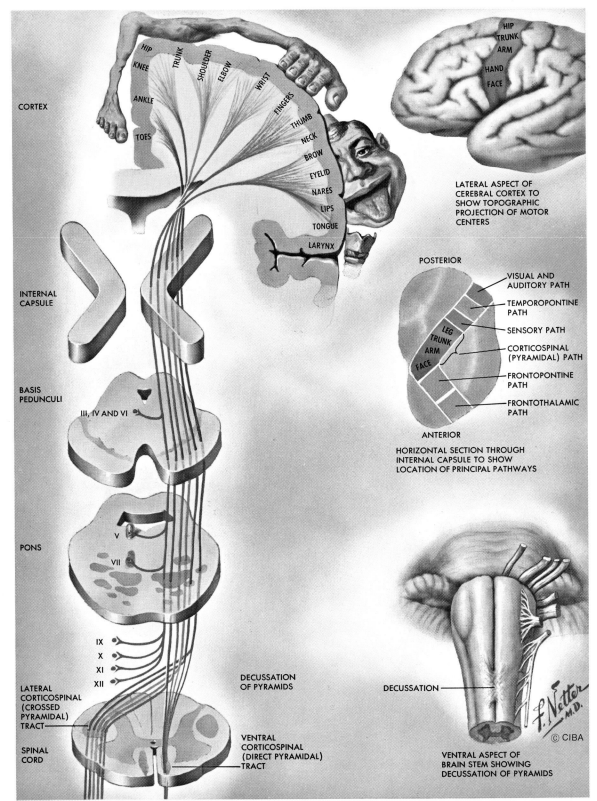

LATERAL ASPECT OF
CEREBRAL CORTEX TO
SHOW TOPOGRAPHIC
PROJECTION OF MOTOR
CENTERS

CORTEX

HIP
KNEE
TRUNK
SHOULDER
ELBOW
WRIST
ANKLE
FINGERS
TOES
THUMB
NECK
BROW
EYELID
NARES
LIPS
TONGUE
LARYNX

HIP
TRUNK
ARM
HAND
FACE

INTERNAL
CAPSULE

POSTERIOR

VISUAL AND
AUDITORY PATH

TEMPOROPONTINE
PATH

SENSORY PATH

CORTICOSPINAL
(PYRAMIDAL) PATH

FRONTOPONTINE
PATH

FRONTOTHALAMIC
PATH

LEG
TRUNK
ARM
FACE

ANTERIOR

HORIZONTAL SECTION THROUGH
INTERNAL CAPSULE TO SHOW
LOCATION OF PRINCIPAL PATHWAYS

BASIS
PEDUNCULI

III, IV AND VI

PONS

V

VII

IX
X
XI
XII

DECUSSATION
OF PYRAMIDS

DECUSSATION

LATERAL
CORTICOSPINAL
(CROSSED
PYRAMIDAL)
TRACT

SPINAL
CORD

VENTRAL
CORTICOSPINAL
(DIRECT PYRAMIDAL)
TRACT

VENTRAL ASPECT OF
BRAIN STEM SHOWING
DECUSSATION OF PYRAMIDS

The pyramidal tracts connect the cortical motor area, shown in the upper right-hand corner, with the final common pathway in the spinal cord (Plate 40, page 65). In the cortex of the precentral gyrus the parts of the body are arranged topographically, roughly as the caricature sprawling over the cross section of the hemisphere indicates. The center for the larynx is close to the Sylvian fissure and may even extend into "Broca's area."

Proceeding upward will be found the center for the face, a large region for the fingers and hand, and a much smaller one for the elbow, shoulder, trunk and hip.

Most of the centers for the foot are on the medial side where the motor area stops about halfway between the dorsal margin and the corpus callosum. In the figure the extent of this area is exaggerated for the sake of clarity.

The pyramidal fibers take their origin from the large pyramidal cells in the fifth layer of the cortex (Plate 48, page 73), some of which attain in the motor cortex a length of over 0.1 mm. These are known as giant pyramidal cells of Betz. The pyramidal fibers twist in their course through the white matter of the hemisphere in such a way that fibers for the

leg (shown in brown) are most posterior in the internal capsule. The fibers for the face, which are shown in red, pass through the knee of the internal capsule (see sketch at right side of illustration).

Descending toward the cerebral peduncle, the twisting continues so that in the pedunculi the fibers for the leg are lateral. The corticobulbar fibers, coming from the area for face and larynx, stream to the motor nuclei of the brain stem. (Nuclei III, IV, and VI are shown in the basis pedunculi.) Nuclei V (mastication), VII (mimetic musculature), IX, X (larynx), XI (trapezius and sternocleidomastoid), and XII (tongue) are shown schematically above the decussation of the pyramids.

Of the pyramidal fibers proper, the corticospinal fibers, about 80 per cent cross over to the opposite

lateral funiculus of the spinal cord at the border between brain stem and spinal cord, while about 20 per cent enter the anterior funiculus on the same side. The lateral pyramidal tract ends in the internuncial pool of the posterior horn and thus acts indirectly on the motor neurons, principally on those of the hand and foot (bottom of Plate 40, page 65). The anterior pyramidal tract ends on the anterior horn, mostly on the motor neurons innervating the musculature of the trunk. Whether these cross over at lower levels of the spinal cord is not certain.

REFERENCES

Bucy, P. C.: *The Precentral Motor Cortex,* 2nd Ed. Urbana, Ill., Univ. of Illinois Press, 1949
Penfield, W., and Rasmussen, T.: *The Cerebral Cortex of Man.* New York, Macmillan, 1950, 248 pp.

PLATE 44

EXTRAPYRAMIDAL SYSTEM

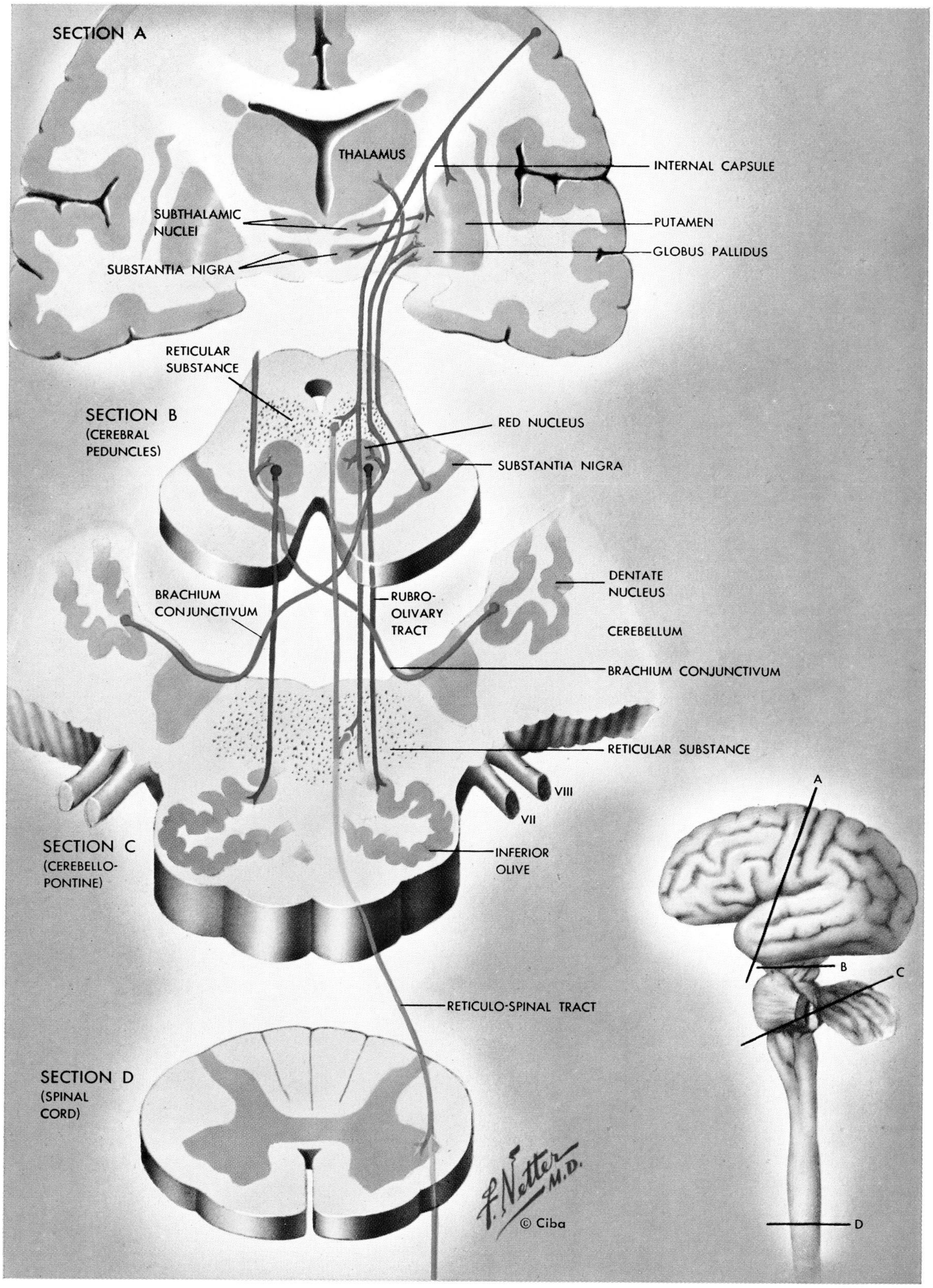

As conventionally defined, the extrapyramidal system comprises all structures other than the cortex sending impulses to the spinal cord from the brain. What we know at present indicates that it is a complicated "servomechanism" for the control of the final common pathway, which is depicted in Plate 40, page 65, by the cerebral cortex. Six nuclear masses belong to the extrapyramidal system: globus pallidus, subthalamic nucleus of Luys, substantia nigra, nucleus ruber, nucleus dentatus, and the inferior olive (all shown on cross sections A, B, and C). These nuclei, and only these, give a positive reaction for iron ions.

The cortex sends fibers (shown in red) to the globus pallidus, the nucleus ruber and, by way of the cerebellum, to the dentate nucleus. Of the connections between the extrapyramidal nuclei (shown in green) the following are known: dentato-

rubral, dentatopallidal, rubro-olival, nigropallidal and subthalamopallidal. The dentatothalamic fibers are not strictly extrapyramidal, although they are part of a "servomechanism," as explained in Plate 46, page 71. The red nucleus and the nuclei of the cerebellum (also shown in Plate 46) discharge into the reticular formation of the brain stem. Rubro-reticular fibers are probably short and diffuse. Dentato- and fastigio-reticular fibers are shown in Plate 46, page 71. The reticular substance also receives cortical fibers as depicted in Plate 50, page 75.

The cranial part of the reticular substance exerts a facilitating influence, the caudal part a suppressing influence on the anterior horn of the spinal cord. Such messages are sent over reticulospinal fibers, which are shown in orange.

The foregoing exposition is certainly not the whole story; the scheme given so far fails to account for all the differences between, e.g., parkinsonian and cerebellar symptoms, although it might be assumed that a disease of the globus pallidus will affect the facilitatory center of the reticular substance almost exclusively while a disease of the cerebellum will affect all of the reticular substance and other mechanisms as well. However, it fails completely to explain the hemiballism after lesions of the body of Luys.

REFERENCES

Magoun, H. W., and Rhines, R.: *Spasticity*. Springfield, Ill., Charles C Thomas, 1947

von Bonin, G.: *Essay on the Cerebral Cortex*. Springfield, Ill., Charles C Thomas, 1950

Whittier, J. R., and Mettler, F. A.: Corpus Subthalamicum, *J. Comp. Neurol*. 90: 211-372, 1949

PLATE 45

CEREBELLUM
Afferent Pathways

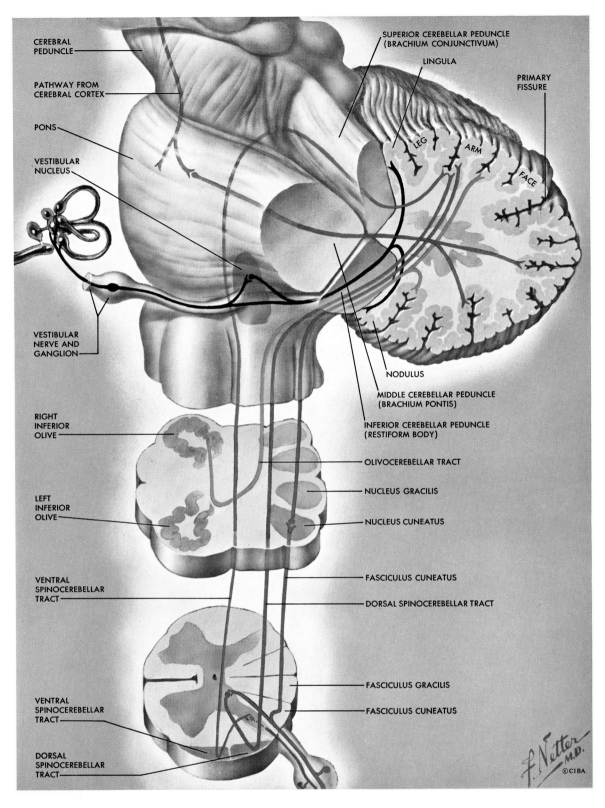

CEREBRAL PEDUNCLE

PATHWAY FROM CEREBRAL CORTEX

PONS

VESTIBULAR NUCLEUS

VESTIBULAR NERVE AND GANGLION

RIGHT INFERIOR OLIVE

LEFT INFERIOR OLIVE

VENTRAL SPINOCEREBELLAR TRACT

VENTRAL SPINOCEREBELLAR TRACT

DORSAL SPINOCEREBELLAR TRACT

SUPERIOR CEREBELLAR PEDUNCLE (BRACHIUM CONJUNCTIVUM)

LINGULA

PRIMARY FISSURE

LEG

ARM

FACE

NODULUS

MIDDLE CEREBELLAR PEDUNCLE (BRACHIUM PONTIS)

INFERIOR CEREBELLAR PEDUNCLE (RESTIFORM BODY)

OLIVOCEREBELLAR TRACT

NUCLEUS GRACILIS

NUCLEUS CUNEATUS

FASCICULUS CUNEATUS

DORSAL SPINOCEREBELLAR TRACT

FASCICULUS GRACILIS

FASCICULUS CUNEATUS

The cerebellum receives somesthetic impulses from the spinal cord, shown in purple and green, and vestibular impulses from the inner ear, shown in black.

Proprioception and touch travel either via Clarke's nucleus in the base of the posterior horn and dorsal spinocerebellar tract, or via posterior funiculus and (para-) cuneate nucleus, to enter the cerebellum via the inferior cerebellar peduncle (restiform body). The dorsal spinocerebellar tract conducts at the high rate of about 150 meters per second. Protopathic sensations are relayed from the posterior column via the ventral spinocerebellar tract. This tract enters the cerebellum by way of the superior cerebellar peduncle (brachium conjunctivum).

Vestibular impulses may go directly to the cerebellum via the inferior cerebellar peduncle (restiform body), or they may be relayed by one of the vestibular nuclei (which are also shown in Plate 41, page 66), particularly by the dorsal one.

The cerebellum also receives optic and acoustic impulses, as the recording of its electrical activity shows. However, the anatomical pathways are not yet known.

The cerebellum is also built into the extrapyramidal system (Plate 44, page 69) by afferents from the contralateral inferior olive, shown in orange, and from the pontine nuclei, shown in red. The latter nuclei relay cortical messages. Some of these afferents end in the deep nuclei of the cerebellum.

Three "stories" have been distinguished in the cerebellum, a lowest one under the influence of the vestibular apparatus, a middle one under the influence of the spinal cord, and a highest portion under the influence of the cerebral cortex, via the pontine nuclei. These "stories" can be recognized on the plate. But in the light of recent advances, it is more fruitful to think of the cerebellum as a center which receives sufficient information, both from the periphery and from the cerebral cortex, to set the "servomechanisms" of the extrapyramidal system for appropriate control of both the postural and dynamic conditions of the body (Plate 50, page 75). Furthermore, the cerebellum acts on the motor cortex via dentatothalamic fibers (Plate 44, page 69), the signals conveyed over these fibers being relayed to the precentral motor cortex, which is delineated in Plate 47, page 72.

NOTE: The ventral spinocerebellar tract is represented as carrying only ipsilateral fibers. Although some authorities think it contains both contralateral and ipsilateral fibers, there is no general agreement about the arrangement in man.

Similarly, some authorities think that the type of sensation conveyed by the ventral spinocerebellar tract is limited to proprioception, while others feel that protopathic sensations are relayed via this tract and that proprioception and touch are relayed via the dorsal spinocerebellar tract. EDITOR

REFERENCES
Bailey, P.: The Cerebellum, in P. C. Bucy: The Precentral Motor Cortex (Plate 43, page 68)
Dow, R. S.: The Evolution and Anatomy of the Cerebellum, Biol. Rev. 17: 179-220, 1942
Snider, R. S., and Stowell, A.: Receiving Areas in the Cerebellum, J. Neurophysiol. 7: 331-357, 1944
Snider, R. S.: Recent Contributions to Our Knowledge of the Cerebellum, Monthly Research Report of the Office of Naval Research, Issue of August, 1950, 15-22

PLATE 46

CEREBELLAR CORTEX

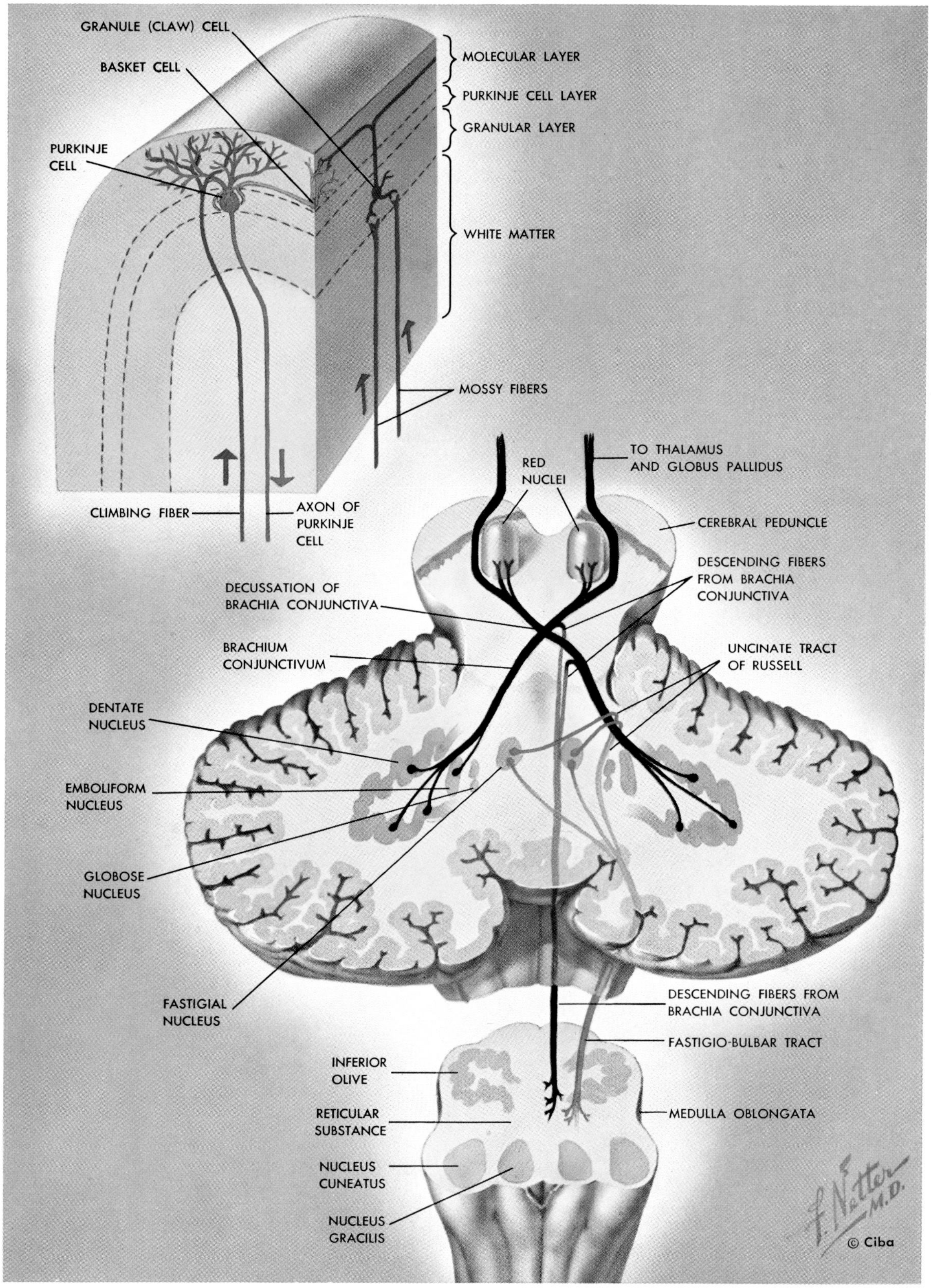

Almost all afferents to the cerebellum, which are shown in blue at the upper left, reach its cortex to end either as "mossy" or "climbing" fibers. The former have their messages relayed twice by claw cells (purple) and basket cells (green) before they reach the cell bodies of Purkinje cells (red) which send their axons out of the cerebellar cortex.

By virtue of the fact that the course of the axons of the claw cells and the basket cells are at right angles to each other, a message coming over one mossy fiber will be delivered to a large number of Purkinje cells.

The climbing fibers end directly on the dendrites of the Purkinje cells where they make extensive contacts. They influence therefore only a few cells.

All messages from the cerebellar cortex are relayed through the deep nuclei of the cerebellum, the dentate in the cerebellar hemispheres, the fastigial in the vermis, and the smaller globose and emboliform nuclei. By far the greatest part of the output goes to the extrapyramidal system. The opposite red nucleus and globus pallidus are reached by fibers of the brachium conjunctivum, which cross immediately on entering the midbrain.

The reticular substance is controlled by cerebellar signals going over both brachium conjunctivum and fastigio-bulbar tract into which the uncinate tract of Russell enters. The latter reaches mainly the inhibitory part of the reticular formation, but there is considerable anatomical overlap. Which part of the reticular substance becomes excited depends also upon the frequency of the impulses sent out by the cerebellum.

Other cerebellar impulses reach the thalamus (Plate 44, page 69), which relays them to the cerebral cortex shown in Plate 47, page 72.

Thus at least two closed circuits run through the cerebellum: a rubro-olivo-cerebello-rubral and a cortico-ponto-cerebello-thalamo-cortical one.

REFERENCES

Bailey, P.: The Cerebellum, in P. C. Bucy: *The Precentral Motor Cortex* (Plate 43, page 68)

Dow, R. S.: The Evolution and Anatomy of the Cerebellum, *Biol. Rev.* 17: 179-220, 1942

Snider, R. S., and Stowell, A.: Receiving Areas in the Cerebellum, *J. Neurophysiol.* 7: 331-357, 1944

PLATE 47

THALAMOCORTICAL RADIATIONS

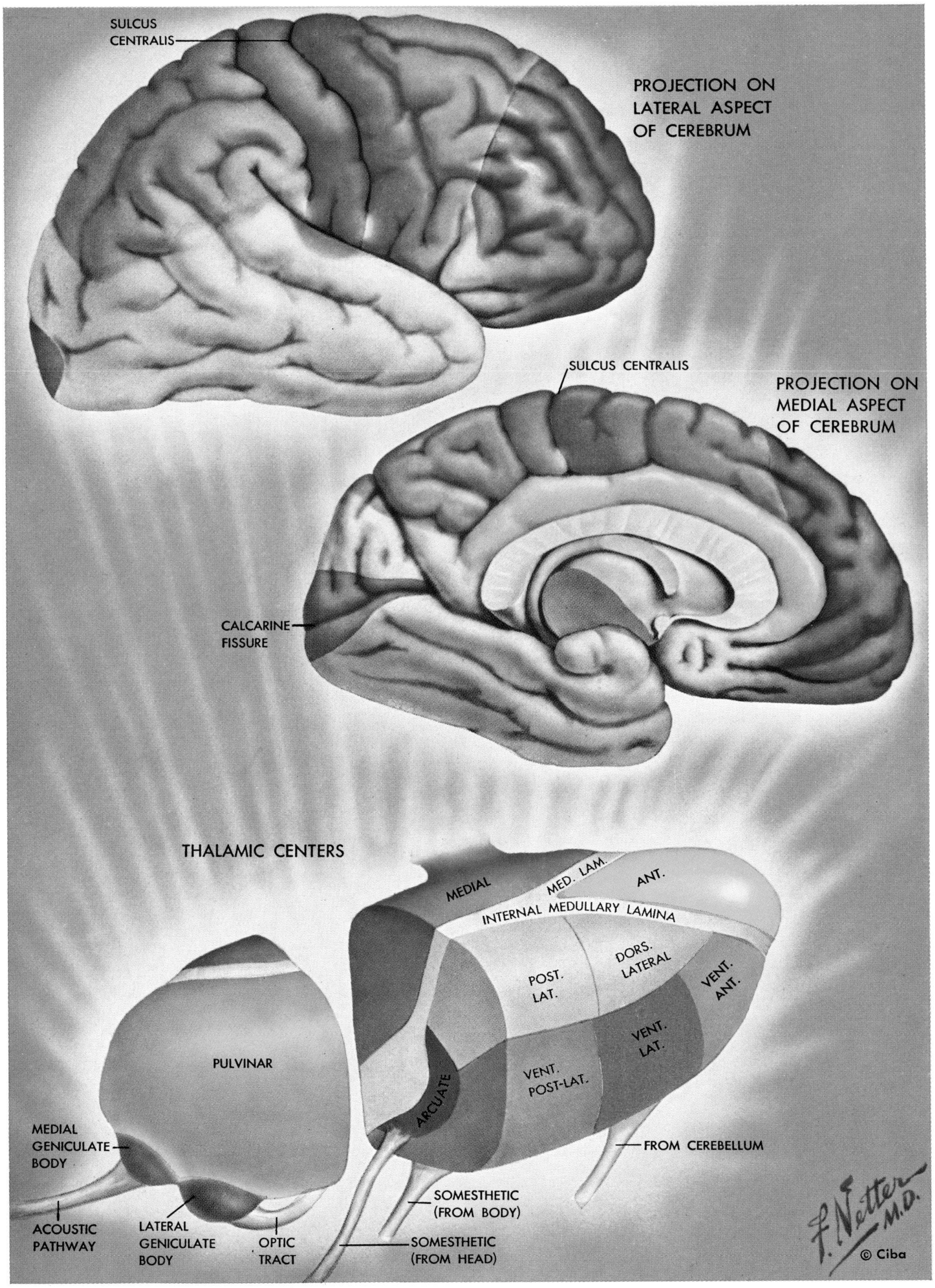

The cerebral cortex receives its afferents exclusively from the thalamic nuclei. Several of these relay sensory messages, however, not all thalamic nuclei send afferents to the cortex.

The important thalamic nuclei are represented diagrammatically in the lower half of the plate. Somesthetic sensations reach the nucleus ventralis posterior lateralis of which the arcuate may be considered a part and are relayed to the postcentral gyrus which is shown in green in the upper drawings.

Acoustic impulses stream to the medial geniculate body and are relayed to the supratemporal transverse gyrus. The uppermost drawing represents the lateral end of this gyrus as just visible over the lower lip of the Sylvian fissure.

The optic tract ends in the lateral geniculate body which sends its fibers to the visual area surrounding the calcarine fissure (see both lateral and medial aspects of hemisphere). Cerebellar impulses reach the nucleus ventralis lateralis and ventralis anterior and are relayed to the precentral motor cortex shown in red in the lateral and medial projections of the cerebrum.

The anterior part of the ventral nucleus receives messages from the pallidum and relays them to the premotor area (light red).

Of the other thalamic nuclei which send radiations to the cerebral cortex, afferents are not well understood. The medial nucleus (blue) sends its radiation to the frontal lobe, into what is often referred to as the "prefrontal field." The pulvinar transmits its radiation to the parietal and temporal lobes. The exact extension of this field is not known; it may reach farther occipitally and ventrally than shown in the illustration. The anterior nucleus of the thalamus sends its radiation to the cingulate gyrus which is shown in yellow on the medial projection of the cerebrum.

The study of thalamocortical relations, so important for an understanding and a rational subdivision of the cortex, has been sadly neglected in studies made of pathological material. Most of our knowledge is derived from experiments on macaques and chimpanzees.

REFERENCES

Chow, K. L.: A Retrograde Cell Degeneration Study of the Cortical Projection Field of the Pulvinar in the Monkey. J. Comp. Neur. 93: 313-340, 1950

Polyak, S.: The Main Afferent Fiber Systems of the Cerebral Cortex in Primates. Berkeley, Calif., Univ. of Calif. Press, 1932

Walker, A. E.: The Primate Thalamus. Chicago, Ill., Univ. of Chicago Press, 1938

Walker, A. E.: The Thalamus of the Chimpanzee. J. Anat. 73: 37-93, 1938

Freeman, W., and Watts, J. W.: Retrograde Degeneration of the Thalamus. . . . J. Comp. Neurol. 86: 65-93, 1947

PLATE 48

CEREBRAL CORTEX
Structure

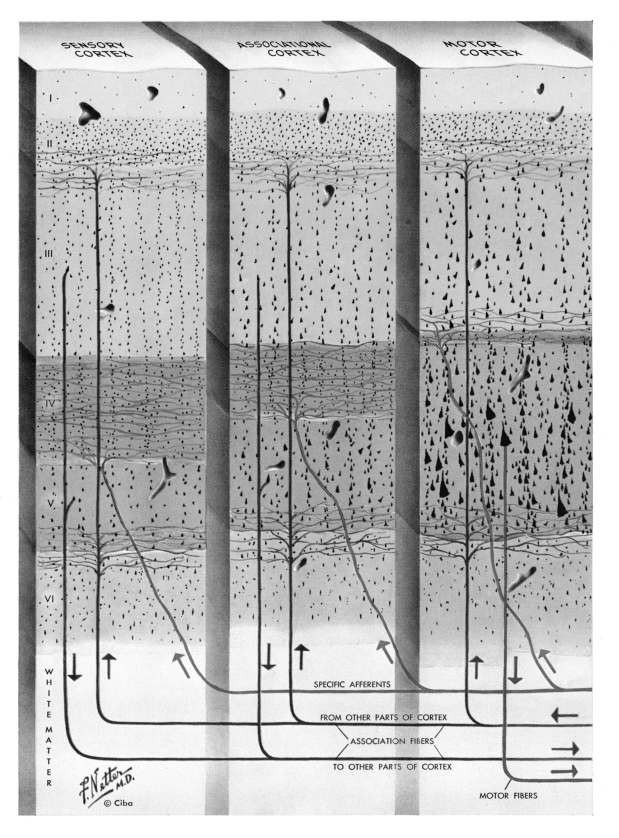

The cerebral cortex contains layers of nerve cells, about 50-100 cells thick, and of glia cells and blood vessels. The nerve cells are arranged in columns and in layers which vary in cell density, size of cells which they contain and sometimes in the degree of "columnization." Six layers are generally recognized. To understand their functional significance — and we are still far from that goal — it is preferable to begin in the middle, with layer IV. It is here that the thalamic radiation (blue) ends. These "specific afferent" fibers split up into a dense feltwork and, reinforced by endogenous fibers, *i.e.,* axons of cells within the cortex, form the outer stripe of Baillarger. It can be seen with the naked eye in the striate area where it has been called the stripe of Gennari or Vicq d'Azyr. The fourth layer also contains a dense population of small cells. Underneath lies a layer, shown in pink, which contains pyramidal cells of varying density, the type most characteristic for the cerebral cortex. The pyramidal and other efferent or projection fibers from the cortex are axons of these cells. A sixth layer contains many spindle-shaped cells. The inner granular layer (IV) is covered by a "third" layer, somewhat sparsely filled with pyramidal and other cells. Above this we encounter an outer granular layer (II) containing a dense population of small pyramidal and granular cells. A first or tangential layer (light yellow) contains mostly fibers, both axonal and dendritic. Each part of the cortex sends out and receives associational or commissural

fibers (dark brown) from other parts of the cortex. These originate in layers III and V, as axons of pyramidal cells. They enter the white matter and upon rising again into the cortex split up into two plexuses, one between layers V and VI, known as the inner stripe of Baillarger; the other between layers II and III, called the stripe of Kaes-Bechterew.

This general structure can be observed in all parts of the cortex though marked areal variations exist. The sensory areas, somesthetic, acoustic and visual, shown in Plate 47, page 72, contain a thinner cortex filled rather densely with small cells, with a rather thick inner granular layer (koniocortex). The motor areas (red and pink in Plate 47, page 72) contain a relatively thick cortex, sparsely filled with larger cells. Here the inner granular layer can be distin-

guished only with difficulty. For the motor area proper (red in Plate 47, page 72), the giant cells of Betz in the fifth layer are characteristic. Most of the rest of the cortex is composed of what has here been labeled "associational cortex." Minor differences from area to area complicate the structure, but they are greatly exaggerated in the cytoarchitectural diagrams in general use.

REFERENCES

Bailey, P., and von Bonin, G.: *The Isocortex of Man.* Urbana, Ill., Univ. of Illinois Press, 1951

Lorente de No, R.: Cerebral Cortex. . . . Chapter XV in J. F. Fulton: *Physiology of the Nervous System,* 2nd Ed. London, New York, Toronto, Oxford University Press, 1943

Ramon y Cajal, S.: *Histologie du système nerveux . . .* t. II. Paris, Maloine, 1911

von Bonin, G.: *Essay on the Cerebral Cortex.* Springfield, Ill., Charles C Thomas, 1950

PLATE 49

CEREBRAL CORTEX

Localization of Function
and Association Pathways

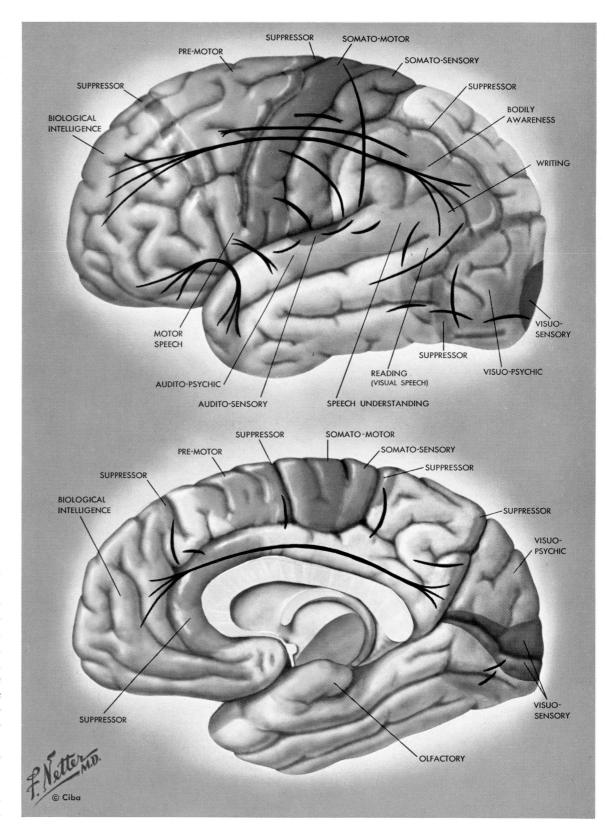

The areas of entry of the various sensory modalities can be located with precision: somatosensory (blue), visuosensory (purple), auditosensory (lavender) and, on the uncus and perhaps a little further back, olfactory impulses, shown in yellow. (The reader is referred also to Plate 37, page 62, and Plate 47, page 72.) The motor area can be mapped with similar precision. Suppressor areas have been found in certain locations in narcotized subhuman primates, but only the precentral suppressor area has been verified in the human brain. Under their stimulation there ensues, among other things, an immediate cessation of any movement of the body musculature. The frontal and occipital suppressor areas also control eye movements. The cortex surrounding both auditosensory and visuosensory areas has to do with the "apperception" or understanding of the information delivered to the sensory areas. The area labeled "premotor" controls the motor area. The lower parietal lobule is concerned with bodily awareness, with the "body scheme" (Schilder). The frontal lobe, the lower part of which is intimately connected with the tip of the temporal lobe, appears to have to do with "biological intelligence," a term borrowed from Halstead.

The areas between the first temporal and the opercular part of the third frontal gyrus are concerned with speech, but a further subdivision into motor and sensory speech centers, etc., is hardly justified and has, although frequently attempted, consistently broken down.

The various cortical areas are connected by associational fibers which have been successfully investigated by physiological methods after a century of unsuccessful anatomical investigations. Some of these results, from experiments on monkeys and apes, have been indicated by black lines. The superior longitudinal bundle consists of long fibers connecting prefrontal with occipital areas as well as of shorter fibers, the shortest ones bridging no more than the central sulcus. The uncinate fasciculus connects the orbitofrontal and temporopolar regions. The wealth and the arrangement of occipital and temporal fibers clearly indicate the importance of the second and third temporal gyri for higher visual functions. The fact (see medial aspect) that all suppressor areas are connected with the cortex on the lips of the cingular sulcus, and that a strong association bundle runs evidently parallel to that sulcus (not the cingulum of older anatomists!) is at the moment only of theoretical interest.

REFERENCES

Bailey, P., von Bonin, G., and McCulloch, W. S.: *The Isocortex of the Chimpanzee*. Urbana, Ill., Univ. of Illinois Press, 1950

Halstead, W.: *Brain and Intelligence*. Chicago, Ill., Univ. of Chicago Press, 1947

Head, H.: *Aphasia and Kindred Disorders of Speech*. Cambridge, The University Press, 1926

McCulloch, W. S.: The Functional Organization of the Cerebral Cortex, *Physiol. Rev.* 24: 390-407, 1944

Schilder, P.: *The Image and Appearance of the Human Body*. London, K. Paul, Trench, Trubner & Company Ltd., 1935

PLATE 50

CEREBRAL CORTEX
Efferent Pathways

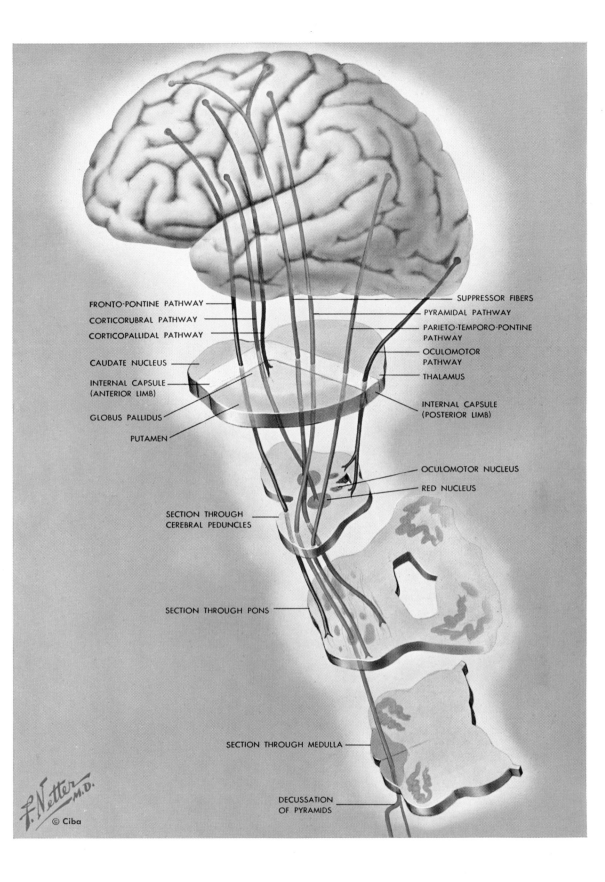

FRONTO-PONTINE PATHWAY
CORTICORUBRAL PATHWAY
CORTICOPALLIDAL PATHWAY
CAUDATE NUCLEUS
INTERNAL CAPSULE (ANTERIOR LIMB)
GLOBUS PALLIDUS
PUTAMEN

SUPPRESSOR FIBERS
PYRAMIDAL PATHWAY
PARIETO-TEMPORO-PONTINE PATHWAY
OCULOMOTOR PATHWAY
THALAMUS
INTERNAL CAPSULE (POSTERIOR LIMB)

OCULOMOTOR NUCLEUS
RED NUCLEUS

SECTION THROUGH CEREBRAL PEDUNCLES

SECTION THROUGH PONS

SECTION THROUGH MEDULLA

DECUSSATION OF PYRAMIDS

F. Netter M.D.
© Ciba

Steering of voluntary movements by the cortex involves at least three types of signals, perhaps even more.

Firstly, the cerebellum, the great regulator of the extrapyramidal system, has to be attuned. The parieto-temporo-pontine fibers, arising in the vicinity of the cortical area concerned with the body scheme, shown in Plate 49, page 74, as well as the fronto-pontine fibers, arising from cortical areas concerned with biological intelligence, carry such signals. Then, the extrapyramidal system proper has to

be informed of what is about to happen. Cortico-pallidal and corticorubral fibers arising from the premotor area or near it carry these signals.

Lastly, pyramidal fibers carry messages to the final common pathway as depicted in Plate 43, page 68.

The cortex also directly influences the inhibitory part of the reticular substance by means of fibers arising in the suppressor areas (green). Only those from frontal and precentral suppressor areas are indicated.

Steering of the eye movements is mediated by pathways arising in the striate area and going to the superior colliculus of the midbrain. The latter, in turn, influences the medial longitudinal fasciculus. Thus,

a part of the output of the cortex is used to regulate its input. Eye movements are also under the influence of the frontal and the occipital suppressor areas as shown in Plate 42, page 67. For the sake of clarity, only the former are shown (green) in the illustration; these fibers go directly to the nuclei of the eye muscles.

REFERENCES

Bucy, P. C.: *The Precentral Motor Cortex*, 2nd Ed. Urbana, Ill., Univ. of Illinois Press, 1949

Magoun, H. W., and Rhines, R.: *Spasticity*. Springfield, Ill., Charles C Thomas, 1947

von Bonin, G.: *Essay on the Cerebral Cortex*. Springfield, Ill., Charles C Thomas, 1950

PLATE 51

HYPOTHALAMUS
Location and Subdivisions

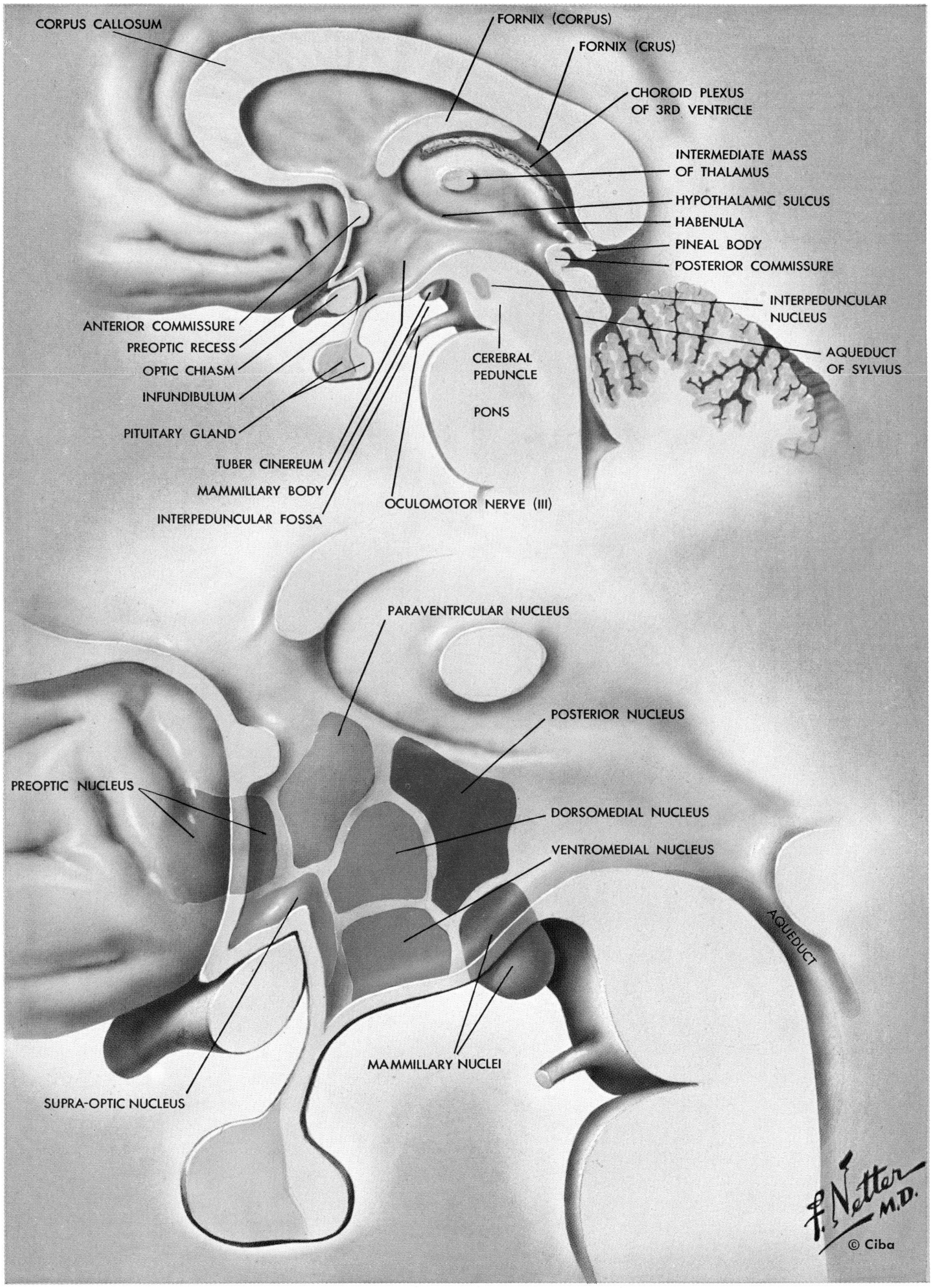

The hypothalamus is the highest vegetative center in the brain, but stands, naturally, in functional relation with both the forebrain and the brain stem. To illustrate these relations, the upper figure shows a part of a midsagittal section through the brain with the hypothalamic region occupying the center of the stage as it were.

Morphologists consider the lamina terminalis and preoptic recess as a part of the endbrain, the structures between the optic chiasm and the mammillary bodies as part of the diencephalon. The dorsal boundary is given by the hypothalamic sulcus.

Of other structures indicated in the upper figure, the interpeduncular nucleus may be in close functional connection with the hypothalamus. It is a small, inconspicuous cluster of cells in man, but a much larger mass in cats, where it appears to play an important role.

The habenula, the main constituent of the epithalamus, is an amazingly constant nucleus in all vertebrates, but has no recognizable function in man.

Within the hypothalamus, a number of nuclei can be distinguished. The main subdivisions are shown in the lower picture. The color scheme is rather arbitrary. Experiments by W. R. Hess and others show that stimulation of the anterior part of the hypothalamus leads to "trophotrop" phenomena, corresponding roughly to parasympathetic responses, while those of the posterior and lateral parts lead to "ergotrop" reactions, roughly resembling sympathetic responses.

It may be important for an understanding of hypothalamic functions that the paraventricular nucleus is quite close to the medial nucleus of the thalamus, as shown in Plate 47, page 72, and that the hypothalamus is fused caudally with the thick central gray around the aqueduct of Sylvius.

The blood supply to the hypothalamic nuclei is extraordinarily rich. In many cells, particularly in those of the paraventricular and the supra-optic nuclei, structures have been observed under the microscope which have been interpreted as signs of a "neurosecretion." This seems constant from fish to man, but has so far remained without physiologic confirmation.

REFERENCES

Clark, W. E. LeGros, et al.: The Hypothalamus. Edinburgh, London, Oliver and Boyd, 1938

Hess, W. R.: Vegetative Funktionen und Zwischenhirn. Helv. Physiol. Acta, Suppl. 4, 1947

Scharrer, E., and Scharrer, B.: Secretory Cells Within the Hypothalamus. Assn. Res. Nerv. & Ment. Dis. 20: 170, 1940

The Hypothalamus and Central Levels of Autonomic Function. Assn. Res. Nerv. & Ment. Dis. 20. Baltimore, Williams and Wilkins, 1940

PLATE 52

HYPOTHALAMUS

Afferent and Efferent

Connections

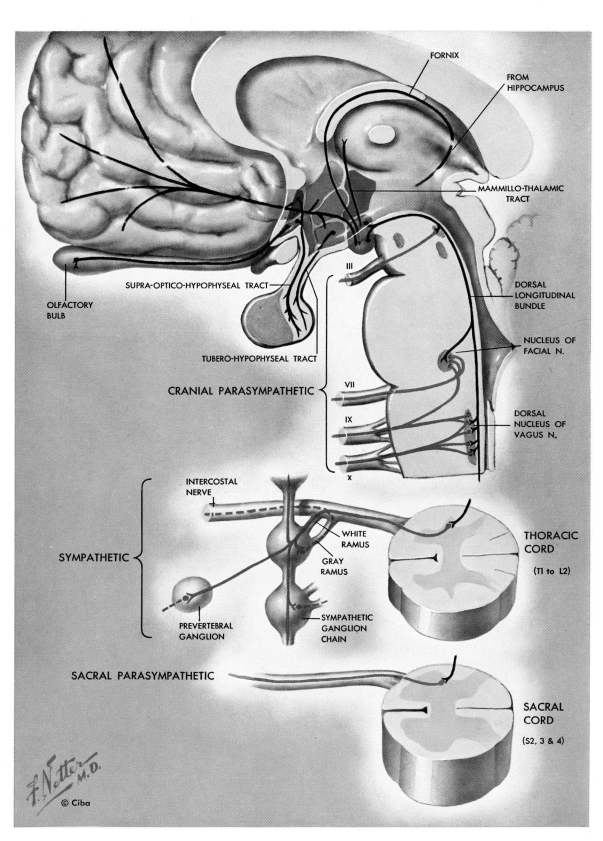

The frontal lobe and the cornu ammonis of the endbrain send messages to the hypothalamus. From the former, pathways have been demonstrated experimentally to various nuclei. The relations appear to be specific: a given locus of the cortex sends messages to only one hypothalamic nucleus. Most of these cortical areas are within the "prefrontal" field, but some are in the premotor area.

The cornu ammonis sends a powerful bundle, known as the fornix, to the mammillary body. Further afferents from the olfactory bulb to the supra-optic nuclei, the medial forebrain bundle, have been described.

The outflow from the hypothalamus goes back toward the cerebral cortex, to the lower vegetative centers and to the hypophysis cerebri. The mammillothalamic tract conveys signals from the mammillary body to the anterior nucleus of the thalamus. It is clear (Plate 47, page 72) that from that nucleus impulses can reach the limbic gyrus, but the pathway from there to the hippocampus does not seem to exist according to Adey *et al*.

Another pathway toward the cortex may be by conduction from the paraventricular to the medial nucleus of the thalamus, to the "prefrontal" field, and back to the hypothalamus. This pathway would be interrupted by prefrontal lobotomy and similar operations.

The outflow toward the lower centers can be followed anatomically through the dorsal longitudinal fasciculus which consists of thin unmyelinated fibers within the central gray. It has been demonstrated only in the brain stem, but its extension into the cord can be inferred. It influences, as its origin from the parasympathetic mammillary body (Plate 51, page 76) would suggest, the parasympathetic centers in the brain stem: III to the eye, VII to face and cerebral vessels, IX to pharynx and the region of the carotid sinus as well as X, which is the medullary cardiovas-

cular center of Plate 6 on page 152. It may be supposed also to influence the sacral parasympathetic center. Its play on the sympathetic centers in the intermediolateral column of the thoracolumbar cord is not so clearly understood, but that these centers are under hypothalamic control has been abundantly shown by physiologists.

The posterior lobe of the pituitary receives direct tracts from supra-optic nucleus (sympathetic?) and the nucleus tuberis (parasympathetic?).

REFERENCES

Adey, W. R., Dunlop and Hendrix: Hippocampal slow waves. *A. M. A. Arch. Neurol.* 3: 74, 1960

Papez, T. W.: Proposed Mechanism of Emotion. *Arch. Neurol. & Psychiat.* 38: 725-743, 1937

Rasmussen, A. T.: Innervation of the Hypophysis. *Endocrinol.* 23: 263-278, 1938

Section IV

THE AUTONOMIC NERVOUS SYSTEM

with descriptive text by

ALBERT KUNTZ, PH.D., M.D.

Professor of Anatomy, Saint Louis University School of Medicine
Saint Louis, Missouri

PLATE 53

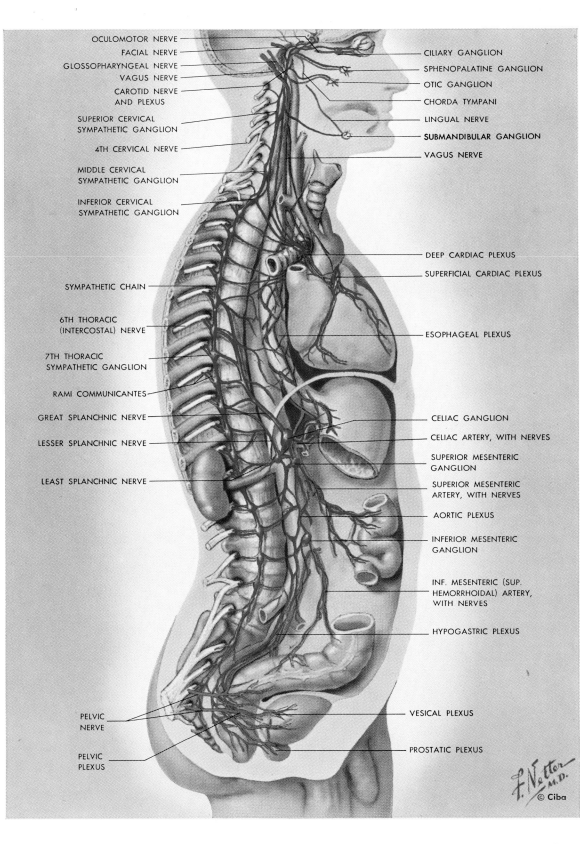

OCULOMOTOR NERVE

FACIAL NERVE

GLOSSOPHARYNGEAL NERVE

VAGUS NERVE

CAROTID NERVE
AND PLEXUS

SUPERIOR CERVICAL
SYMPATHETIC GANGLION

4TH CERVICAL NERVE

MIDDLE CERVICAL
SYMPATHETIC GANGLION

INFERIOR CERVICAL
SYMPATHETIC GANGLION

SYMPATHETIC CHAIN

6TH THORACIC
(INTERCOSTAL) NERVE

7TH THORACIC
SYMPATHETIC GANGLION

RAMI COMMUNICANTES

GREAT SPLANCHNIC NERVE

LESSER SPLANCHNIC NERVE

LEAST SPLANCHNIC NERVE

PELVIC
NERVE

PELVIC
PLEXUS

CILIARY GANGLION

SPHENOPALATINE GANGLION

OTIC GANGLION

CHORDA TYMPANI

LINGUAL NERVE

SUBMANDIBULAR GANGLION

VAGUS NERVE

DEEP CARDIAC PLEXUS

SUPERFICIAL CARDIAC PLEXUS

ESOPHAGEAL PLEXUS

CELIAC GANGLION

CELIAC ARTERY, WITH NERVES

SUPERIOR MESENTERIC
GANGLION

SUPERIOR MESENTERIC
ARTERY, WITH NERVES

AORTIC PLEXUS

INFERIOR MESENTERIC
GANGLION

INF. MESENTERIC (SUP.
HEMORRHOIDAL) ARTERY,
WITH NERVES

HYPOGASTRIC PLEXUS

VESICAL PLEXUS

PROSTATIC PLEXUS

F. Netter
M.D.
© Ciba

GENERAL TOPOGRAPHY

The autonomic nervous system comprises all the efferent nerves through which the visceral organs, including the cardiovascular system, the glands and the peripheral involuntary muscles, such as the intrinsic muscles of the eyes and those associated with the hair follicles, are innervated. It includes all the nerve cells, or neurons, located outside the spinal cord and the brain stem, excepting those which are associated with the sensory roots of the spinal and the cranial nerves and the special sense organs, and the efferent neurons located in the spinal cord and the brain stem which send their axons peripherad to make anatomic and functional contacts with the outlying autonomic neurons. The neurons in question in the spinal cord and the brain stem are known as preganglionic neurons. The outlying ones are the autonomic ganglionic neurons or ganglion cells. The conduction pathways from the central nervous system to the visceral organs, consequently, are made up of preganglionic and ganglionic neurons. The cell bodies of the ganglionic neurons are arranged in aggregates which are known as autonomic ganglia. Some of these ganglia are incorporated in a pair of longitudinal cords, the sympathetic trunks. Some are located in relation to the thoracic, the abdominal and the pelvic viscera, and some in the cephalic area.

The sympathetic trunks extend from the base of the cranium to the coccyx. In general, the ganglia in each sympathetic trunk are arranged segmentally except in the cervical region. Deviations from a strictly segmental arrangement occur frequently, particularly in the lumbar region. The interganglionic portions of each sympathetic trunk consist mainly of nerve fibers which run longitudinally. In the cervical region, the trunk lies ventral to the transverse proc-

esses of the cervical vertebrae and dorsal to the carotid arteries. In the thorax, it lies ventral to the necks of the ribs. At the level of the twelfth thoracic vertebra it tends ventrad until it reaches the ventrolateral aspect of the bodies of the vertebrae at the caudal border of the first lumbar segment. From this level to the sacral prominence, it lies along the medial border of the psoas muscle. In the pelvic region, it lies on the ventral surface of the sacrum medial to the sacral foramina. In this region, it tends mesad and terminates in the ganglion impar, or coccygeal ganglion, which is common to both sympathetic trunks.

Each sympathetic trunk is connected with every spinal nerve on the same side by strands of nerve fibers, the communicating rami. In the thoracic and the rostral two or three lumbar segments, the communicating rami are made up of the axons of preganglionic neurons which deviate from the spinal nerves to join the sympathetic trunk, the axons of ganglionic neurons which join the spinal nerves, and afferent spinal nerve fibers which traverse the sympathetic trunks. The communicating rami in

other segments do not include axons of preganglionic neurons or preganglionic fibers.

Some of the autonomic ganglia which are located in relation to the thoracic, the abdominal and the pelvic organs are located within the walls of the organs. Others are located in nerve plexuses which are closely associated with the visceral organs. These plexuses are connected with the sympathetic trunks through nerves which are made up of fibers which arise in the sympathetic trunk ganglia and of spinal nerve fibers which traverse these ganglia. The pelvic nerves convey sacral spinal nerve fibers into the plexuses associated with the pelvic organs without traversing the sympathetic trunks. The autonomic ganglia, which are located in the cephalic region, are connected with the brain stem through cranial nerve fibers. Fibers which arise in the cervical sympathetic trunk ganglia also extend into the cephalic region. Cranial nerve fibers, furthermore, extend into the plexuses associated with the thoracic and the abdominal viscera through the vagus nerves.

PLATE 54

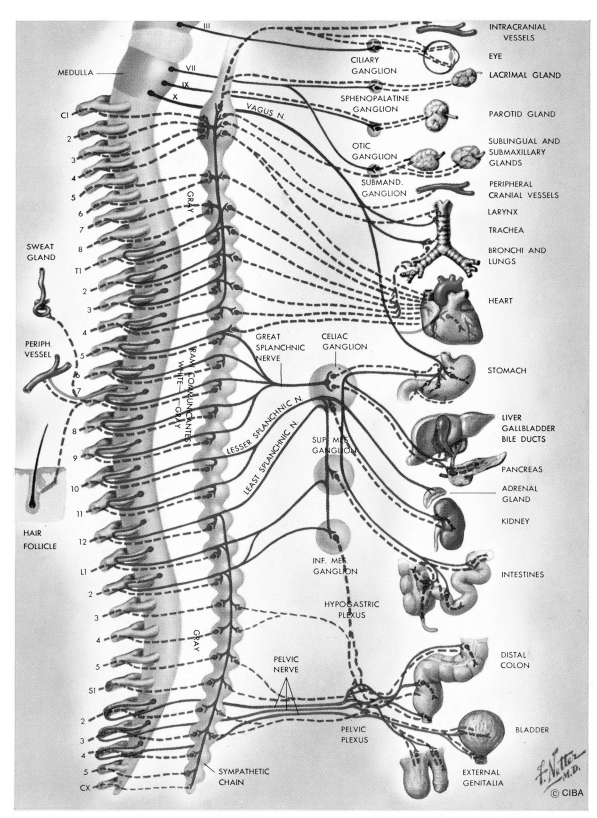

SCHEMA

The tissues of the body which require autonomic innervation are supplied with nerve fibers arising from autonomic ganglion cells. These ganglion cells are activated mainly by impulses received through preganglionic neurons. The contact of the axon of a preganglionic neuron with a ganglion cell, like that of the axon of any neuron with a dendrite or the cell body of another, and through which nerve impulses are transmitted, is called the synapse. A single preganglionic neuron, through the terminal branches of its axon, makes synaptic contacts with more than one ganglion cell. A single ganglion cell may also be synaptically related to more than one preganglionic neuron.

The preganglionic neurons are located in the spinal cord and the brain stem. Those in the spinal cord are localized in the lateral portion of the intermediate zone of the gray matter throughout the thoracic and the first two lumbar segments, and in a less clearly delimited portion of the gray matter in the second, the third and the fourth sacral segments. Those in the brain stem are aggregated in groups called nuclei which are located respectively at the levels of the cranial nerve roots through which the preganglionic nerve fibers emerge. These nuclei constitute the paired visceral efferent nuclear columns in the brain stem. Each column includes the motor nucleus of the vagus nerve, the salivatory nuclei and a group of visceral efferent neurons, called the Edinger-Westphal nucleus, which is a part of the nucleus of the oculomotor nerve.

Since the preganglionic neurons are limited to certain segmental levels of the spinal cord and the brain stem, some of the spinal and some of the cranial nerves include no preganglionic autonomic nerve fibers. Pre-

ganglionic fibers are present in the third, the seventh, the ninth, the tenth and the eleventh cranial, all of the thoracic, the first and second lumbar, and the second, third and fourth sacral spinal nerves. The autonomic nervous system, therefore, may be said to comprise a cranial, a thoracolumbar and a sacral division. The preganglionic fibers which emerge from the spinal cord in the thoracic and the first two lumbar nerves traverse the ventral roots and the white communicating rami of these nerves and join the sympathetic trunk. Those concerned with the innervation of peripheral structures and the thoracic viscera terminate in sympathetic trunk ganglia. Those concerned with the innervation of the abdominal and the pelvic viscera, in general, traverse the sympathetic trunk, without making synaptic contacts in its ganglia, and extend via the splanchnic nerves to ganglia located in closer proximity to the abdominal and the pelvic viscera. The preganglionic fibers which emerge from the brain stem in cranial nerves and from the spinal cord in sacral nerves do not join the sympathetic trunk, but

extend through rami of the respective nerves into the ganglia in which they make synaptic contacts. From the sympathetic trunk ganglia and the other ganglia in which preganglionic components of the thoracic and the lumbar nerves terminate, postganglionic fibers are distributed to all parts of the body. The thoracolumbar preganglionic neurons and all the ganglionic neurons with which they make synaptic contacts constitute the sympathetic division of the autonomic nervous system which is shown in red. The cranial and the sacral preganglionic neurons and the ganglionic neurons with which they make synaptic contacts constitute the parasympathetic division which is depicted in blue. The parasympathetic nerves are less widely distributed in the body than the sympathetic nerves. They are limited mainly to the thoracic, the abdominal and the pelvic viscera and to smooth muscle and glands in the cephalic region. Some autonomically innervated tissues, consequently, are supplied with both sympathetic and parasympathetic nerves, and others only with sympathetic nerves.

PLATE 55

AUTONOMIC
REFLEX PATHWAYS

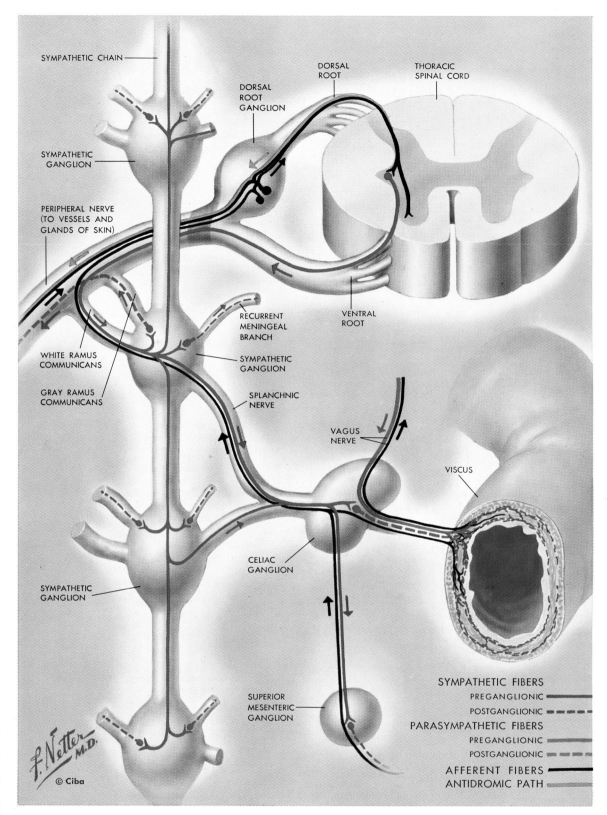

SYMPATHETIC CHAIN

DORSAL ROOT GANGLION

DORSAL ROOT

THORACIC SPINAL CORD

SYMPATHETIC GANGLION

PERIPHERAL NERVE (TO VESSELS AND GLANDS OF SKIN)

RECURRENT MENINGEAL BRANCH

VENTRAL ROOT

WHITE RAMUS COMMUNICANS

SYMPATHETIC GANGLION

GRAY RAMUS COMMUNICANS

SPLANCHNIC NERVE

VAGUS NERVE

VISCUS

CELIAC GANGLION

SYMPATHETIC GANGLION

SUPERIOR MESENTERIC GANGLION

F. Netter M.D.

© Ciba

SYMPATHETIC FIBERS
PREGANGLIONIC ▬▬▬
POSTGANGLIONIC ▬ ▬ ▬
PARASYMPATHETIC FIBERS
PREGANGLIONIC ▬▬▬
POSTGANGLIONIC ▬ ▬ ▬
AFFERENT FIBERS ▬▬▬
ANTIDROMIC PATH ▬▬▬

The autonomic nervous system, as illustrated in Plate 53, page 80, and Plate 54, page 81, does not include nerve components which conduct impulses into the central nervous system. The afferent neurons which conduct impulses from visceral organs to the spinal cord and the brain stem are visceral afferent components of the spinal and the cranial nerves. The cell bodies of these neurons, like those of the somatic afferent neurons, are located in the ganglia associated with the sensory roots of the respective nerves. The visceral afferent nerve fibers in general traverse the autonomic ganglia but make no synaptic contacts in them. They enter the spinal cord or the brain stem in association with the somatic afferent fibers of the same nerves. Both visceral and somatic afferent nerve fibers make reflex connections with preganglionic autonomic neurons in the spinal cord and the brain stem. They are, therefore, functionally related to the autonomic nerves, but are not anatomic components of them.

The major portion of the neural regulation of visceral functions is carried out through reflex mechanisms with their central connections in the spinal cord and the brain stem. The simplest autonomic reflex arc consists of an afferent conductor which may be either a visceral or a somatic afferent neuron, a connecting mechanism located in the central nervous system and an efferent conducting chain made up of a preganglionic and a ganglionic neuron. Autonomic and somatic reflex arcs differ anatomically

mainly in the efferent limb. In the former, this limb comprises two neurons. In the latter, it comprises only a single neuron. In either case, the transmission of the impulse from the afferent to the efferent limb of the reflex arc probably involves one or more intercalated neurons. The portion of the reflex arc located within the central nervous system may be limited to a single segment or it may involve several segments. Some preganglionic neurons terminate in a single ganglion. Others make synaptic contacts in more than one ganglion.

Located within the brain stem are certain reflex and correlation mechanisms of higher orders than those described above which are concerned primarily with autonomic functions. They comprise neuron aggregates in the medulla oblongata, such as the respiratory and the vasomotor centers, the center for carbohydrate metabolism and certain others, and the major portion of the hypothalamus, which is the ventral portion of the diencephalon. Impulses emanating from the cerebral cortex also exert a regulatory influence on autonomic functions. Impulses

which arise in the visceral organs are conducted to the higher autonomic centers mainly through pathways in the spinal cord and the brain stem which are made up of short neurons and frequent synaptic relays. Somatic afferent impulses reach them through collaterals from the ascending somatic conduction pathways and through fibers which extend into the hypothalamus from the diencephalic nuclei in which the sensory conduction systems from the spinal cord and the brain stem terminate. Impulses emanating from the higher autonomic centers are conducted downward mainly through pathways which comprise short neurons and frequent synaptic relays. The reticulospinal tracts, which are made up of long fibers, are related in part to the autonomic nerves. Impulses conducted downward from the higher autonomic centers are transmitted to both preganglionic autonomic and somatic efferent neurons. Impulses emanating from the cerebral cortex exert their influence on autonomic functions mainly through the hypothalamus and the other autonomic centers in the brain stem.

PLATE 56

CHOLINERGIC AND ADRENERGIC NERVES

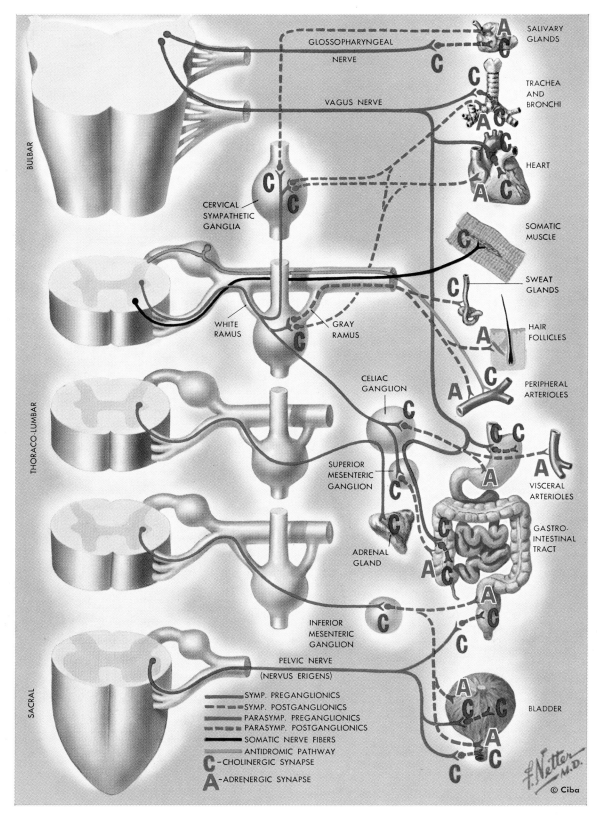

Stimulation of autonomic ganglion cells or their axons results in the liberation of chemical substances which play essential roles in the transmission of the nerve impulses from the nerve fibers to the effector tissues. The substance liberated most commonly at the neuroeffector junctions, due to stimulation of sympathetic ganglion cells or sympathetic postganglionic fibers (A in plate), possesses properties of adrenin. This substance has been called sympathin. The substance liberated at the neuroeffector junctions most commonly, due to stimulation of parasympathetic ganglion cells or postganglionic fibers (C in plate), possesses properties of acetylcholine. It has been called parasympathin.

Stimulation of some sympathetic ganglion cells results not in the liberation of sympathin, but in the liberation of an acetylcholine-like substance which probably is identical with parasympathin. Stimulation of some parasympathetic ganglion cells likewise results not in the liberation of parasympathin, but in the liberation of an adrenin-like substance which probably is identical with sympathin. These facts show clearly that neither the sympathetic nor the parasympathetic ganglion cells fall into single functional categories; consequently, those which liberate an adrenin-like substance when stimulated have been classified as adrenergic, and those which liberate an acetylcholine-like substance when stimulated have been classified as cholinergic. This classification is more significant than one based solely on the anatomic relationships of the autonomic ganglion cells and the nerve fibers. Stimulation of the preganglionic neurons or nerve fibers results in the liberation at the synaptic junctions within

the ganglia of a chemical substance with properties of acetylcholine, which probably plays an essential role in the transmission of impulses from the preganglionic fibers to the ganglion cells.

Impulses conducted by adrenergic nerve fibers in general elicit reactions in the effector organs which are the opposite of those elicited by impulses conducted by cholinergic fibers. For example, stimulation of the sympathetic cardiac nerves, which are adrenergic, elicits acceleration of the heart rate, whereas stimulation of the parasympathetic cardiac nerves, which are cholinergic, results in retardation of the heart rate. In most instances the stimulation of adrenergic nerve fibers results in excitation of the effector organ, and stimulation of the cholinergic fibers results in inhibition. In some instances, as illustrated by the nerves to the gastrointestinal tract, stimulation of the sympathetic nerves, which are predominantly adrenergic, results in retardation of gastrointestinal motility; and stimulation of the parasympathetic nerves, which are predominantly cholinergic, results in accelera-

tion of gastrointestinal motility and increased tonus of the gastrointestinal musculature. In many instances nerves of either sympathetic or parasympathetic origin include both adrenergic and cholinergic fibers.

The autonomic innervation of certain organs and tissues, e.g., most of the blood vessels, the sweat glands and the smooth muscle of the nictitating membrane, is solely sympathetic. The sympathetic nerves in question may comprise both adrenergic and cholinergic fibers or fibers of only one of these categories. In general, the nerves which supply blood vessels include adrenergic vasoconstrictor fibers and cholinergic vasodilator fibers. The sympathetic nerves to the sweat glands, with certain possible exceptions, are cholinergic. Those to the nictitating membrane are adrenergic. The chromaffin tissue of the adrenal medulla is innervated directly through sympathetic preganglionic fibers which are cholinergic. The occurrence of adrenergic fibers in parasympathetic nerves appears to be less common than the occurrence of cholinergic fibers in sympathetic nerves.

PLATE 57

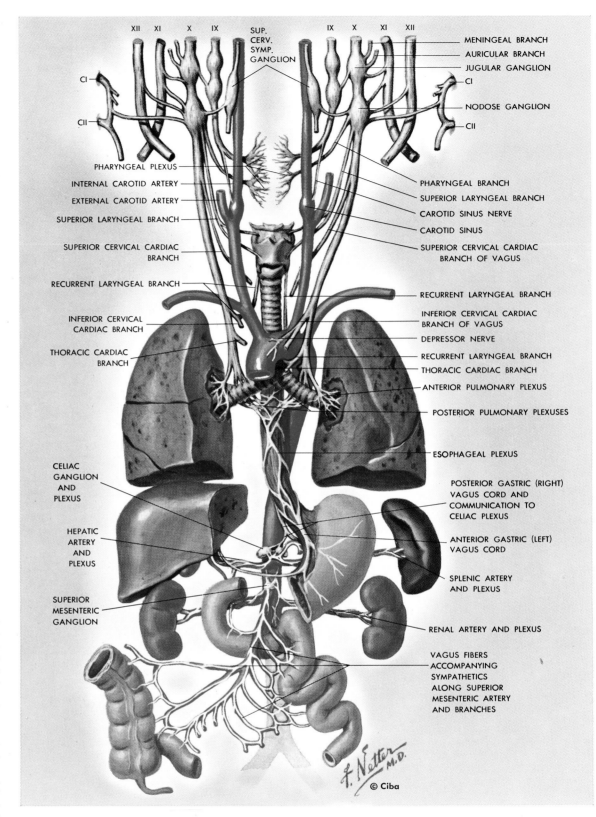

THE VAGUS NERVE

The vagus nerve includes general and special visceral efferent and both visceral and somatic afferent fibers. It is attached to the medulla oblongata by eight to ten radicles and traverses the jugular foramen. The general visceral efferent fibers arise in the dorsal motor nucleus of the vagus. They are the parasympathetic preganglionic fibers to the respiratory tract, pharynx, esophagus, and thoracic and abdominal viscera. They terminate in small ganglia near the viscera or within them in synaptic contacts with parasympathetic ganglion cells. The special visceral efferent fibers, which are few in number, arise in the nucleus ambiguus. The afferent fibers arise in the jugular and the nodose vagus ganglia. The visceral afferent fibers enter the medulla oblongata and bifurcate in the tractus solitarius. Their terminal branches end in the nucleus of this tract. The somatic afferent fibers terminate in the nucleus of the trigeminospinal tract.

The vagus nerve extends through the neck and the thorax into the abdomen. In the neck it lies within the carotid sheath. The right vagus passes across the subclavian artery and descends along the lateral surface of the trachea to the root of the lung where it spreads out in the posterior pulmonary plexus. From this plexus two rami descend along the esophagus and divide to form, with branches of the left vagus, the esophageal plexus. From the lower border of this plexus a single ramus descends along the dorsal surface of the esophagus and enters the abdomen where it gives off several branches which are distributed to the stomach and others which join the celiac plexus. The left vagus enters the thorax between the left subclavian and the left carotid arter-

ies, crosses the aortic arch and descends along the anterior surface of the esophagus, unites with the right vagus in the esophageal plexus and continues to the stomach. Some filaments arising from its gastric branches enter the lesser omentum; others join the hepatic plexus.

Both the jugular and the nodose ganglia are connected with the superior cervical sympathetic ganglion through intercommunicating rami. The jugular ganglion is also connected through rami with the accessory, the glossopharyngeal and the facial nerves. The nodose ganglion is connected with the hypoglossal nerve and with the loop between the first and the second cervical nerves. In the jugular fossa, the vagus nerve gives off a meningeal and an auricular branch. In the neck, it gives off a pharyngeal branch, the superior laryngeal nerve, the recurrent nerve and the cervical cardiac branches. The upper cervical cardiac branches extend into the deep cardiac plexus. The lower cervical cardiac branch of the right vagus joins the deep cardiac plexus; that of the left vagus joins the superficial cardiac plexus.

In the thorax, the vagus nerve gives rise to thoracic cardiac, anterior and posterior bronchial and esophageal branches. The cardiac branches, two or three in number, join filaments from the sympathetic trunks to form the anterior pulmonary plexus. The posterior bronchial branches, more numerous than the anterior ones, join filaments from the third and the fourth thoracic sympathetic trunk ganglia and enter the posterior pulmonary plexus. Esophageal branches arise both above and below the bronchial branches.

In the abdomen the vagus nerve gives rise to gastric, celiac and hepatic branches. The gastric branches of the right vagus are distributed to the posterior-inferior surface of the stomach. Those of the left vagus are distributed to the anterior-superior surface. The celiac branches arise mainly from the right vagus. They join the celiac plexus. From this plexus vagus fibers reach the pancreas, the spleen and the intestine. The hepatic branches are derived mainly from the left vagus and join the hepatic plexus through which they are distributed to the biliary tract.

PLATE 58

SYMPATHETIC TRUNK IN THE THORAX

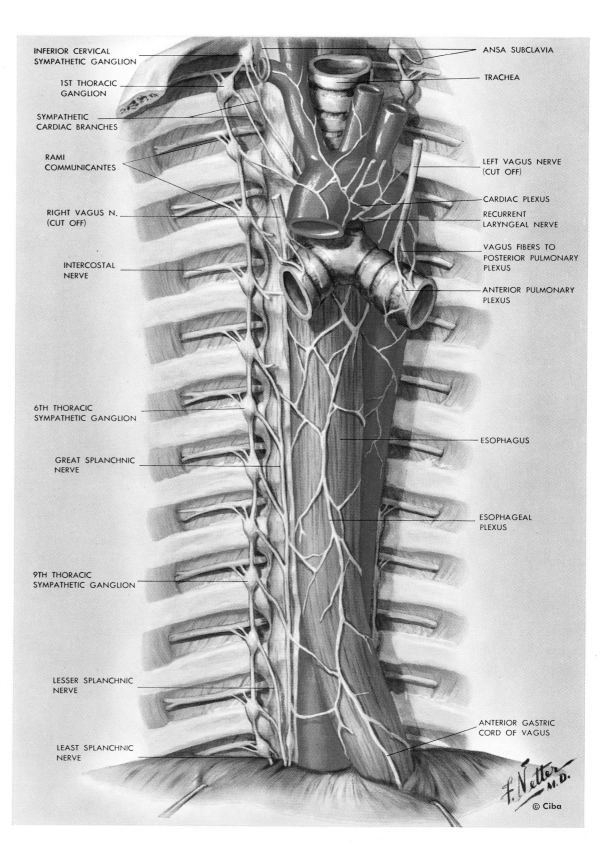

INFERIOR CERVICAL SYMPATHETIC GANGLION

1ST THORACIC GANGLION

SYMPATHETIC CARDIAC BRANCHES

RAMI COMMUNICANTES

RIGHT VAGUS N. (CUT OFF)

INTERCOSTAL NERVE

6TH THORACIC SYMPATHETIC GANGLION

GREAT SPLANCHNIC NERVE

9TH THORACIC SYMPATHETIC GANGLION

LESSER SPLANCHNIC NERVE

LEAST SPLANCHNIC NERVE

ANSA SUBCLAVIA

TRACHEA

LEFT VAGUS NERVE (CUT OFF)

CARDIAC PLEXUS

RECURRENT LARYNGEAL NERVE

VAGUS FIBERS TO POSTERIOR PULMONARY PLEXUS

ANTERIOR PULMONARY PLEXUS

ESOPHAGUS

ESOPHAGEAL PLEXUS

ANTERIOR GASTRIC CORD OF VAGUS

F. Netter M.D.
© Ciba

The thoracic portion of the sympathetic trunk lies ventral to the necks of the ribs and is covered by the pleura. It includes ten or eleven ganglia. In many instances the first thoracic ganglion is fused with the inferior cervical to form the stellate, or cervicothoracic, ganglion. In some instances other thoracic ganglia also are fused. Every thoracic sympathetic trunk ganglion is connected with the corresponding spinal nerve by means of a white communicating ramus and a sympathetic root. The white communicating rami consist of preganglionic and visceral afferent fibers which deviate from the spinal nerves and join the sympathetic trunk. The sympathetic roots are made up of fibers which arise in the sympathetic trunk ganglia and join the spinal nerves. Since these fibers are mainly unmyelinated, the bundle appears gray. The sympathetic roots, consequently, have been called the gray communicating rami. Since fibers of spinal cord origin join the sympathetic trunk only in the thoracic and the first and second lumbar segments, white communicating rami are limited to the spinal nerves in these segments. Since fibers of sympathetic trunk origin join all the spinal nerves, every spinal nerve is connected with the sympathetic trunk by one or more sympathetic roots. In general, the white communicating ramus arises from the nerve trunk distal to the point at which the sympathetic root joins it. In some instances the white

communicating ramus and the sympathetic root are enveloped by a common sheath. Occasionally, a thoracic sympathetic trunk ganglion is connected with more than one spinal nerve. Some preganglionic fibers make synaptic contacts only in the sympathetic trunk ganglion which is joined directly by the white ramus of which they are components. Others run longitudinally in the sympathetic trunk through a number of segments to reach the trunk ganglia in which they make synaptic contacts or the roots of the splanchnic nerves through which they reach ganglia in abdominal or pelvic plexuses.

The fibers which join the spinal nerves through their sympathetic roots extend peripherad in their somatic rami to be distributed to the structures within the area of distribution of every spinal nerve which requires sympathetic innervation, particularly the blood vessels, the sweat glands and the erector pili muscles. Some extend centralward along the roots of the spinal nerves to innervate the blood vessels within the vertebral canal.

In the upper five or six thoracic segments, rami which

arise from the sympathetic trunk join the plexus on the aorta. Other rami extend into the cardiac and the pulmonary plexuses. The splanchnic nerves, through which the abdominal and the pelvic viscera receive their sympathetic innervation, arise from the thoracic and the lumbar segments of the sympathetic trunk and join the plexuses in the abdomen and the pelvis which are associated with the aorta and its branches. Rami which arise from the sympathetic trunk in the fifth to the ninth or the tenth thoracic segments unite to form the greater splanchnic nerve. It traverses the mediastinum, passes through the diaphragm and joins the celiac plexus, which is located in relation to the celiac artery. Rami which arise from the sympathetic trunk in the ninth and the tenth thoracic segments unite to form the lesser splanchnic nerve, which also joins the celiac plexus but terminates mainly in the aorticorenal plexus. The least splanchnic nerve, when present, is derived from the most caudal portion of the thoracic sympathetic trunk or from the lesser splanchnic nerve. It terminates in the renal plexus.

PLATE 59

AUTONOMIC NERVES IN THE NECK

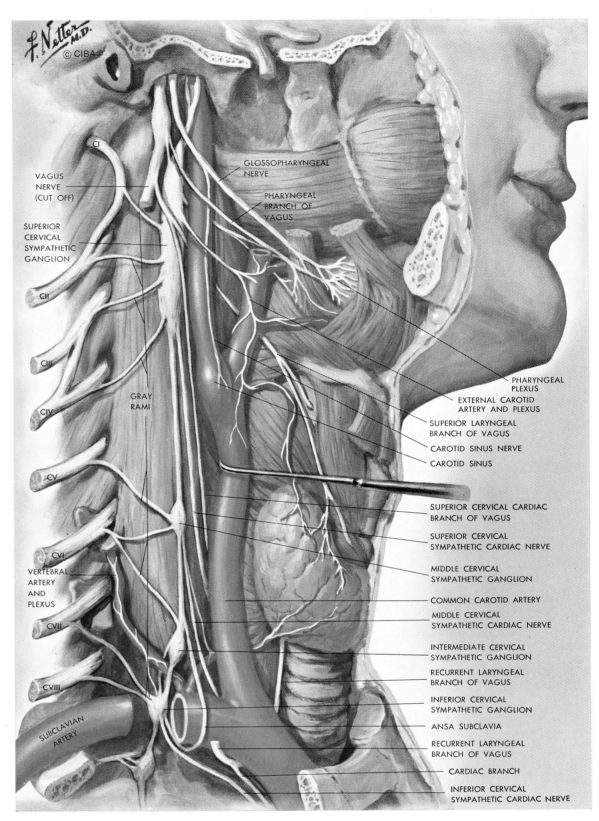

The cervical portion of the sympathetic trunk lies in the dorsal wall of the carotid sheath. It includes the inferior, the intermediate, the middle (frequently absent) and the superior cervical sympathetic ganglia. The inferior cervical ganglion is located on the ventral aspect of the head of the first rib. Frequently it is fused with the first thoracic ganglion to form the stellate, or cervicothoracic, ganglion. It is joined by the white communicating ramus of the first thoracic nerve and is connected with the seventh and the eighth cervical and the first thoracic nerves and sometimes also with the sixth cervical by sympathetic roots. The inferior cervical sympathetic cardiac nerve extends from the inferior cervical or the stellate ganglion to the cardiac plexus. Slender rami which arise from this ganglion also join the plexuses on the common carotid, the vertebral and the subclavian arteries. Fibers which arise in it also join the phrenic nerve and the plexus on the internal mammary artery through the ansa subclavia.

The intermediate cervical sympathetic ganglion is located medial to the vertebral artery approximately at the level of the eighth cervical nerve. It is joined by a large ramus which arises from the inferior cervi-

cal ganglion and passes ventral to the vertebral artery. In most instances it is also connected with the inferior cervical ganglion through the ansa subclavia. Sympathetic roots arising from this ganglion join the sixth and sometimes the first or seventh cervical nerve.

The middle cervical sympathetic ganglion usually lies approximately at the level of the body of the sixth cervical vertebra. Sympathetic roots arising from it join the fifth and sixth and sometimes the fourth and seventh cervical nerves. The middle cervical sympathetic cardiac nerve extends from this ganglion or, in the absence of the ganglion, directly from the sympathetic trunk to the deep portion of the cardiac plexus. Slender rami arising at this level also accompany the inferior thyroid artery.

The superior cervical sympathetic ganglion is located between the internal carotid artery and the jugular vein on the ventral aspects of the transverse processes of the second, the third and the fourth cervical vertebrae. It is the largest of the sympathetic trunk ganglia. It receives preganglionic fibers through the sympathetic trunk from

the first four or more thoracic nerves. Sympathetic roots arising from this ganglion join the first and the second cervical nerves, frequently the third and occasionally the fourth. It is also connected through sympathetic roots with the superior laryngeal and the hypoglossal nerves and through intercommunicating rami, with the jugular and the nodose ganglia of the vagus nerve and the petrosal ganglion of the glossopharyngeal nerve. Fibers arising in it also join the pharyngeal plexus and the phrenic nerve. The superior cervical sympathetic cardiac nerve arises near its caudal border. The internal carotid nerve is formed by the union of several rami which arise from the rostral portion of the superior cervical ganglion. Fibers derived from this ganglion make up the major portion of the internal carotid plexus. Other rami extend rostrad along the external carotid artery and form the external carotid plexus. The rami which extend rostrad from the superior cervical sympathetic ganglion represent the major portion of the extension of the sympathetic nerves into the cephalic region.

PLATE 60

AUTONOMIC NERVES IN THE HEAD

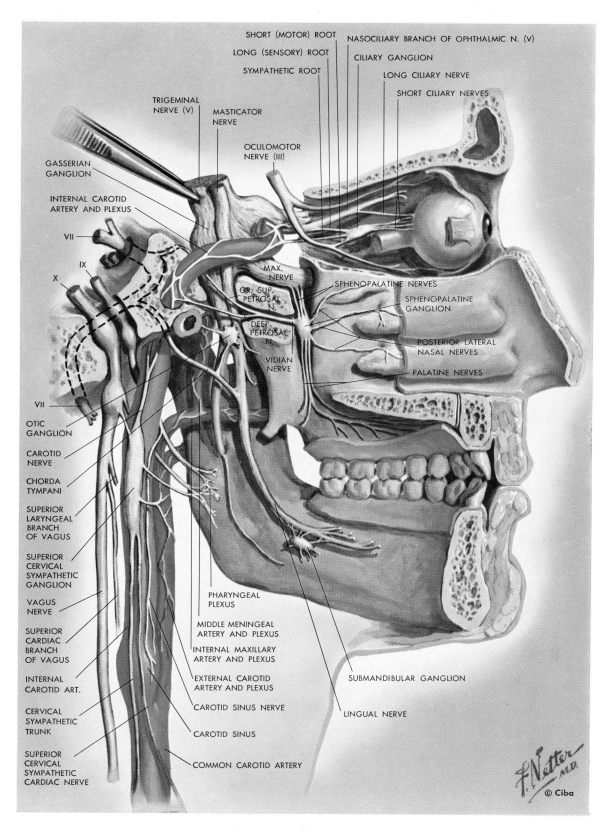

SHORT (MOTOR) ROOT
LONG (SENSORY) ROOT
SYMPATHETIC ROOT
NASOCILIARY BRANCH OF OPHTHALMIC N. (V)
CILIARY GANGLION
LONG CILIARY NERVE
SHORT CILIARY NERVES
TRIGEMINAL NERVE (V)
MASTICATOR NERVE
OCULOMOTOR NERVE (III)
GASSERIAN GANGLION
INTERNAL CAROTID ARTERY AND PLEXUS
VII
IX
X
MAX. NERVE
GR. SUP. PETROSAL N.
DEEP PETROSAL
VIDIAN NERVE
SPHENOPALATINE NERVES
SPHENOPALATINE GANGLION
POSTERIOR LATERAL NASAL NERVES
PALATINE NERVES
VII
OTIC GANGLION
CAROTID NERVE
CHORDA TYMPANI
SUPERIOR LARYNGEAL BRANCH OF VAGUS
SUPERIOR CERVICAL SYMPATHETIC GANGLION
VAGUS NERVE
SUPERIOR CARDIAC BRANCH OF VAGUS
INTERNAL CAROTID ART.
CERVICAL SYMPATHETIC TRUNK
SUPERIOR CERVICAL SYMPATHETIC CARDIAC NERVE
PHARYNGEAL PLEXUS
MIDDLE MENINGEAL ARTERY AND PLEXUS
INTERNAL MAXILLARY ARTERY AND PLEXUS
EXTERNAL CAROTID ARTERY AND PLEXUS
CAROTID SINUS NERVE
CAROTID SINUS
COMMON CAROTID ARTERY
SUBMANDIBULAR GANGLION
LINGUAL NERVE
F. Netter M.D.
© Ciba

The sympathetic nerves which extend into the cephalic region are distributed to all parts of the head. In addition to these nerves, the autonomic innervation of the head includes parasympathetic ganglia and nerves. The major cephalic parasympathetic ganglia are located in relation to the oculomotor nerve and the several divisions of the trigeminal nerve.

In addition to the nerve fibers which extend rostrad from the superior cervical sympathetic ganglion, the sympathetic innervation of the head includes some fibers which join the plexus on the common carotid and the one on the vertebral artery from the middle, the intermediate and the inferior cervical sympathetic trunk ganglia. The plexus on the common carotid artery is continuous with those on the internal and the external carotid arteries. The one on the vertebral artery is continuous with the plexus on the basilar artery. Most of the fibers which extend rostrad from the superior cervical ganglion join the plexuses on the internal and the external carotid arteries. Rami derived from the internal carotid plexus join the abducens, the trigeminal, the deep petrosal and the caroticotympanic nerves and the cavernous plexus. From the cavernous plexus, located in the middle cranial fossa, sympathetic fibers join the oculomotor, the trochlear and the ophthalmic nerves. Fibers from this plexus also accompany blood vessels into the hypophysis. The external carotid plexus gives rise to subordinate plexuses on the branches of the external carotid artery through which the fibers reach their peripheral distribution.

The otic ganglion is located on the medial aspect of the mandibular nerve just below the foramen ovale. It receives pre-

ganglionic fibers from the glossopharyngeal nerve via the lesser superficial petrosal nerve, and is traversed by afferent components of the glossopharyngeal nerve and by sympathetic fibers derived from the plexus on the middle meningeal artery. It gives rise to rami which join the auriculotemporal nerve, the chorda tympani and the nerve of the pterygoid canal. It is traversed by rami of the mandibular nerve which supply the tensor tympani and the tensor veli palatini muscles.

The submandibular (submaxillary) ganglion is located in relation to the duct of the submandibular gland and the lingual nerve. It receives preganglionic fibers from the facial nerve via the chorda tympani and the lingual nerve and is traversed by afferent components of the nervus intermedius and by sympathetic fibers derived from the plexus on the external maxillary artery. Rami which arise from this ganglion are distributed to the submandibular gland and its duct, the sublingual gland and the anterior portion of the tongue.

The sphenopalatine ganglion is located in the pterygo-

palatine fossa, close to the sphenopalatine foramen and beneath the maxillary nerve. It receives preganglionic fibers from the facial nerve via the greater superficial petrosal nerve and the nerve of the pterygoid canal, and is traversed by afferent components of the maxillary nerve and by sympathetic fibers derived from the internal carotid plexus which join the nerve of the pterygoid canal through the deep petrosal nerve. Rami which arise from this ganglion are distributed mainly to the mucous membranes of the nares, the mouth and the pharynx and to certain orbital structures.

The ciliary ganglion is located in the deep portion of the orbit between the optic nerve and the lateral rectus muscle. It receives preganglionic fibers through the inferior division of the oculomotor nerve, with which it is connected by a short ramus. It is traversed by afferent components of the ophthalmic nerve and by sympathetic fibers derived from the cavernous plexus. The short ciliary nerves, twelve to fifteen in number, extend forward from this ganglion above and below the optic nerve.

PLATE 61

SYMPATHETIC NERVES IN THE ABDOMEN

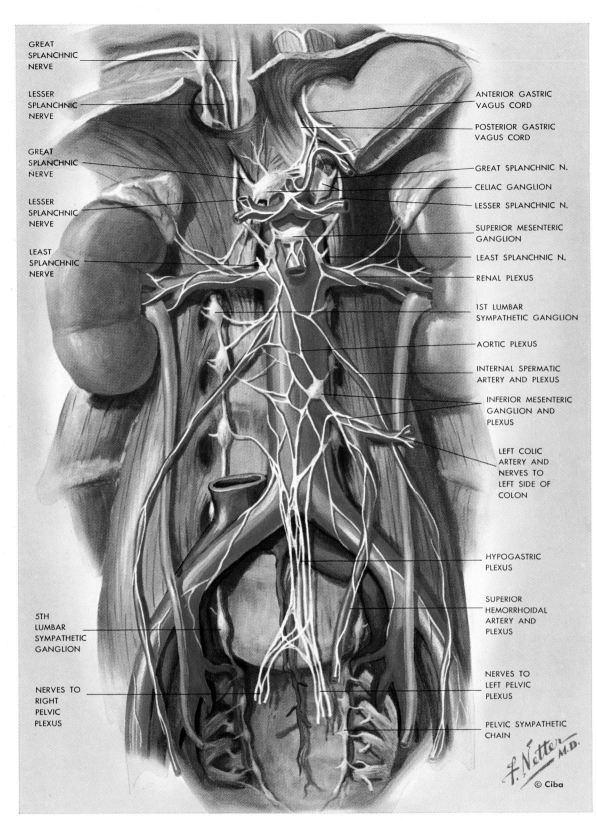

GREAT SPLANCHNIC NERVE

LESSER SPLANCHNIC NERVE

GREAT SPLANCHNIC NERVE

LESSER SPLANCHNIC NERVE

LEAST SPLANCHNIC NERVE

5TH LUMBAR SYMPATHETIC GANGLION

NERVES TO RIGHT PELVIC PLEXUS

ANTERIOR GASTRIC VAGUS CORD

POSTERIOR GASTRIC VAGUS CORD

GREAT SPLANCHNIC N.

CELIAC GANGLION

LESSER SPLANCHNIC N.

SUPERIOR MESENTERIC GANGLION

LEAST SPLANCHNIC N.

RENAL PLEXUS

1ST LUMBAR SYMPATHETIC GANGLION

AORTIC PLEXUS

INTERNAL SPERMATIC ARTERY AND PLEXUS

INFERIOR MESENTERIC GANGLION AND PLEXUS

LEFT COLIC ARTERY AND NERVES TO LEFT SIDE OF COLON

HYPOGASTRIC PLEXUS

SUPERIOR HEMORRHOIDAL ARTERY AND PLEXUS

NERVES TO LEFT PELVIC PLEXUS

PELVIC SYMPATHETIC CHAIN

f. Netter M.D.

© Ciba

The sympathetic trunk extends from the thorax into the abdomen between the lateral and the medial crura of the diaphragm. Here it tends ventrad until it reaches the ventrolateral surface of the body of the second lumbar vertebra. From this level to the sacral prominence, it lies adjacent to the bodies of the vertebrae along the medial border of the psoas muscle. The communicating rami in this region are relatively long. The most caudad white communicating ramus usually is that of the second lumbar nerve. In some instances the third lumbar nerve also gives rise to a white communicating ramus. In general, the white communicating rami take oblique courses from the spinal nerves to the sympathetic trunk. The sympathetic roots, or gray communicating rami, usually lie more nearly horizontal. Every lumbar nerve is connected with the sympathetic trunk by at least one sympathetic root. The lumbar portion of the sympathetic trunk is highly variable both with respect to the number of ganglia present and with respect to their exact locations. Fusion of two or more of the lumbar sympathetic trunk ganglia occurs frequently. A ganglion in every lumbar segment of the sympathetic trunk occurs but rarely, if at all. Rami arising from the sympathetic trunk in the lumbar segments join the plexus on the aorta, through which some of their fibers enter intermesenteric nerves.

The celiac plexus lies on the ventral surfaces of the aorta and the crura of the diaphragm. It surrounds the origins of the celiac and the superior mesenteric arteries and extends caudad as far as the level of origin of the renal arteries. It is continuous both rostrally and caudally with the aortic plexus. It comprises a large ganglion on either side, the semilunar ganglion, and a variable number of smaller ones. Usually there is a discrete ganglion, the superior mesenteric ganglion, located in relation to the superior mesenteric artery. The ganglia in the celiac plexus receive preganglionic fibers through the splanchnic nerves. This plexus is traversed by visceral afferent components of the vagus nerves and by some preganglionic vagus components. The sympathetic plexuses in the abdomen which are subsidiary to the celiac plexus and continuous with it include the left gastric, the hepatic, the phrenic, the adrenal and the renal plexuses. Rami which arise from the celiac plexus also join the spermatic (or ovarian) plexuses. Nerves which arise from it also accompany the intermesenteric arteries into the small intestine and the

large intestine approximately to the left colic flexure.

The inferior mesenteric plexus, located in relation to the inferior mesenteric artery, is connected with the celiac plexus through the aortic plexus which comprises both preganglionic and visceral afferent fibers. Plexuses which may be regarded as subsidiary to the inferior mesenteric plexus are associated with the inferior mesenteric artery and its branches. They include the colic, the sigmoid, and the superior hemorrhoidal plexuses. The nerves arising from the inferior mesenteric plexus, like those which arise from the other abdominal plexuses, comprise both postganglionic and afferent fibers.

The hypogastric plexus extends from the inferior mesenteric plexus into the pelvis. It includes preganglionic and postganglionic sympathetic and visceral afferent fibers. It consists of numerous bundles of nerve fibers which form a plexiform structure and serve to connect the pelvic plexuses with the inferior mesenteric plexus. The term presacral nerve, frequently used by surgeons, refers to the hypogastric plexus.

PLATE 62

AUTONOMIC NERVES AND GANGLIA IN THE PELVIS

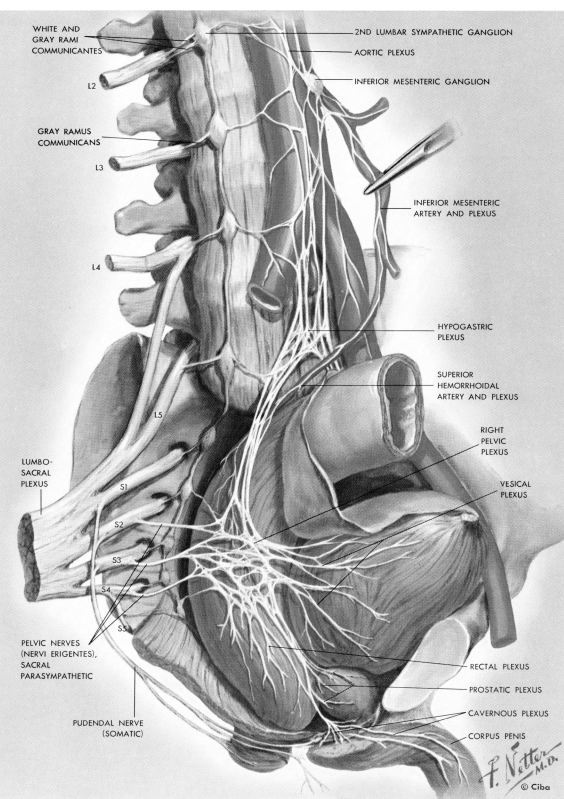

WHITE AND GRAY RAMI COMMUNICANTES

L2

GRAY RAMUS COMMUNICANS

L3

L4

L5

LUMBO-SACRAL PLEXUS

S1

S2

S3

S4

S5

PELVIC NERVES (NERVI ERIGENTES), SACRAL PARASYMPATHETIC

PUDENDAL NERVE (SOMATIC)

2ND LUMBAR SYMPATHETIC GANGLION

AORTIC PLEXUS

INFERIOR MESENTERIC GANGLION

INFERIOR MESENTERIC ARTERY AND PLEXUS

HYPOGASTRIC PLEXUS

SUPERIOR HEMORRHOIDAL ARTERY AND PLEXUS

RIGHT PELVIC PLEXUS

VESICAL PLEXUS

RECTAL PLEXUS

PROSTATIC PLEXUS

CAVERNOUS PLEXUS

CORPUS PENIS

F. Netter M.D.

© Ciba

As the sympathetic trunk extends from the lumbar region into the pelvis it lies on the pelvic surface of the sacrum medial to the anterior sacral foramina. In the lower sacral segments both trunks converge toward the median plane and terminate in a common ganglion, the ganglion impar or coccygeal ganglion, on the surface of the coccyx. The sacral portion of the sympathetic trunk usually includes four small ganglia. Sympathetic roots arising from them join all the sacral and the coccygeal spinal nerves. Slender rami also extend into the pelvic plexuses.

The pelvic plexuses are located along the lateral aspects of the pelvic viscera. They are continuous with the hypogastric plexus rostrally. Each pelvic plexus comprises an extensive meshwork of nerve fiber bundles which spreads out between the viscera and the pelvic wall. It is joined by the visceral rami of the sacral nerves which include the preganglionic fibers of the sacral parasympathetic outflow.

Each pelvic plexus may be subdivided into regional parts named according to the organs with which they are associated, but these subdivisions, or subordinate plexuses, are not sharply delimited. Two of them, the medial hemorrhoidal plexus and the vesical plexus, are common to both sexes. The medial hemorrhoidal plexus is located in relation to the medial hemorrhoidal artery. It receives fibers from the superior hemorrhoidal plexus and sends fibers into the rectum. The vesical plexus lies on the lateral surface of the urinary bladder. Rami derived from this plexus penetrate into the bladder wall. Some also become associated with the ureter, and some with the urethra.

In the male, the prostatic plexus lies on the dorsolateral aspect of the prostate gland, to which it gives off rami. Other rami derived from this plexus join the plexus on the ductus deferens. The cavernous plexus is continuous with the prostatic plexus. It gives off rami which extend into the penis. These rami, with the dorsal nerve of the penis, supply the membranous portion of the urethra and the corpora cavernosa.

In the female, the uterovaginal plexus is located in relation to the cervix of the uterus and to the upper part of the vagina. It is a more extensive structure than the prostatic plexus. Rami derived from this plexus penetrate into the walls of the uterus and the vagina to innervate the musculature and the blood vessels of these organs.

The pelvic plexuses include numerous small ganglia. Many comprise both parasympathetic and sympathetic ganglion cells, some comprise only parasympathetic, and others only sympathetic ganglion cells. The parasympathetic preganglionic fibers concerned with the pelvic plexuses are components of the sacral nerves. They reach the pelvic plexuses through the pelvic nerves. The sympathetic preganglionic fibers are components of the splanchnic nerves. They traverse the celiac roots of the inferior mesenteric plexus and reach the pelvic plexus through the hypogastric plexus.

Both the parasympathetic and the sympathetic components of the pelvic plexuses are accompanied by visceral afferent nerve fibers. Those associated with the parasympathetic nerves are components of the sacral spinal nerves. Those associated with the sympathetic nerves are mainly components of the tenth thoracic to the second lumbar spinal nerves. They accompany the preganglionic sympathetic fibers throughout their courses to the pelvic organs.

PLATE 63

INNERVATION OF THE HEART

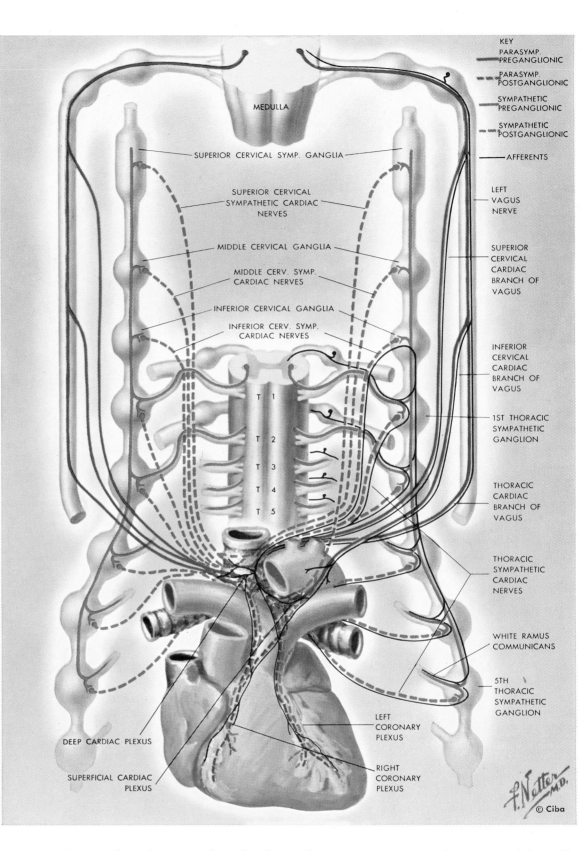

The heart is innervated through sympathetic, parasympathetic and afferent fibers. All of the nerve components concerned mingle to some extent in the cardiac plexus, located in relation to the base of the heart. It consists of a superficial portion, the superficial cardiac plexus; and a deep portion, the deep cardiac plexus.

The superficial cardiac plexus lies mainly in the concavity of the arch of the aorta and superficial to the pericardium.

The deep cardiac plexus is situated mainly behind the arch of the aorta and in part between the aorta and the pulmonary veins. It consists of two lateral parts which are joined together by numerous bundles of nerve fibers. It is also connected with the superficial cardiac plexus by numerous nerve fiber bundles. Extensions along the coronary arteries are known as the right and the left coronary plexuses.

The cardiac plexus includes numerous ganglia, all of which are parasympathetic. The preganglionic fibers which connect them with the central nervous system are components of the vagus nerves. Most of the cardiac ganglia are located in relation to the walls of the atria. They lie mainly in the subepicardial connective tissue. A single ganglion of somewhat larger size than most of the ganglia in the cardiac plexus, the cardiac ganglion of Wrisberg, is usually located in the concavity of the aortic arch.

The sympathetic nerves of the heart include the superior, the middle and the inferior cervical, and the thoracic sympathetic cardiac nerves.

The superior cervical sympathetic cardiac nerve regularly arises from the superior cer-

vical sympathetic ganglion either as a single trunk or by several roots from the ganglion and one or more from the sympathetic trunk.

The middle cardiac nerve arises singly or by several roots from the middle cervical ganglion or, in the absence of this ganglion, directly from the sympathetic trunk.

The inferior cervical sympathetic cardiac nerve arises by several roots from the lower cervical portion of the sympathetic trunk and the inferior cervical or the stellate ganglion.

The thoracic sympathetic cardiac nerves vary in number. They arise from the rostral four or five thoracic segments of the sympathetic trunk. Occasionally, a ramus arising from the sixth thoracic segment of the sympathetic trunk joins the cardiac plexus.

The left superior cervical cardiac nerve joins the superficial cardiac plexus. All other sympathetic cardiac nerves join the deep cardiac plexus. The efferent nerve fibers extending from the sympathetic trunk into the cardiac plexus all arise in sympathetic trunk ganglia. The sympa-

thetic cardiac nerves except the superior and the middle cervical are accompanied by afferent spinal nerve components which conduct sensory impulses from the heart and the coronary blood vessels.

The parasympathetic innervation of the heart involves three branches of the vagus nerve on either side. The superior cervical cardiac branch arises from the vagus trunk just distal to the origin of the superior laryngeal nerve. The inferior cervical cardiac branch usually arises from the recurrent nerve. The third, or thoracic, cardiac branch arises from the vagus nerve within the thorax.

On the left side, the inferior cervical cardiac branch of the vagus joins the superficial cardiac plexus. All the other cardiac branches of the vagi join the deep cardiac plexus.

The efferent fibers in the cardiac branches of the vagus nerves are preganglionic parasympathetic fibers which make synaptic connections in the cardiac ganglia. The socalled depressor nerves consist of afferent vagus components which are connected with receptors in the proximal parts of the aorta and the adjacent cardiac wall.

PLATE 64

INNERVATION OF THE BLOOD VESSELS

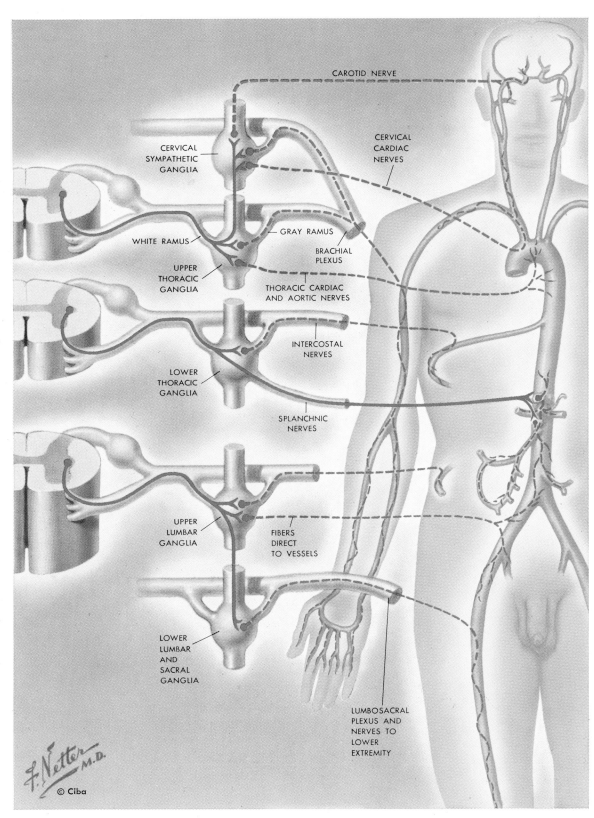

CAROTID NERVE

CERVICAL SYMPATHETIC GANGLIA

CERVICAL CARDIAC NERVES

WHITE RAMUS

GRAY RAMUS

UPPER THORACIC GANGLIA

BRACHIAL PLEXUS

THORACIC CARDIAC AND AORTIC NERVES

INTERCOSTAL NERVES

LOWER THORACIC GANGLIA

SPLANCHNIC NERVES

UPPER LUMBAR GANGLIA

FIBERS DIRECT TO VESSELS

LOWER LUMBAR AND SACRAL GANGLIA

LUMBOSACRAL PLEXUS AND NERVES TO LOWER EXTREMITY

F. Netter M.D.
© Ciba

The blood vessels are innervated through both efferent and afferent nerves. The efferent nerves include both vasoconstrictor and vasodilator fibers. They are mainly sympathetic. Limited vascular areas are innervated through both sympathetic and parasympathetic nerves. The afferent nerve fibers concerned in the innervation of the blood vessels are sensory root components of the cerebrospinal nerves.

The large blood vessels in the trunk, such as the aorta and the venae cavae, receive nerves directly from the sympathetic trunks. In the thorax, these vessels are innervated in part through the cardiac plexus which also innervates the coronary vessels. The pulmonary vessels are innervated through the pulmonary plexuses.

The nerve plexus on the aorta is relatively meager in the thorax. It is somewhat more abundant in the abdomen. From the aortic plexus, nerve plexuses extend distad on all the major branches of the aorta, but fibers derived from the aortic plexus extend only short distances along the arteries arising from the aorta.

The blood vessels of the abdominal viscera are innervated through nerves which accompany them from the plexuses associated with the celiac and the intermesenteric arteries, particularly the celiac and the inferior mesenteric plexuses. Preganglionic sympathetic fibers reach these plexuses through the splanchnic nerves.

The blood vessels of the pelvic organs are innervated through the inferior mesenteric, the hypogastric and the pelvic plexuses. Preganglionic sympathetic fibers reach

the pelvic plexuses through the inferior mesenteric and the hypogastric plexuses.

The blood vessels in the cervical and the cephalic regions derive their innervation mainly from the cervical portions of the sympathetic trunks. The preganglionic fibers concerned are components of the rostral two or three thoracic nerves.

The major portion of the vasomotor innervation of the head is derived from the superior cervical sympathetic ganglion through the plexuses on the internal and the external carotid arteries. It receives fibers from all the upper thoracic sympathetic trunk ganglia. Most of these fibers do not extend into the internal and the external carotid plexuses.

The plexus on the vertebral artery also receives fibers from the cervical sympathetic trunk ganglia. The vertebral plexuses are continuous with the plexus on the basilar artery which extends into the cranial cavity. This plexus appears to play a role in the innervation of the vascular bed associated with the brain stem.

The peripheral blood vessels, including those which supply the extremities and the somatic tissues of the trunk, are innervated through sympathetic fibers derived from the sympathetic trunk ganglia. These fibers join the spinal nerves through their sympathetic roots and reach the blood vessels through branches which join them at intervals along their courses.

The nerve branches which join the arteries become more frequent in the more distal parts of the branching arterial trees.

The nerves which innervate veins have an arrangement comparable to the arrangement of those which innervate arteries, but the nerve supply of the veins is less abundant than that of the arteries. The nerve branches which join the peripheral blood vessels convey afferent as well as sympathetic fibers. Although the nerve plexus in the adventitial layers of an artery or a vein is continuous throughout the length of the vessel, individual nerve fibers do not extend longitudinally along the vessel except for short distances.

PLATE 65

INNERVATION OF THE INTRINSIC EYE MUSCLES

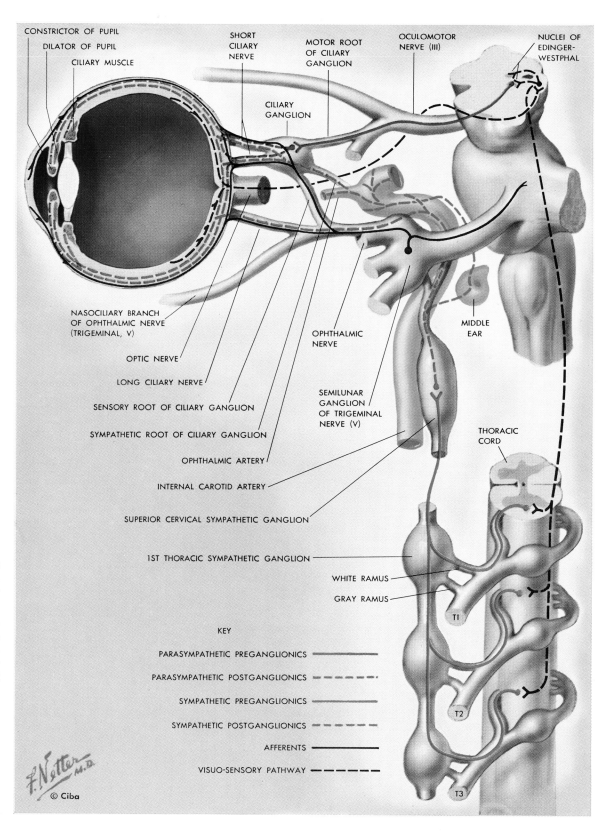

The intrinsic muscles of the eye are innervated mainly through parasympathetic nerves. Sympathetic nerves are distributed only to the blood vessels and the radial muscles of the iris.

The sympathetic nerve fibers which reach the eye are derived from the superior cervical sympathetic trunk ganglion. The preganglionic sympathetic fibers concerned emerge from the spinal cord in the first, the second and the third thoracic nerves. Most of those concerned with the innervation of the radial muscles of the iris emerge in the second thoracic nerve.

The preganglionic sympathetic fibers ascend through the cervical portion of the sympathetic trunk without making synaptic contacts with ganglion cells except in the superior cervical ganglion.

The postganglionic sympathetic fibers to the eye, in general, extend rostrad in the internal carotid plexus to the cavernous plexus which is located in the middle cranial fossa. Those which innervate the radial muscles of the iris do not traverse the internal carotid plexus all the way to the cavernous plexus. A short distance from the superior cervical ganglion, they deviate into the middle ear with the caroticotympanic fibers and traverse the tympanic plexus. After emerging from the middle ear, they pass into the cranium lateral to the nerve of the pterygoid canal and enter the cavernous plexus.

From the cavernous plexus, sympathetic fibers enter the orbit through the superior orbital fissure. Some of them traverse the sympathetic root of the ciliary ganglion and become incorporated in the short ciliary nerves. Others reach the eye through the long ciliary nerves. The latter do not communicate with the ciliary ganglion, but extend directly to the eyeball.

The long ciliary nerves are made up chiefly of afferent fibers derived from the

nasociliary nerve and sympathetic fibers derived directly from the plexus on the ophthalmic artery. The sympathetic fibers which reach the iris traverse the long ciliary nerves.

Parasympathetic nerve fibers reach the eye from the ciliary ganglion via the short ciliary nerves. The preganglionic neurons concerned with the parasympathetic innervation of the eye are located in the Edinger-Westphal nucleus which is incorporated in the nucleus of the oculomotor nerve. Their axons reach the ciliary ganglion through the oculomotor nerve. Postganglionic parasympathetic fibers derived from the ciliary ganglion are distributed to the muscles of the ciliary body and the circular muscles of the iris.

The visual reflex centers are located in the tectum of the mesencephalon and in the pretectal area. Reflex movements of the eyes or of the head in response to stimulation of receptors in the retina are carried out through reflex connections in the superior colliculus.

The light reflex, i.e., constriction of the pupil in re-

sponse to illumination of the retina, and the accommodation reflex are carried out through reflex connections in the pretectal area. The afferent limbs of the reflex arcs concerned in these reflexes include optic nerve fibers. The efferent limbs are composed of parasympathetic preganglionic neurons in the Edinger-Westphal nucleus and ganglion cells in the ciliary ganglion.

From the superior colliculus, conduction pathways lead downward through the brain stem and the spinal cord through which both sympathetic and somatic reflex responses to retinal stimulation may be carried out. Reflex responses through the sympathetic innervation of the eye involve mainly the ocular blood vessels and the radial muscles of the iris.

Afferent impulses from the extraretinal portions of the eye are conducted into the brain stem through afferent components of the trigeminal nerve. These fibers terminate in the sensory nuclei of the trigeminal nerve from which reflex connections are made with both somatic and autonomic nerves.

PLATE 66

INNERVATION
OF THE STOMACH

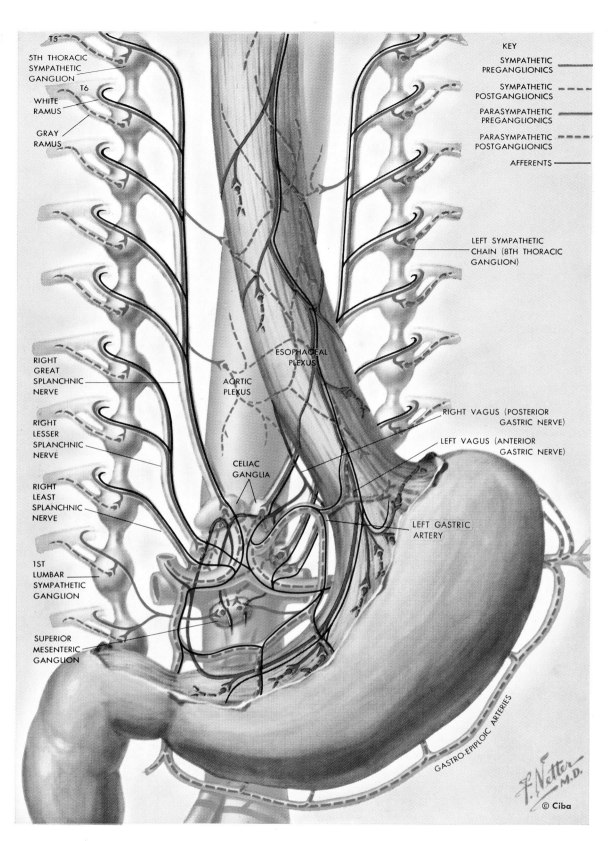

KEY

SYMPATHETIC PREGANGLIONICS	——
SYMPATHETIC POSTGANGLIONICS	----
PARASYMPATHETIC PREGANGLIONICS	——
PARASYMPATHETIC POSTGANGLIONICS	----
AFFERENTS	——

T5

5TH THORACIC SYMPATHETIC GANGLION

T6

WHITE RAMUS

GRAY RAMUS

RIGHT GREAT SPLANCHNIC NERVE

RIGHT LESSER SPLANCHNIC NERVE

RIGHT LEAST SPLANCHNIC NERVE

1ST LUMBAR SYMPATHETIC GANGLION

SUPERIOR MESENTERIC GANGLION

ESOPHAGEAL PLEXUS

AORTIC PLEXUS

CELIAC GANGLIA

LEFT SYMPATHETIC CHAIN (8TH THORACIC GANGLION)

RIGHT VAGUS (POSTERIOR GASTRIC NERVE)

LEFT VAGUS (ANTERIOR GASTRIC NERVE)

LEFT GASTRIC ARTERY

GASTRO-EPIPLOIC ARTERIES

F. Netter M.D.

© Ciba

The innervation of the stomach is derived through the vagus and sympathetic nerves. The vagus nerves include afferent components. Afferent spinal nerve components also reach the stomach in association with the sympathetic nerves.

In the thorax, both vagus nerves lie close to the esophagus and give off branches to it. Communications between the right and the left vagus also occur. The esophageal branches of each vagus nerve are not limited to one side of the organ, but some are distributed to the opposite side. In general, branches of the left vagus are distributed mainly on the ventral surface, and branches of the right vagus on the dorsal surface of the esophagus. The branches of the vagus nerves, with their intercommunicating rami, form a plexus around the esophagus.

The anatomic relationships of the vagus nerves from the esophageal plexus to the stomach are highly variable. As each nerve reaches the stomach, it commonly gives rise to a left, a middle and a right gastric ramus. As the left vagus extends caudad on the ventral surface of the stomach, its left ramus gives off branches to the fundus and approximately the rostral two-thirds of the corpus. Its middle ramus gives off branches to the prepyloric region. Its right ramus

extends to the liver. As the right vagus extends caudad on the dorsal surface of the stomach, its left ramus supplies branches to the cardia, the lesser curvature and a limited portion of the corpus. Its middle ramus sends branches into the prepyloric region. Its right ramus joins the celiac plexus. In the prepyloric region, branches of the middle gastric ramus of each vagus nerve enter the hepatogastric ligament. All efferent components of the vagus nerves which terminate in the stomach make synaptic contacts with ganglionic neurons in the myenteric and the submucous plexuses.

The sympathetic nerves of the stomach are derived mainly from the celiac plexus. The preganglionic fibers concerned reach the celiac ganglia through the splanchnic nerves. Most of the postganglionic fibers accompany the arteries to the stomach. The proximal portion of the stomach also receives sympathetic fibers from the left phrenic plexus and occasionally from the right, the left gastric plexus and the hepatic plexus. Slender rami which arise from the sympathetic trunk in the upper lumbar seg-

ments join the stomach directly. In the hepatogastric ligament, sympathetic fibers derived from the celiac plexus become associated with vagus fibers as they approach the stomach, but in general the vagus and the sympathetic fibers are conveyed in separate bundles, the hepatogastric nerves, which lie parallel to each other.

The intramural ganglia of the stomach receive preganglionic fibers only through the vagus nerves. Fibers which arise in these ganglia are distributed in the gastric musculature and in the glands of the mucosa. The sympathetic fibers which enter the gastric wall may traverse intramural ganglia, but they make no functional connections in them. They are distributed mainly to the gastric musculature and the blood vessels. Afferent spinal nerve fibers which accompany the sympathetic nerves of the stomach and afferent vagus components are distributed to receptors in the gastric serosa and throughout the gastric wall. Terminal branches of afferent fibers also take part in the formation of a delicate subepithelial plexus in the gastric mucosa.

PLATE 67

INNERVATION
OF THE INTESTINE

The nerves of the small intestine, like those of the stomach, include sympathetic, parasympathetic and afferent components. The parasympathetic innervation is derived mainly through the branch of the right vagus (posterior vagal trunk), which joins the celiac plexus. The preganglionic sympathetic fibers concerned in the innervation of the small intestine originate chiefly in the ninth and tenth spinal cord segments, but some may also come from the eighth and eleventh segments. They emerge with the spinal nerves and pass through the white rami communicantes to the sympathetic trunks. They reach the celiac, aorticorenal and superior mesenteric ganglia by way of the thoracic splanchnic nerves and here synapse with postganglionic neurons.

Both the vagus and postganglionic sympathetic fibers reach the small intestine through the mesenteric nerves which, in general, accompany the intestinal (jejunal and ileal) arteries. The sympathetic fiber bundles lie usually in close proximity to the blood vessels in the mesentery. As they enter the intestinal wall, many of them remain associated with the intramural blood vessels; others ramify in the muscle layers. The bundles in which the vagus fibers traverse the mesentery are less intimately associated with the mesenteric blood vessels. Some of these pursue courses, through the mesentery, which are not obviously related to blood vessels. Within the intestinal wall they enter the myenteric and submucous plexuses, in the ganglia of which they make synaptic contacts with postganglionic fibers.

The sympathetic nerve supply to the cecum, vermiform appendix and ascending and transverse portions of the colon originates in the twelfth thoracic and first lumbar segments and sometimes also in the eleventh thoracic segment of the spinal cord. The pathway then traverses the white rami communicantes, sympathetic trunks and the thoracic splanchnic nerves (lesser and least) to the celiac, aorticorenal and superior mesenteric ganglia, where synapses take place. The postganglionic fibers then accompany the superior mesenteric artery and its branches of distribution to the cecum, appendix, ascending colon and transverse colon. The parasympathetic supply to these portions of the large bowel, like that to the small intestine, is derived from the vagus nerves, chiefly the branch of the right vagus to the celiac plexus. From here, they accompany the sympathetic fibers along the course of the superior mesenteric artery and its branches to the bowel.

The sympathetic innervation of the descending colon, sigmoid colon and rectum originates in the first and second lumbar spinal segments. It traverses the white rami communicantes, the sympathetic trunks, the lumbar splanchnic nerves, the superior mesenteric and the intermesenteric (preaortic) plexuses to the inferior mesenteric ganglion and plexus, where some of the fibers make synapses. Some of the postganglionic fibers then pass out along the inferior mesenteric artery and its branches to the descending colon, sigmoid colon and upper portion of the rectum. Some preganglionic and some postganglionic fibers continue downward in the superior hypogastric plexus and hypogastric (presacral) nerves to the pelvic (inferior hypogastric) plexuses, where the remaining preganglionic fibers synapse. The postganglionics are then dis-

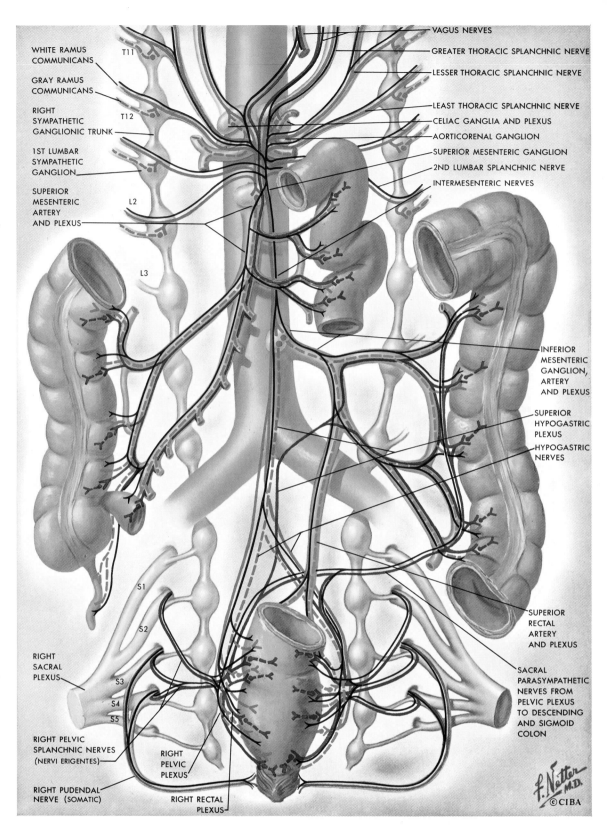

tributed through the rectal plexuses to the rectal wall.

The parasympathetic supply to the descending colon, sigmoid colon and rectum derives from the second, third and fourth sacral segments of the spinal cord and then goes via the pelvic splanchnic nerves (nervi erigentes) to the pelvic (inferior hypogastric) plexuses. The fibers to the middle and lower rectum then go via the rectal plexus to the rectal wall. The fibers to the descending colon, sigmoid colon and upper rectum, however, mostly emerge from the pelvic plexuses or from the hypogastric nerves, pass to the right and ascend in nerves which course in front of the sigmoid arteries on the medial side of the left colon. In some cases, however, the fibers to these parts of the bowel follow an alternative course, ascending from the pelvic plexus in the hypogastric nerves to the superior hypogastric plexus and thence shunting, via a short communicating branch or branches, to the inferior mesenteric plexus, to be distributed with the latter.

All the parasympathetic preganglionic fibers to the large bowel, like those to the small bowel, synapse with

postganglionic neurons in the myenteric and submucous plexuses of the intestinal wall.

Afferent pathways, in general, follow (in reverse direction) both the sympathetic and the parasympathetic supplies to the small and large bowel. The afferent components of the vagus and pelvic nerves and of the sympathetic subserve reflex activity, but most localizable sensations (pain, distention, etc.), referable to the gastrointestinal tract, appear to be mediated through the sympathetic afferents.

The external anal sphincter and the skin of the lower anal canal and the perianal skin are supplied by the pudendal nerves, which are somatic and which include both efferent and afferent components.

NOTE: The above description has been modified from Dr. Kuntz's original description for previous printings of this volume, based upon the work of Mitchell (*Edinb. med. J.* 42: 11, 1935), Rankin and Learmonth (*Ann. Surg.* 92: 710, 1930) and Telford and Stopford (*Brit. med. J.* 1: 572, 1934)

PLATE 68

THE ENTERIC NERVOUS SYSTEM

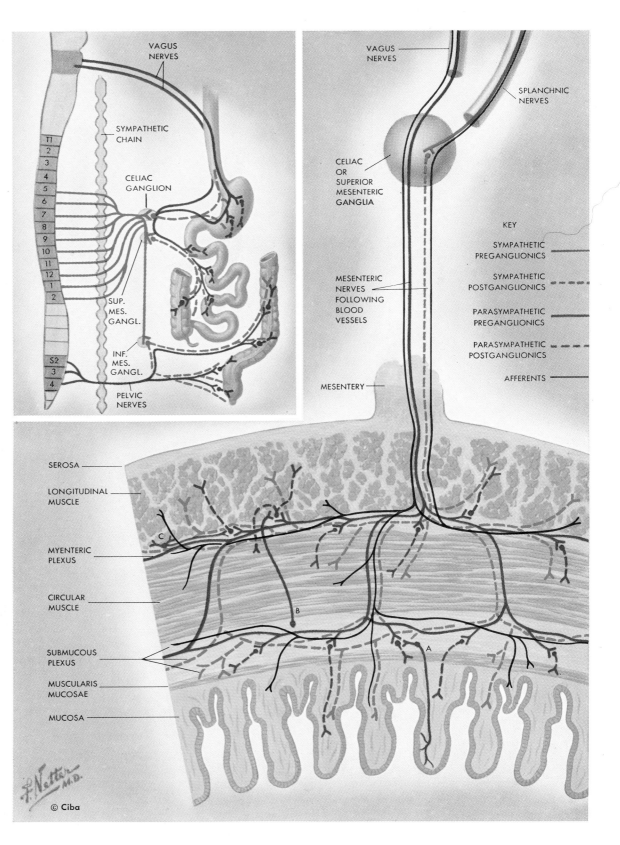

The intramural nerves of the enteric canal comprise the myenteric plexus, which is situated chiefly between the longitudinal and the circular muscle layers, and the submucous plexus, which is situated in the submucosa. These plexuses are continuous from a level 3 to 4 cm. below the larynx to the anal canal. They include numerous small ganglia which are functionally connected with the central nervous system through preganglionic components of the vagus and the pelvic nerves. They are also traversed by sympathetic nerve fibers, afferent spinal nerve components which are associated with the sympathetic nerves, and afferent components of the vagus and the pelvic nerves.

The myenteric plexus consists essentially of an abundant meshwork of bundles of nerve fibers in which ganglia are located chiefly at nodal points. The ganglia vary within a wide range both with respect to size and to the number of their constituent ganglion cells.

Branches of the extrinsic nerves enter the myenteric ganglia by penetrating the longitudinal muscle layer. Some of the preganglionic fibers in these nerves make synaptic contacts with ganglion cells at this level. Others continue into the submucous plexus. The ganglia in the myenteric plexus are intimately interconnected by numerous fiber bundles which lie between the muscle layers. They are also connected with the ganglia in the submucous plexus by fiber bundles which, in general, lie between bundles of circular muscle fibers.

The fiber bundles which make up the meshwork of the myenteric plexus and those which interconnect this plexus with the sub-

mucous plexus include both fibers of extrinsic origin and fibers which arise in the intramural ganglia.

The submucous plexus comprises a meshwork of relatively slender bundles of nerve fibers with ganglia located at nodal points. The rami which connect the submucous with the myenteric plexus include preganglionic fibers which make synaptic contacts in the submucous ganglia, and sympathetic and afferent fibers which traverse the plexus.

Slender bundles of nerve fibers extend from the submucous plexus into the muscularis mucosae, into relationship with the glands in the mucosa and into relationship with the gastrointestinal epithelium.

The fibers which approach the epithelium most closely form a subepithelial plexus from which fibers approach the epithelial cells. In the esophagus, the submucous plexus appears to be devoid of ganglia. The major portion of the plexus in this region lies close to the muscularis. It is intimately connected with the myenteric plexus and is traversed by many fibers of relatively large caliber which

appear to be afferent components of the vagus and the thoracic spinal nerves which are connected with receptors in the mucosa. Some afferent nerve fibers also terminate in the esophageal musculature.

The subepithelial plexus throughout the enteric canal probably is essentially receptive. In addition to the terminal branches of afferent fibers of extrinsic origin, it includes receptive processes of ganglion cells in the submucous plexus.

The enteric plexuses, unlike most other parts of the autonomic nervous system, include local reflex arcs. The existence of local reflex mechanisms in the wall of the enteric canal is demonstrated by abundant physiologic data. Some of these mechanisms involve ganglion cells only in the myenteric or only in the submucous plexus. Others involve one or more ganglion cells in each plexus. By virtue of the intramural reflex mechanisms, coordinated reflex activity may take place in the enteric canal independently of impulses received through the extrinsic nerves.

PLATE 69

INNERVATION OF THE BILIARY SYSTEM

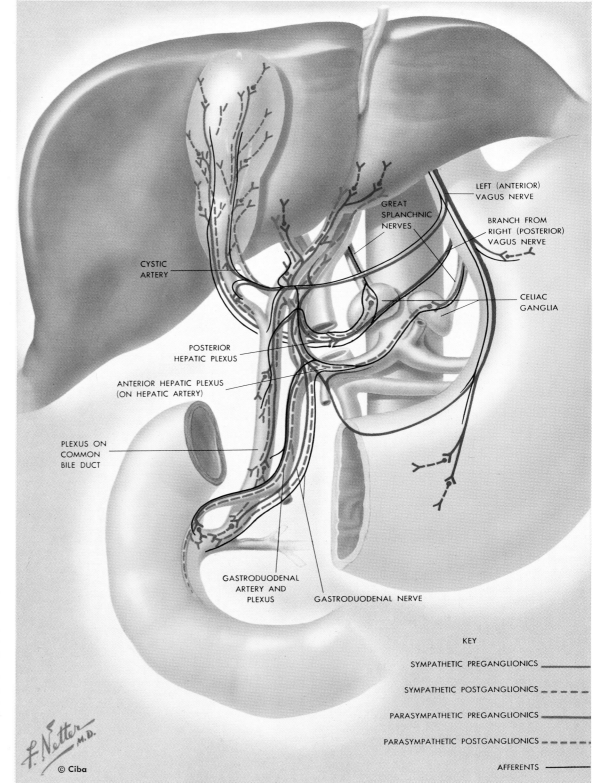

The nerves through which the biliary system is innervated include sympathetic, parasympathetic and afferent components.

The sympathetic nerves are mainly derived from the celiac plexus. Some sympathetic fibers derived from the inferior phrenic plexus join the biliary nerves in some cases. The preganglionic sympathetic fibers concerned traverse the splanchnic nerves. The ganglion cells concerned in the parasympathetic innervation of the biliary system are located in proximity to the bile ducts and in part within the walls of these ducts and the wall of the gallbladder. The preganglionic parasympathetic neurons are components of the vagus nerves.

Extending from the celiac plexus into the hepatic portal is a plexiform structure which comprises the anterior hepatic plexus, located in relation to the hepatic artery, and the posterior hepatic plexus, located in relation to the portal vein and the bile duct.

The anterior hepatic plexus consists chiefly of fibers derived from the left portion of the celiac plexus and the right abdominal branch of the left vagus nerve. It includes the internal nerve of the cystic duct and the gallbladder and the nervus pancreaticocholedochus.

The posterior hepatic plexus is derived mainly from the right portion of the celiac plexus and branches of the right vagus nerve. It comprises three or four main fiber bundles which pass transversely behind the portal vein to reach the posterior surfaces of the bile ducts. The right lateral bundle extends along the posterior surface of the common bile duct. It supplies fibers to the bile duct and gives off slender rami to the lateral nerve of the gallbladder and

to the anterior hepatic plexus.

The major portion of the sympathetic fibers in the biliary nerves appears to be derived from the left celiac ganglia. Fibers derived from the right celiac ganglia also traverse these nerves. In cases in which the phrenic nerves contribute to the innervation of the biliary system, branches of these nerves join the sympathetic rami which enter the liver. In some instances, branches of the phrenic nerve join hepatic rami of the left vagus nerve. Sympathetic nerve fibers are distributed to the blood vessels and the bile ducts throughout the liver, the extrahepatic bile ducts and the blood vessels associated with them. The liver cells are not innervated directly.

The choledochoduodenal junction receives fibers through the gastroduodenal nerve and through the gastroduodenal plexus. The gastroduodenal nerve includes fibers derived from both the right and the left celiac ganglia and the right vagus nerve. It divides into two main branches, one of which terminates at the junction of the common bile duct with the intestine. The gastroduodenal

plexus is intimately associated with the gastroduodenal artery. It is made up mainly of fibers derived from the hepatic plexus. At the junction of the bile duct with the duodenum, the fibers derived from the gastroduodenal plexus tend to follow the superior pancreaticoduodenal artery and its duodenal branch. Those derived from the duodenal nerve terminate mainly in the intramural plexuses of the adjacent portion of the intestine.

The bile ducts and the gallbladder are subject to direct neural regulation through both sympathetic and parasympathetic nerves. In general, the parasympathetic nerves conduct tonic and motor impulses, whereas the sympathetic nerves conduct inhibitory impulses. Experimental data, however, indicate that both the sympathetic and the parasympathetic biliary nerves include both motor and inhibitory fibers. The afferent components of the biliary nerves play a significant role in the reflex activity of the biliary system. Those associated with the sympathetic nerves include the fibers which mediate pain arising in this system.

PLATE 70

INNERVATION OF THE ADRENAL GLANDS AND THE KIDNEYS

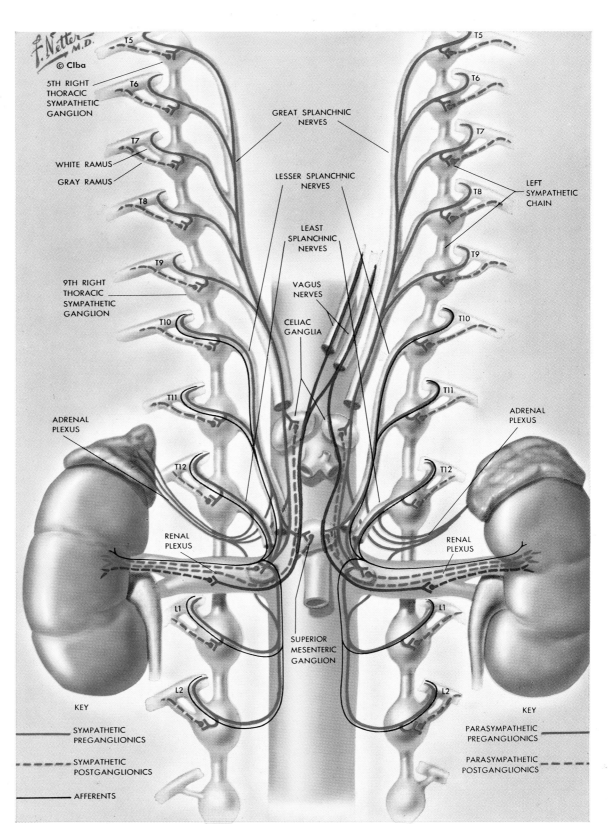

The nerves of the adrenal gland reach the organ through the adrenal plexus. This plexus extends from the celiac plexus to the adrenal body along the adrenal artery. It is connected with the inferior phrenic plexus rostrally and with the renal plexus caudally. It includes preganglionic and afferent components of the splanchnic nerves, components of the phrenic nerve and postganglionic fibers with their cells of origin in celiac ganglia.

Some splanchnic nerve components join the adrenal plexus or enter the gland without traversing the celiac plexus. The innervation of the chromaffin tissue in the adrenal medulla is effected through preganglionic sympathetic fibers, derived mainly from the lower thoracic and the upper lumbar spinal nerves, without the intervention of ganglion cells. The absence of ganglion cells in these sympathetic conduction pathways undoubtedly may be explained on the basis of the neural origin of the chromaffin cells. The postganglionic sympathetic fibers in the adrenal nerves are distributed to the vascular bed throughout the medullary and the cortical portions of the gland. The cortical tissue probably is devoid of direct innervation.

Some of the nerve fiber bundles derived from the adrenal plexus enter the adrenal medulla through the hilus. Others enter the cortex of the gland along the blood vessels. The postganglionic fibers in these nerves are distributed to the blood vessels.

The secretory activity of the adrenal me-

dulla is regulated in a large measure through its sympathetic innervation. The regulatory control of the secretory activity of the adrenal cortex is essentially hormonal.

The renal nerves enter the kidney through the renal plexus. This plexus extends from the aortic plexus into the hilus of the kidney. It is made up mainly of fibers derived from the celiac and the aortic plexuses. It usually includes a ganglion near the origin of the renal artery and one or more in the hilus of the kidney. Other ganglia may be located irregularly at nodal points throughout the plexus.

The preganglionic sympathetic fibers concerned traverse the splanchnic nerves, and most of the synaptic relays are made in celiac ganglia. The least splanchnic nerve and, in some instances, at least one branch of the lesser splanchnic join the renal plexus directly. Their preganglionic fibers make synaptic connection in ganglia within the plexus. The renal plexus is connected with the adrenal plexus and also receives fibers through one or more slender rami from lumbar segments of the sym-

pathetic trunk and from intermesenteric nerves. Vagus fibers also enter the renal plexus both directly and through the celiac plexus. They probably are afferent. The afferent spinal nerve fibers which reach the kidney are chiefly components of the tenth, eleventh and twelfth thoracic nerves.

Within the kidney the renal nerves accompany the renal artery and its branches around which they form plexuses. These plexuses continue along the branches of arteries even to those of small size. The efferent fibers are distributed to the vascular musculature, the smooth muscle in the renal pelvis and any smooth muscle which may be associated with the renal calyces. The renal tubules probably are not directly innervated. Any parasympathetic fibers which may be present in the renal nerves probably are distributed to the smooth muscle in the renal pelvis and the proximal portion of the ureter. Afferent nerve fiber terminations have been reported in the kidney, particularly in the adventitia of the renal vessels, the glomerular capsules and the musculature of the renal pelvis.

PLATE 71

INNERVATION OF THE MALE GENITAL SYSTEM

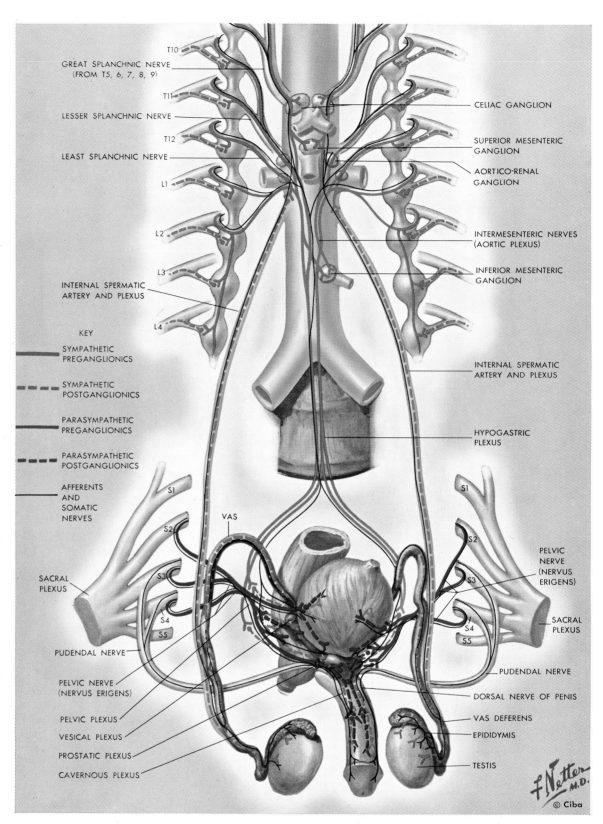

The testis and the spermatic cord are innervated through the internal spermatic, the hypogastric, and the vesical plexuses. The internal spermatic plexus is associated with the internal spermatic artery. It is derived mainly from the aortic plexus, but it also receives fibers from the renal plexus. It comprises sympathetic postganglionic and visceral afferent fibers.

The preganglionic fibers are components of the splanchnic nerves. Those innervating the testis emerge from the spinal cord through the tenth and higher thoracic nerves; others emerge at somewhat lower levels.

The afferent spinal nerve fibers which traverse the internal spermatic plexus are components of the spinal nerves through which the preganglionic fibers emerge. Those which terminate in relation to the epididymis are chiefly components of the eleventh and the twelfth thoracic and the first lumbar nerves.

The nerves of the vas deferens and the seminal vesicle are derived chiefly from the hypogastric and the vesical plexus. Those derived from the hypogastric plexus include sympathetic and visceral afferent components. The synaptic relays in the sympathetic pathways are located in part in the inferior mesenteric ganglia and in part in ganglia located at more caudal levels. Some of them are included in the vesical plexus. The preganglionic sympathetic fibers concerned in these pathways are components of the splanchnic nerves which traverse the celiac roots of the inferior mesenteric plexus. Those which extend into the pelvic plexus also traverse the hypogastric plexus.

The nerves derived from the vesical plexus are mainly parasympathetic, but they include some sympathetic fibers. The preganglionic parasympathetic fibers innervating

the vas deferens and the seminal vesicle are components of the pelvic nerve.

In the spermatic cord, the internal spermatic plexus gives off numerous slender rami which are closely associated with the blood vessels. Slender rami derived from this plexus also join the plexus on the vas deferens. Nerve fibers also become associated with the ductus epididymidis and the ductuli efferentes where they make functional contacts with the smooth muscle in the walls of these ducts. The seminiferous epithelium and the interstitial cells in the testis are not directly innervated. Afferent components of the spermatic plexus extend into the testis where many of them are distributed to the tunica albuginea. The sympathetic fibers in the nerves of the vas deferens are distributed to the musculature of the duct and the blood vessels associated with it. The parasympathetic fibers probably are distributed solely to the musculature of the vas deferens and the ductus epididymidis. The afferent fibers are distributed to the vas deferens and adjacent tissues.

Located on both sides of the prostate gland is the prostatic plexus. It is intimately connected with the vesical plexus and is continuous with the cavernous plexus of the penis. The prostate gland and the prostatic urethra are innervated through the prostatic plexus. The corpora cavernosa and the penile portion of the urethra are innervated mainly through the cavernous plexus. These plexuses include sympathetic, parasympathetic and afferent components. The sympathetic preganglionic fibers concerned traverse the hypogastric plexus. The parasympathetic preganglionic fibers are components of the pelvic nerve.

The glans and the skin of the penis are innervated through the dorsal nerve of the penis. This nerve arises from the pudendal nerves. Its constituent fibers are derived from the third and the fourth sacral nerves. The voluntary muscles employed in the act of ejaculation, i.e., the compressor urethrae and the ischiocavernosus and bulbocavernosus muscles are also innervated through branches of the pudendal nerve.

PLATE 72

INNERVATION OF THE FEMALE GENITAL SYSTEM

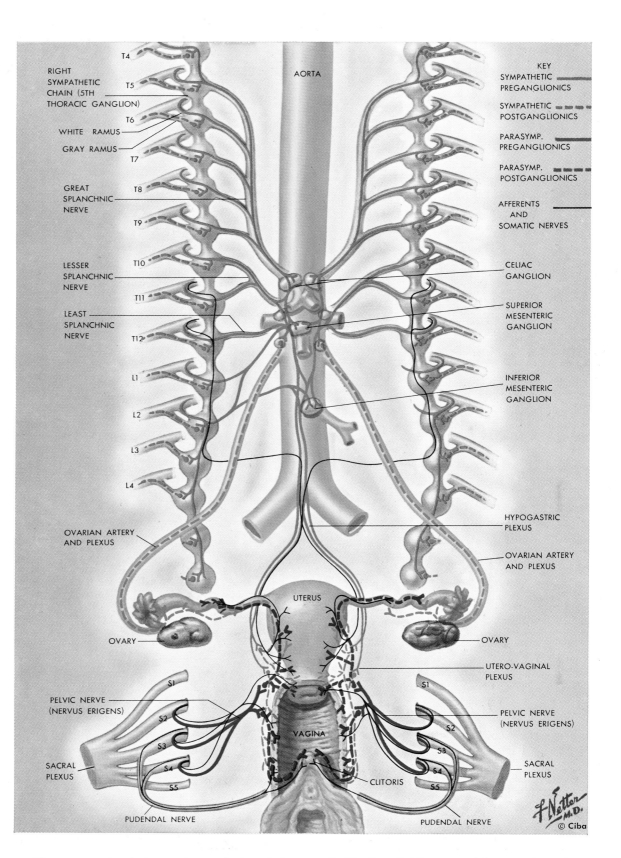

The major portion of the ovarian plexus is derived from the aortic plexus, but it also receives fibers from the renal plexus. It includes sympathetic postganglionic and visceral afferent nerve fibers. Many of the sympathetic fibers arise in the ovarian ganglion, which is located near the origin of the ovarian artery. Others arise in ganglia in the celiac and the renal plexuses. The preganglionic sympathetic fibers concerned and the afferent fibers which traverse the ovarian plexus are components of the splanchnic nerves. The ovarian plexus invests the ovarian artery and the ovarian vein. It supplies fibers to the ovary, the fallopian tube and the broad ligament. In the broad ligament it communicates with the uterine plexus through which it also supplies fibers to the uterus. The afferent fibers which are distributed to the ovary are mainly components of the tenth thoracic nerve.

The ovary is devoid of parasympathetic nerves. The sympathetic fibers within the ovary accompany the blood vessels. They innervate the vascular and other smooth muscle fibers in the gonad. The ovarian follicles and the interstitial tissue are not directly innervated.

The fallopian tube is innervated mainly through the uterine plexus. It also receives fibers from the ovarian plexus, the hypogastric plexus and intermesenteric nerves. Most of the efferent fibers derived from the uterine plexus are parasympathetic. Those from the other sources are sympathetic. The afferent fibers to the fallopian tube which accompany its sympathetic nerves are components of the eleventh and the twelfth thoracic and the upper lumbar nerves.

The uterus receives its innervation mainly through the uterine portion of the uterovaginal plexus. This plexus receives preganglionic sympathetic and visceral afferent fibers through the hypogastric plexus and preganglionic parasympathetic and visceral afferent fibers through the pelvic nerves. It also receives sympathetic fibers directly from the lower lumbar and the sacral segments of the sympathetic trunk. It usually includes one large ganglion and a variable number of smaller ones. The afferent fibers which accompany the sympathetic nerves to the uterus are chiefly components of the eleventh and the twelfth thoracic nerves.

Fibers derived from the vaginal portion of the uterovaginal plexus are distributed to the vaginal wall, including the mucous membrane, to the urethra and to the clitoris. Those which innervate the clitoris mingle with fibers derived from the dorsal nerve of the clitoris which, in turn, is derived from the pudendal nerves. The larger nerves in the uterus are limited to the myometrium. Smaller ones extend into the endometrium where they are distributed to the blood vessels. The nerves of the vagina form a loose plexiform structure in the vaginal wall. The intrinsic nerves of the clitoris form a plexiform structure, the cavernous plexus, in relation to the cavernous tissue. The afferent fibers which are connected with sensory receptors in the clitoris are components of the pudendal nerves.

The labia are innervated through both autonomic and somatic nerves. The autonomic nerves are derived almost exclusively through the vesical and the vaginal plexuses. They include mainly sympathetic fibers which are distributed to the blood vessels. The somatic innervation of the anterior portion of each labium is derived through branches of the ilio-inguinal nerve. The posterior portion of each labium receives its somatic innervation through branches of the pudendal nerve and the perineal branch of the posterior cutaneous nerve of the thigh. The labia minora are abundantly supplied with receptive end organs. Receptive organs in the labia majora are less abundant. The afferent fibers connected with the receptors in the labia are components of the pudendal nerves.

Section V

PATHOLOGY OF THE BRAIN
AND SPINAL CORD

with descriptive text by

ABRAHAM KAPLAN, M.D., F.A.C.S., D.N.S.
Clinical Professor of Neurosurgery
New York Polyclinic Medical School and Hospital
New York, N. Y.

PLATE 73

HYDROCEPHALUS

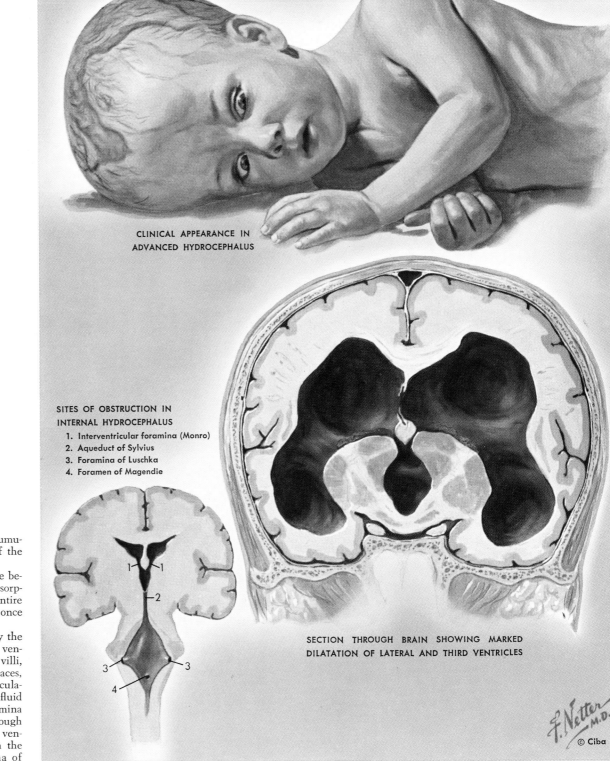

CLINICAL APPEARANCE IN
ADVANCED HYDROCEPHALUS

SITES OF OBSTRUCTION IN
INTERNAL HYDROCEPHALUS

1. Interventricular foramina (Monro)
2. Aqueduct of Sylvius
3. Foramina of Luschka
4. Foramen of Magendie

SECTION THROUGH BRAIN SHOWING MARKED
DILATATION OF LATERAL AND THIRD VENTRICLES

Hydrocephalus is an abnormal accumulation of fluid within the ventricles of the brain.

Normally, there is a delicate balance between the rate of formation and of absorption of the cerebrospinal fluid, the entire volume being absorbed and replaced once every twelve to twenty-four hours.

The cerebrospinal fluid is formed by the choroid plexus mainly in the lateral ventricles. It is absorbed by the arachnoid villi, the perivascular and subarachnoid spaces, and eventually reaches the venous circulation. From the lateral ventricles the fluid passes through the interventricular foramina (Monro) to the third ventricle, then through the aqueduct of Sylvius to the fourth ventricle where it makes its exit through the foramen of Magendie and foramina of Luschka, and spreads along the base of the brain through the various basilar cisternae and then over the cerebral surface. In 1913, Blackfan and Dandy proved that hydrocephalus could be produced by occlusion of the aqueduct of Sylvius. Subsequently, Dandy also demonstrated a unilateral hydrocephalus following obstruction of one foramen of Monro. This failed to occur after removal of the choroid plexus from that side.

Hydrocephalus may be either communicating or noncommunicating (obstructive). When phenolsulfonphthalein or indigo carmine is injected into the lumbar subarachnoid space and the head tilted downward, the dye will appear in the lateral ventricles within twenty to thirty minutes if there is no obstruction. In the event the dye fails to appear in the ventricles, one must conclude that there exists either a partial or a complete obstruction of the circulation of the cerebrospinal fluid. The obstruction may be due to atresia of the aqueduct, nonpatency of the foramina, or obliteration of the subarachnoid spaces by an inflammatory process or neoplasm. Ventriculography will determine the site and nature of the obstruction and indicate the advisability of surgical intervention.

The communicating (infantile) type of hydrocephalus is due to a faulty absorption of the cerebrospinal fluid, rarely to excessive fluid formation. As fluid accumulates, the intracranial pressure increases, producing a symmetrical dilatation of the ventricular system. As a result, the cerebral cortex becomes thinner, the convolutions widen, the venous pressure within the dural sinuses rises, the scalp veins dilate and finally the skull sutures begin to separate. In advanced cases, the base of the brain also shows evidence of pressure but the basal ganglia seem to resist the damaging effect of such prolonged increase of tension.

If an infant begins to show a tense or bulging anterior fontanelle, a steady increase in the size of the head, or the beginning separation of cranial sutures, hydrocephalus must be suspected. Vomiting and irritability may be the earliest symptoms. The child has a frightened expression and the eyes bulge, showing the upper sclerae. However, the pulse, respiration, and color of the child appear normal. Vision and hearing are undisturbed and motor and sensory functions remain surprisingly intact. After the third or fourth month, there is definite evidence of mental retardation. X-rays of the skull show a widening of the frontoparietal and parieto-occipital sutures.

Communicating hydrocephalus must be differentiated from the obstructive type and from chronic subdural hematoma of infancy.

Medical treatment of communicating hydrocephalus has been unsuccessful. The rare cases in which the hydrocephalus becomes arrested are explained by an increase in the rate of absorption of the cerebrospinal fluid, permitting a balance to be established between formation and absorption. The most successful surgical procedure for arresting the hydrocephalus is the removal or fulguration of the choroid plexus of the lateral ventricles.

PLATE 74

CRANIOSYNOSTOSES AND ENCEPHALOCELE

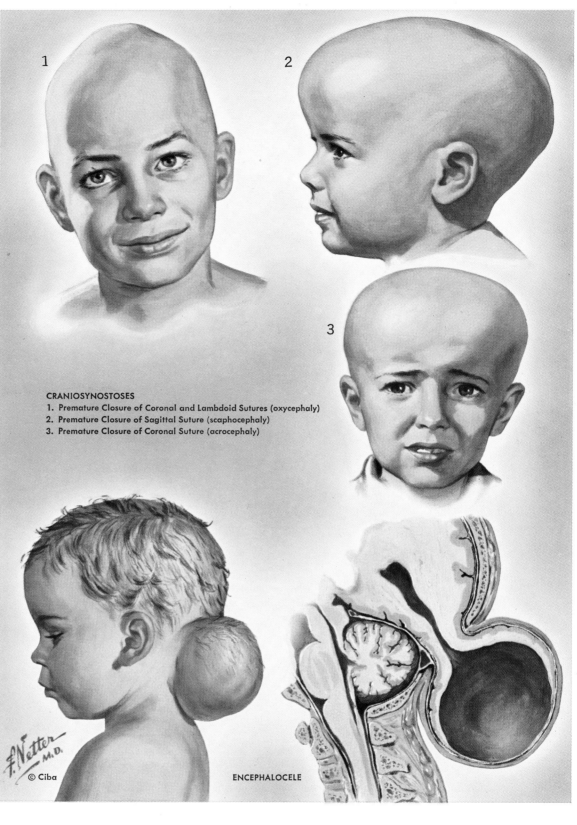

CRANIOSYNOSTOSES
1. Premature Closure of Coronal and Lambdoid Sutures (oxycephaly)
2. Premature Closure of Sagittal Suture (scaphocephaly)
3. Premature Closure of Coronal Suture (acrocephaly)

ENCEPHALOCELE

Craniosynostoses

If all cranial sutures close prematurely, microcephalus results. However, if, during the latter part of fetal life or shortly after birth, certain sutures of the calvarium fuse prematurely while others remain open, a variety of skull deformities develop. These are called craniosynostoses. (Normally, the cranial sutures do not begin to close until the brain approaches full growth and growth of the brain and skull keep pace thereafter.)

The etiology of these congenital anomalies is unknown, though the theory of a defective germ plasm is the one most often accepted. However, heredity plays no part.

The most common deformity, oxycephaly, "Turmschadel," "turrecephaly" or "tower head," in which the head elongates upward, occurs during the first year and is frequently associated with other congenital defects of the face, neck, arms, and particularly the fingers — syndactylism.

The head is characteristically dome-shaped, narrow in the anteroposterior diameter, with a broad forehead and depressed temporal fossae. The eyes set in shallow orbits show exophthalmos, strabismus, and most often optic atrophy. The optic foramina are frequently distorted, resulting in compression or constriction of the optic nerve, leading to atrophy and poor vision, which in some patients progress to blindness. Although the brain is prevented from expanding normally, the mentality of these patients is normal.

X-rays of the skull are diagnostic. The tall dome with scalloping of the inner table of the frontal bones, and the distortion and narrowing of the foramina of the skull, particularly the optic foramina, are all the result of closure of the coronal and lambdoid sutures. In some cases, the cervical vertebrae may fuse producing a short neck (Klippel-Feil syndrome).

The life span of these patients is not affected by the skull deformity. To save vision and to allow for brain expansion, treatment must be undertaken during the first year of life. The King operation, which consists of removal of one or two longitudinal strips of bone which are cut in short lengths and replaced in a geometric arrangement resulting in a mosaic pattern, allowing for brain expansion, or linear craniectomy with the insertion of a tantalum foil or polyethylene strips over the cut bony edges have given the best results.

Other skull deformities due to synostosis are (1) scaphocephaly—elongated or boat-shaped skull—in which the skull expands in an anteroposterior diameter. This occurs following premature closure of the sagittal suture only. Operation during the first few weeks of life will improve the skull contour, (2) acrocephaly with a high, wide and prominent forehead. This occurs when there has been premature closure of the coronal sutures only. Coronal craniectomy has given encouraging results.

Encephalocele

Skull defects present at birth are usually in the midline. They occur most frequently in the occipital region, but may also be found over the foramen magnum or as far forward as the nose or the orbit. Over the defect a sac is formed into which herniate the meninges, cerebrospinal fluid, choroid plexus or cerebral tissue.

The sac is covered by atrophic skin and not infrequently by only a thin layer of meninges. This congenital abnormality is called an encephalocele and may be associated with other neurologic or visceral abnormalities. Unless an intracranial obstruction exists, pressure applied to the sac will readily be reflected by bulging of the anterior fontanelle. If the sac remains small, it is best to wait a year before undertaking a plastic repair. However, if the mass over the defect is very large or if danger of rupture exists, an early repair should be attempted to prevent certain fatality from meningitis.

PLATE 75

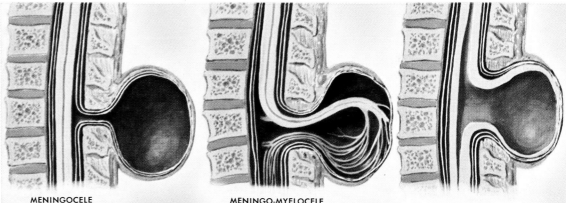

MENINGOCELE   MENINGO-MYELOCELE   SYRINGO-MYELOCELE

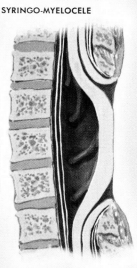

SPINA BIFIDA WITH
CENTRAL CICATRIX

MYELOCELE

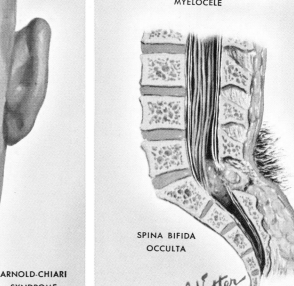

ARNOLD-CHIARI
SYNDROME
DECOMPRESSION

SPINA BIFIDA
OCCULTA

f. Netter
M.D.
© Ciba

SPINA BIFIDA

Spina Bifida

Failure of the vertebral arches to unite in the midline results in a defect called spina bifida. In spina bifida *occulta* the defect is small and marked only by a dimple in the skin or a tuft of hair overlying a small fatty mass in the lumbosacral region. The roots of the cauda equina may be matted together at the level of the bony defect, and sometimes there is a small lipoma or dermoid cyst nearby. The only symptoms may be mild saddle hypalgesia and intermittent urinary disturbances. X-rays show a small defect in the lumbosacral area. Operation is advisable only in selected cases.

Larger defects in the laminae, which begin about the fourth month of fetal life, are due to a failure of normal separation of the mesoblastic tissue from the neural canal. Such midline defects occur posteriorly in any part of the spinal column. When the sac overlying the defect contains only dura, arachnoid and cerebrospinal fluid, it is called a *meningocele*. If the sac also contains nerve roots and portions of the spinal cord, it is called a *meningomyelocele*. When portions of the spinal cord herniate into the sac and also cause a dilatation of the central canal, we have a *syringomyelocele*. If the spinal cord completely fills the sac, the malformation is known as a *myelocele*. The sac is usually covered by atrophic skin with a central cicatrix. However, not infrequently the only covering is a transparent layer of arachnoidal membrane.

Spina bifida and the accompanying disability is easily recognized at birth. The paresis and disturbance of sphincter function are dependent upon the extent of abnormality of the nerve roots and spinal cord. Paralysis may be partial or complete. Sensation and sphincter control may be partially or completely lost. Reflexes may be absent.

Clubfoot is frequently present at birth in patients who have spina bifida, and hydrocephalus may develop later.

The presence of nerve roots or spinal cord in the sac can be detected by transillumination. X-rays show the location and degree of the laminar defect.

If the neck of the sac is small, repair can easily be done; but surgery should be withheld if the sac is ruptured, if meningitis is present, if paralysis is complete, or if other serious congenital abnormalities are present. In infants with slight or no paralysis, and with good sphincter function, plastic repair should be carried out without delay, preferably under local anesthesia, during the first few days of life. Every attempt should be made to preserve all neurogenic elements as well as portions of the herniated dural sac.

Arnold-Chiari Syndrome

The Arnold-Chiari syndrome is due to a congenital malformation of the occipitocervical region. The pathology consists of a herniation of the cerebellar tonsils and adjacent structures into a funnel-shaped enlargement of the upper cervical canal and a swelling and posterior displacement of the medulla against the upper spinal cord.

The symptoms and signs accompanying this abnormality depend upon the degree and duration of compression of the upper cervical cord, cerebellum and medulla oblongata. Mild symptoms may be present during early childhood, but these become more pronounced and disabling during the second and third decades of life. Although variable, the symptoms consist mainly of stiffness of the neck, headaches, dizziness, thickness of speech, unsteadiness of gait, and paresis of the lower extremities. The chief neurological abnormalities found are nystagmus, hypotonia, ataxia, paresis of the lower extremities, and a positive Babinski reflex.

X-rays show a shortening of the upper cervical canal, fusion of the atlas and occiput, some posterior displacement of the odontoid, and a funnel-shaped foramen magnum with a shallow basiocciput.

Manometric test frequently shows subarachnoid block, which may be sufficient to cause ventricular dilatation. If this syndrome is recognized early and the signs and symptoms are progressive, a generous decompression as shown in the illustration will usually bring great symptomatic relief.

PLATE 76

CEREBRAL BIRTH INJURIES, CEPHALHEMATOMA

Birth injuries to the cranium may vary in degree from very simple to very serious. During labor, the scalp, skull, and brain are exposed to so many stresses and strains that it is really rather surprising that most human beings are born uninjured.

During birth, trauma may produce bleeding between the skull and pericranium. This produces a cephalhematoma which may appear within the first few days.

This condition occurs about once in two hundred births, is usually unilateral, and is found most frequently over the occipital region. The tense, smooth, convex swelling is limited by pericranial attachments at the suture line and is absorbed within a week or ten days. However, it may last several months and occasionally it calcifies. Aspiration of the blood clot is inadvisable and surgical removal is rarely necessary.

Intracranial Hemorrhage

Less than one per cent of all infants sustain any cerebral trauma at birth. However, about sixty per cent of the infant mortality that occurs within the first three days of life is due to intracranial hemorrhage. Such hemorrhage may result from indirect cerebral trauma during spontaneous labor, either normal or abnormal, as well as from the trauma imposed by forceps or such manipulations as the extraction of the aftercoming head.

The pathological findings are tears in the cerebral vessels, rupture of the great vein of Galen or its tributaries, or lacerations of the falx or tentorium. These conditions produce subarachnoid, pial, subpial and intracerebral hemorrhage, mainly located over the cerebral cortex. Petechial hemorrhages may also be scattered throughout the white matter and basal ganglia. The aftermath of the hemorrhage is atrophy, degeneration and sclerosis of the motor cortical cells, the basal ganglia, and the lateral columns of the spinal cord.

Cerebral birth injuries of mild degree may produce no ill effects, but if the cerebral trauma is severe, abnormal signs appear very quickly. With less extensive injuries, abnormal neurologic signs may be delayed for weeks or months.

It is not an easy task to differentiate abnormalities due to cerebral birth injury from those caused by prenatal cerebral defects such as cerebral agenesis, atrophic cerebral sclerosis, porencephaly, and the like. Some of these latter cerebral disorders are caused by abnormal conditions existing during pregnancy, such as infectious diseases, syphilis, tuberculosis, encephalitis, eclampsia, alcoholism, or blood dyscrasias.

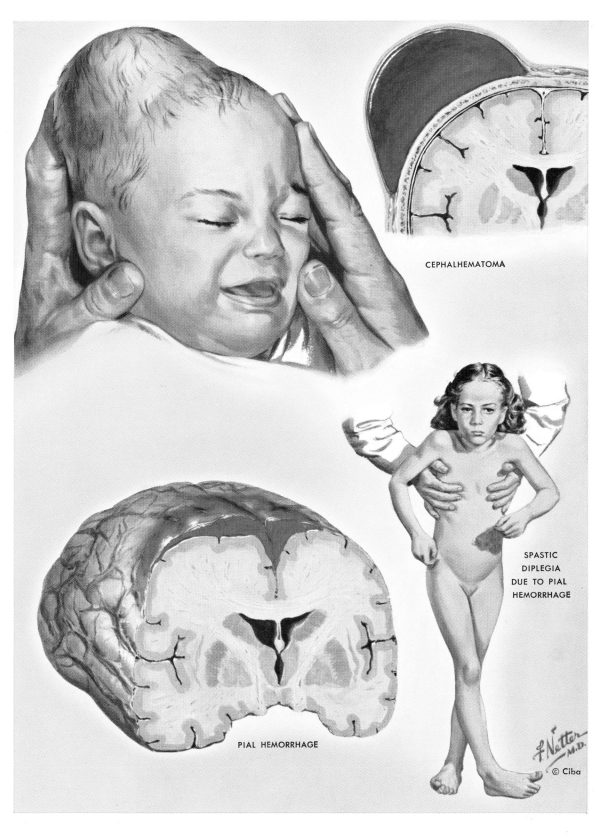

CEPHALHEMATOMA

PIAL HEMORRHAGE

SPASTIC DIPLEGIA DUE TO PIAL HEMORRHAGE

The early clinical findings, which are noted during the first twenty-four hours, depend upon the degree of cerebral damage. These findings are mainly irregularity of respiration, cyanosis or extreme pallor, a weak cry, marked drowsiness, fretfulness on handling, intermittent fever, poor food intake, convulsions, bulging of the anterior fontanelle, dilated pupils, and bloody or xanthochromic spinal fluid.

The late symptoms of cerebral damage may not be recognizable at first, but usually they manifest themselves during the first year of life. Delay in standing or walking, mental retardation, spasticity of the extremities, crosslegged progression and athetoid movements, all develop gradually. The chief abnormal neurologic findings are hyperactive deep reflexes, Babinski signs, ankle clonus, somewhat delayed speech, and mental retardation. This condition has been called Little's disease, because as far back as 1861 William John Little recognized the relationship between difficult labor and signs and symptoms.

The early treatment of cerebral birth trauma consists mainly of the administration of oxygen and blood transfusion, as well as lumbar and ventricular punctures which are carried out to remove blood from the subarachnoid space and ventricle, and to decrease the intracranial pressure.

The late treatment of these patients presents difficult, complicated, prolonged, and at times disheartening, problems. One must first determine whether the pathological changes are stationary or progressive, and then evaluate the residual physiological and intellectual function of the individual patient. In other words, one must estimate what can be accomplished with the remaining mental, motor, and intellectual functions. It would be futile to expect much if the cerebral condition points to idiocy. However, many of these patients have excellent minds and the problem of their rehabilitation has recently aroused much interest and gained considerable public support. Intensive training programs are already under way for improvement of physical defects, speech rehabilitation, family readjustment, and occupational and social integration.

PLATE 77

CHRONIC SUBDURAL HEMATOMA IN INFANTS

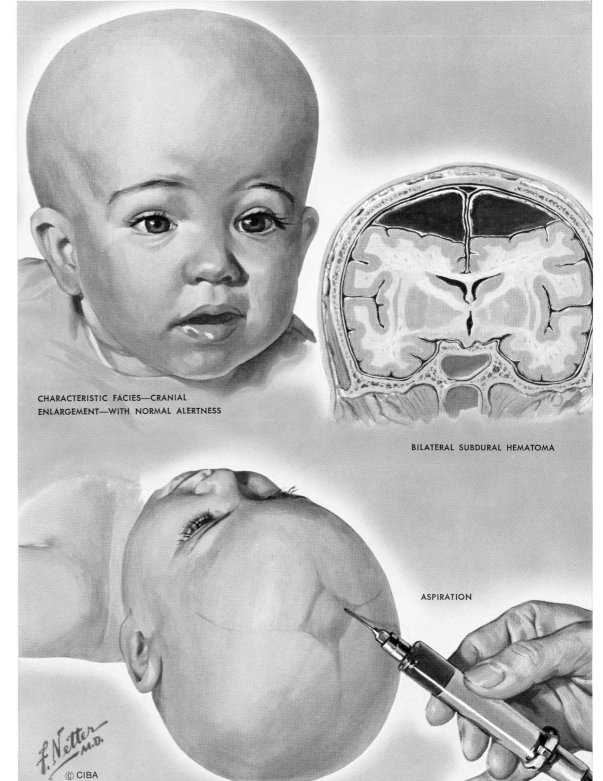

CHARACTERISTIC FACIES—CRANIAL
ENLARGEMENT—WITH NORMAL ALERTNESS

BILATERAL SUBDURAL HEMATOMA

ASPIRATION

Chronic subdural hematoma of infancy occurs most frequently between the ages of six months and two years. It is not a very rare condition. It is essential that such a hematoma be recognized early because it is amenable to proper treatment and must be differentiated from internal hydrocephalus.

The etiology of chronic subdural hematoma in infants is still obscure in many cases, but trauma is the most likely cause. Chronic subdural hematoma occurs most frequently in malnourished children having a vitamin C deficiency which predisposes to hemorrhage. A mild head trauma in an anteroposterior direction may tear a vein traversing the subdural space which is anchored to the superior longitudinal sinus. Such a tear is followed by recurrent venous bleeding into the subdural space where it is trapped and cannot be absorbed.

The clot gradually increases in size. Within two or more weeks, a capsule is formed which arises in part from the under-surface of the dura and also from the meso-

thelial lining of the arachnoid. The capsule gradually becomes thicker and reaches a thickness of one or two millimeters. The hematoma may cover the greater part of the fronto-parieto-temporal surfaces of the cortex and not infrequently may be bilateral.

The earliest clinical symptoms may be unexplained irritability, mild fever, recurrent vomiting, some difficulty in feeding, or a generalized or focal convulsion. As a rule, the child appears bright, cheerful and alert, and does not have a frightened appearance or downward protrusion of the eyeballs with sclerae showing as seen in communicating hydrocephalus. Gradually the head enlarges, the anterior fontanelle begins to bulge, and the percussion tone over the skull is not "cracked-pot" but, instead, is dull or flat. Bilateral papilledema may also be present.

The only dependable diagnostic measure, which should be performed without hesitation, is a subdural puncture at the most extreme lateral angle of the anterior fontanelle. Just beneath the dura, gentle aspiration will yield varying quantities of dark pinkish blood or xanthochromic

fluid. This diagnostic puncture must always be carried out on both sides.

Treatment. In some patients, repeated bilateral aspiration for several weeks may be sufficient to allow for brain expansion and for complete disappearance and organization of the hematoma capsule. As the patient improves clinically, the anterior fontanelle may be found to be flattened or sunken, bloody fluid can no longer be obtained from the subdural space, and the circumference of the head is decreased or remains stationary.

As Ingraham has advocated, bilateral temporal trephine will determine with certainty the presence and thickness of the subdural hematoma and the necessity for surgical removal of the clot. In many instances, the subdural hematoma and greater portion of the capsule have to be removed through an osteoplastic craniotomy in order to allow for complete brain expansion. In patients with bilateral subdural hematoma, an interval of two or three weeks should pass before the craniotomy is done on the contralateral side.

PLATE 78

CHRONIC SUBDURAL HEMATOMA IN ADULTS

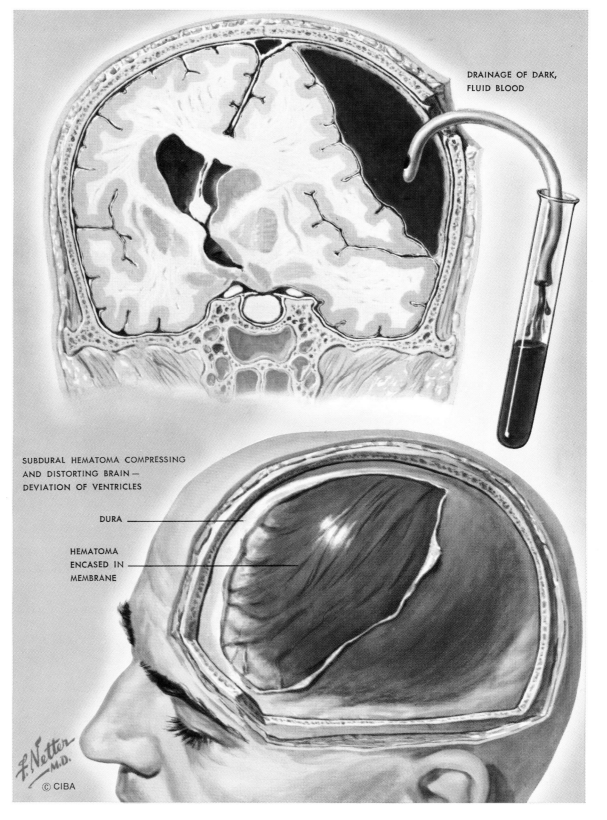

DRAINAGE OF DARK, FLUID BLOOD

SUBDURAL HEMATOMA COMPRESSING AND DISTORTING BRAIN — DEVIATION OF VENTRICLES

DURA

HEMATOMA ENCASED IN MEMBRANE

Chronic subdural hematoma in adults has only recently become a clinical entity that is frequently recognized. Virchow, in 1857, labeled this condition pachymeningitis hemorrhagica interna and believed it was due to insanity, chronic alcoholism, syphilis, or advanced arteriosclerosis. Sperling, in 1872, and Spiller, in 1899, independently reproduced subdural hematoma with membrane formation in dogs and cats by introducing blood into the subdural space.

However, it was not until 1914 when Trotter reported four cases of chronic subdural hematoma, two of which were bilateral, that the mechanism of this clinical syndrome became more clearly understood. Chronic subdural hematoma is due to trauma and is about ten times as frequent as extradural bleeding from an injury to the middle meningeal artery.

The trauma that is responsible for the hematoma is frequently trivial, often forgotten, and in only twenty-five per cent of patients is it sufficiently severe to produce unconsciousness. The trauma usually causes the brain to be displaced in its anteroposterior diameter as from a blow to the jaw or to the forehead.

As a result of the blow, a venous tear occurs at a point where the vein traverses the subdural space from the cerebral cortex to the undersurface of the dura. From the injured vein, blood oozes into the subdural space which has practically no absorbing power. Organization of the blood clot takes place mainly from the undersurface of the dura and some from the outer mesothelial layer of the arachnoid.

Gradually, a cyst lining is formed around the hematoma. When the pressure within the cyst falls below the venous pressure, bleeding recurs and ceases only when the intracystic pressure rises above the venous pressure. These pressure alterations within the cyst, which are largely produced by variations in intracranial pressure, account for the clinical variability of the signs and symptoms and also explain the laminated appearance of the hematoma as revealed by histological studies.

The usual symptoms are headache, di-

plopia, and dizziness, frequently followed by drowsiness, lethargy, mental torpor, and confusion. Paresis of one side of the body is often associated with a dilated pupil on the side corresponding to the lesion. The patient gradually becomes more lethargic and then comatose.

The frequent fluctuations in the clinical findings often produce doubt concerning the diagnosis. And yet, these fluctuations of signs and symptoms are most characteristic of chronic subdural hematoma. These patients are often suspected of cerebral neoplasm, post-traumatic neurosis, encephalitis, cerebral arteriosclerosis, cerebral thrombosis and psychoneurosis.

X-rays of the skull may, at times, show a shift of a calcified pineal shadow away from the side of the lesion. The spinal fluid is frequently under increased pressure; in only fifty per cent of the cases is it xanthochromic.

Electroencephalograms in many instances have been inconsistent, but more recently reports show low voltage and slow waves on the side of the lesion. In some instances, if the patient's condition is not too critical,

pneumoencephalograms or ventriculograms should be performed. These frequently show ventricular deformity and displacement out of harmony with the objective neurological findings. The diagnosis of chronic subdural hematoma often rests on very few signs and at times has to be made on the basis of exclusion. In about fifteen per cent of patients, the subdural hematoma is bilateral.

Once the diagnosis is suspected, surgical intervention becomes mandatory. Expectant medical treatment will only lead to a deterioration of the patient's condition. The treatment advocated is a bilateral trephine over both postparietal regions to be done under local anesthesia. The dura is opened and the clot is removed by suction and irrigation until the compressed brain rises to the undersurface of the dura. Bilateral subtemporal decompression with clot removal is another operative approach. Occasionally, when the hematoma is solid or highly organized, craniotomy may be necessary for complete removal of the clot in order for the brain to expand properly.

PLATE 79

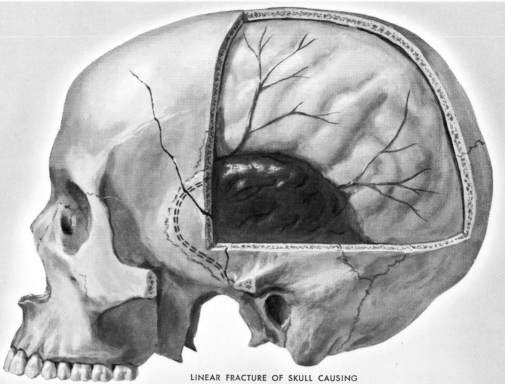

LINEAR FRACTURE OF SKULL CAUSING
MIDDLE MENINGEAL HEMORRHAGE

EXTRADURAL HEMATOMA

A blood clot between the dura and the inner table of the skull is known as an extradural hematoma. It results from arterial bleeding or, more rarely, is due to a rupture or tear in a large venous sinus. Bleeding is continuous and persistent, producing rapid compression of the dura and the brain. Therefore, unless the diagnosis is made early, coma and death will ensue. To prevent such an outcome, the presence and site of the hematoma must be recognized before coma sets in, the extradural clot completely removed, and the bleeding point controlled.

An extradural hematoma is most often the result of a serious head injury which fractures the skull, tearing the middle meningeal artery. Less frequently, injury to the anterior meningeal artery, a large venous sinus, or a fracture through a large diploic lake may result in extradural bleeding. In the classical case, the fracture starts at the parietal region and extends downward toward the middle fossa crossing the middle meningeal artery or one of its branches. The force of the fracture will displace the artery from its groove and by its shearing action will cause a rupture of the vessel. The nearer the tear is to the foramen spinosum, the more rapid the bleeding and the greater the emergency.

An extradural hematoma is rare in children and in the aged. In children, the meningeal groove is very shallow and the artery can be readily displaced without damage. In the aged, the dura is so adherent to the inner surface of the calvarium that it cannot be readily displaced.

Although an extradural hematoma is most commonly found in the temporoparietal area, such an accumulation of blood may also occur in the frontal region where it is produced by a tear in the anterior meningeal artery, or over the occipital and cerebellar lobes when a tear has occurred in the superior longitudinal or lateral sinus.

Whereas the symptoms of compression usually appear within hours after injury, in very rare instances a tear of one of the small terminal branches of the middle meningeal artery will be followed by a small extradural hematoma, producing delayed symptoms which do not manifest themselves until after ten days or possibly two weeks. An extradural hematoma unfortunately may be overshadowed by severe cerebral laceration with arachnoid and subdural bleeding or by alcoholism.

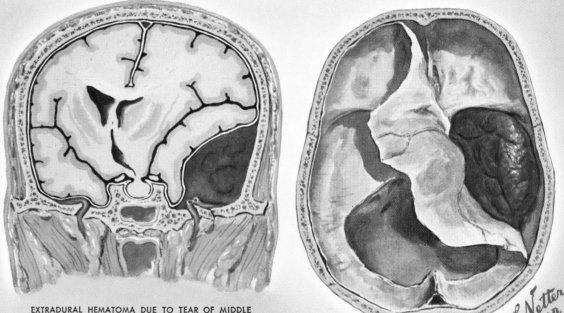

EXTRADURAL HEMATOMA DUE TO TEAR OF MIDDLE
MENINGEAL ARTERY AT THE FORAMEN SPINOSUM
BY FRACTURE OF THE BASE OF THE SKULL

CLOT EXPOSED ON SKULL BASE
BY REFLECTION OF DURA

Although the typical symptomatology of an extradural hematoma is rather widely recognized, it must be emphasized that symptoms do not always run true to form. Usually the head trauma is followed by a transient loss of consciousness which is followed by a lucid interval of a few minutes to several hours during which the patient complains of headache, nausea, and vomiting. The headache increases, the patient becomes drowsy, then stuporous, and eventually comatose. It cannot be stressed too strongly that the most important and dependable sign of an extradural hematoma is the presence of increasing stupor. The rate of pulse and respirations is frequently slowed. Dilation of the pupil on the side of the lesion appears, and in right-handed persons, if the hematoma is on the left side, signs of aphasia may be found. Facial weakness and the paresis of the contralateral arm and leg usually progress to a total paralysis with increase of deep reflexes and a positive Babinski sign. Focal convulsions may help localize the lesion. In the later or near terminal phase of an extradural hematoma, decerebrate rigidity may set in.

X-ray of the skull almost invariably shows a linear fracture crossing the middle meningeal artery or one of its branches, or the fracture may be in the vicinity of a large venous sinus. On occasion, x-ray evidence of a displaced calcified pineal shadow will help in the localization of the lesion. Unless concomitant cerebral laceration with subarachnoid bleeding has occurred, the spinal fluid is clear and colorless and under increased pressure.

Because the source of the intracranial bleeding is arterial, brain compression is rapid. The diagnosis of an extradural hematoma must therefore be made long before coma sets in; otherwise irreversible damage may occur. Operation consists of an enlarged trephine over the point where the fracture crosses the bleeding vessel, a complete removal of the hematoma by suction, and the identification and control of the bleeding point. The bleeding is controlled by coagulation, suture or with the use of a silver clip. If the laceration involves the large venous sinus, muscle grafts or Gelfoam® is used to arrest the hemorrhage.

PLATE 80

FRACTURES OF THE SKULL

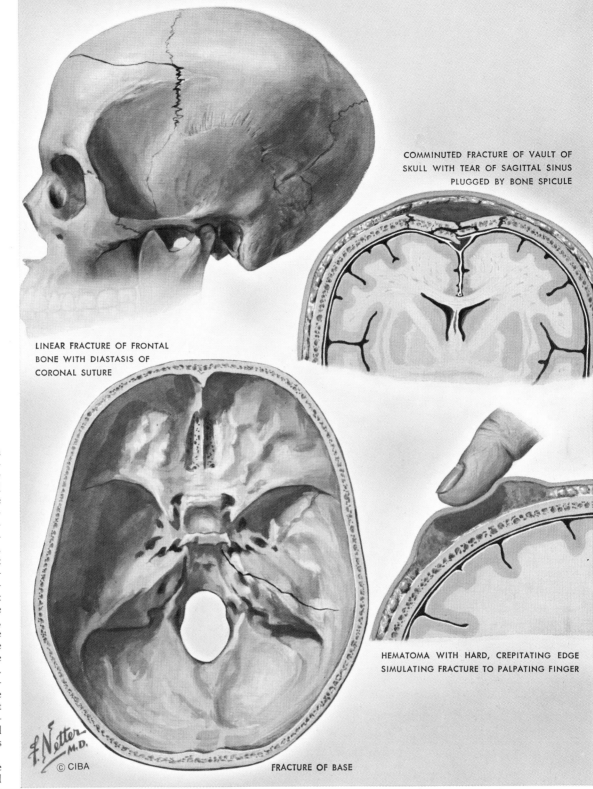

COMMINUTED FRACTURE OF VAULT OF SKULL WITH TEAR OF SAGITTAL SINUS PLUGGED BY BONE SPICULE

LINEAR FRACTURE OF FRONTAL BONE WITH DIASTASIS OF CORONAL SUTURE

HEMATOMA WITH HARD, CREPITATING EDGE SIMULATING FRACTURE TO PALPATING FINGER

FRACTURE OF BASE

Skull fracture must not be considered a separate clinical entity. It is only one component of a craniocerebral injury which may also involve injury to the scalp, dura, cranial nerves, and cerebral tissue, and produce alterations in the intracranial, arterial, venous, and cerebrospinal fluid circulation. Indeed, a patient may suffer serious craniocerebral injury *without* a fracture of the skull.

Skull fractures occur at all ages, even at birth. Invariably there is damage to underlying intracranial structures even if abnormal signs are not present upon first examination. The type and location of the skull fracture depend upon the patient's age, the thickness and contour of the skull, the instrument of injury, the power and the point of the blow, and whether or not the head was in motion at the time of impact.

Several generalizations about skull fractures are well worth keeping in mind. The prominence of the parietal bone makes it the most common site of fracture. Following in frequency of fracture are the frontal and temporal bones; least often fractured is the occipital bone.

Basilar fractures frequently involve the petrous portion of the temporal bone and frontal sinus and tend to extend toward the sella turcica or foramen magnum. At times, such fractures involve the olfactory and optic nerves. X-rays for diagnosis of skull fracture may be wisely postponed in most craniocerebral injuries, but should always be taken if operation is contemplated.

Surgical shock is rare even in severe craniocerebral injuries unless there was profuse scalp bleeding, or injury to viscera or bones.

Skull fractures are either nonoperative or operative and treatment should be individualized and fitted to the underlying intracranial damage as well as other bodily injuries. The nonoperative group is by far the larger. A subperiosteal hematoma producing a sharp crepitating margin with a central depression is frequently suspected of being a depressed skull fracture, but the exact diagnosis can be readily verified by x-ray films.

A simple linear or comminuted nondepressed skull fracture, when revealed by x-ray, may come as a complete surprise. If the fracture line crosses the middle meningeal artery or superior longitudinal sinus, hemorrhage must be watched for; if it communicates with the frontal sinus or middle ear, infection may be prevented by the generous use of antibiotics.

The operative group of skull fractures constitutes only about ten per cent of all craniocerebral injuries. The optimal time for surgery is within three to six hours after injury, but in cases of surgical shock, operation may be delayed twenty-four hours or longer with the generous use of antibiotics.

Scalp lacerations must not be regarded lightly. A scalp infection may lead to cellulitis or osteomyelitis and thus delay or even prevent intracranial surgery that is urgently required.

Simple depressed skull fractures, comminuted or otherwise, should be elevated particularly if they produce symptoms, overlie vital areas, or appear to behave like foreign bodies. Loose skull fragments with poor blood supply are better removed. However, operation in such cases is not an emergency procedure.

A compound depressed comminuted skull fracture should be operated without delay. A thorough débridement of the wound with removal of driven-in dirt, hair, and devitalized skull fragments must be carried out to prevent chronic osteomyelitis. The depressed viable portion of both tables of the skull must be elevated.

If, in addition, the dura is torn, the risk of meningitis is serious. All devitalized cerebral tissue, blood clot, and foreign material must be removed with great care, and the hemostasis must be perfect before the dura and scalp are closed tightly in layers. Plastic repair of the cranial defect is a secondary consideration.

The treatment of a compound depressed skull fracture involving the superior longitudinal or transverse sinus is a hazardous undertaking. A depressed bone spicule which has pierced the sinus may also serve to plug it, and unless adequate preparations have been made for control of hemorrhage, the removal of the bone spicule may be followed by exsanguination.

PLATE 81

INTRACEREBRAL HEMATOMA

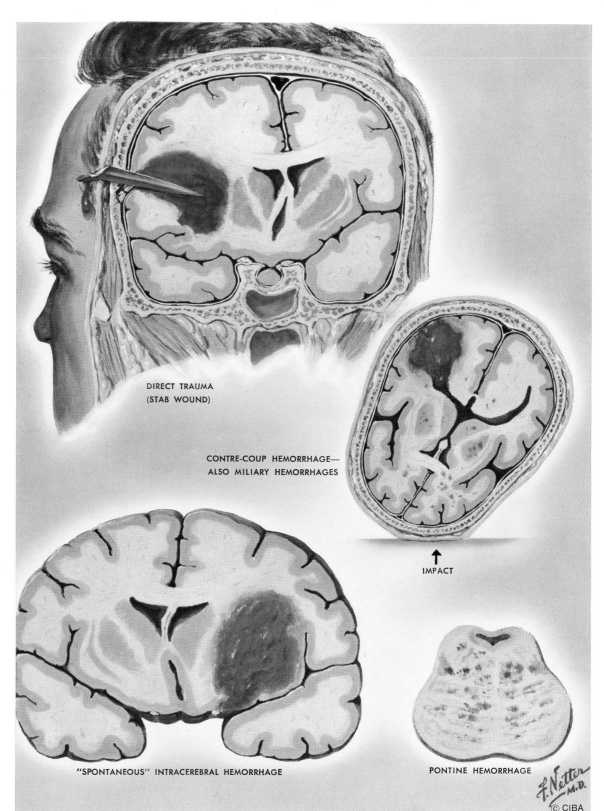

DIRECT TRAUMA
(STAB WOUND)

CONTRE-COUP HEMORRHAGE—
ALSO MILIARY HEMORRHAGES

IMPACT

"SPONTANEOUS" INTRACEREBRAL HEMORRHAGE

PONTINE HEMORRHAGE

Intracerebral hematomas are of two kinds: traumatic and nontraumatic.

The traumatic variety may follow a severe or a mild head injury. The bleeding is venous or arterial, but may be capillary, and is chiefly restricted to the white matter. Rupture of the clot into the ventricle or petechial hemorrhages within the pons are rapidly fatal.

The diagnosis of a traumatic intracerebral hematoma may be easy or most difficult, depending on its location and size. The intracerebral hematoma following a stab or bullet wound can easily be traced from the wound or localized by x-ray evidence of a small skull depression, a broken-off knife blade, or bullet fragments. However, recognition of an intracerebral hematoma following a contrecoup cerebral injury is difficult. The signs of increasing intracranial pressure and focal cerebral irritation will depend upon the increasing size and location of the hematoma. Headaches, dizziness, vomiting, and drowsiness may not set in for 36 to 72 hours following the injury. Shortly thereafter, generalized or focal convulsions, aphasia, hemiparesis, hemianopsia, and Babinski's sign appear. The cerebrospinal fluid is under increased pressure, frequently clear or xanthochromic and, very rarely, grossly bloody. Ventricular air studies may be necessary for accurate diagnosis and localization.

Treatment of traumatic intracerebral hematoma is a major surgical procedure requiring all available measures for control of hemorrhage and infection. All foreign material and skull fragments are removed before the rent in the dura is enlarged. The discolored and contused cerebral surface will readily lead to the tract of perforation and the hematoma, which is removed by gentle suction and irrigation with penicillin solution. All skull fragments, foreign material, and devitalized cerebral tissue are removed; but if metallic fragments are deeply or critically situated, it is wiser not to disturb them. After complete hemostasis, the dura must be repaired and the wound closed in layers without drainage. Antibiotics must be administered generously.

Intracerebral hematoma following a mild head trauma is rare. In such cases, it is due to a rupture of a diseased blood vessel in an area of cerebral softening. The temporal, occipital, and frontal lobes are the most frequent sites of intracerebral hematoma. Symptoms may be abrupt in onset but progress slowly. Headaches, dizziness, vomiting, and drowsiness may be overshadowed by the focal signs of aphasia, hemiparesis, hemianopsia, dilated pupil, and pathological toe signs. The spinal fluid pressure is increased and slightly xanthochromic. It is difficult to differentiate intracerebral hematoma from chronic subdural hematoma, cerebral abscess, or a neoplasm. Ventriculography may be necessary for localization. Early removal of an intracerebral hematoma offers a good prognosis.

The nontraumatic intracerebral hematoma, usually found in the internal capsule, is due to bleeding secondary to hypertensive or atheromatous vascular changes which produce areas of cerebral edema, softening and degeneration with cyst formation. The initial rupture may produce mild symptoms and clear up, but years later a recurrent apoplectic hemorrhage is often fatal. This is marked by a violent bursting headache, then hemiplegia, drowsiness and coma, and grossly bloody spinal fluid. Surgical attempts at clot removal from this area, on rare occasions, have been successful.

An intracerebral hematoma secondary to degenerating malignant gliomas of the brain occurs in only four per cent of all brain neoplasms. The treatment, of course, is the same as that of a primary neoplasm.

There are other causes of intracerebral hematoma such as ruptured basilar aneurysm, blood dyscrasias, polycythemia, and operative exploration, each calling for special consideration and therapy.

PLATE 82

TRAUMATIC PNEUMOCEPHALUS

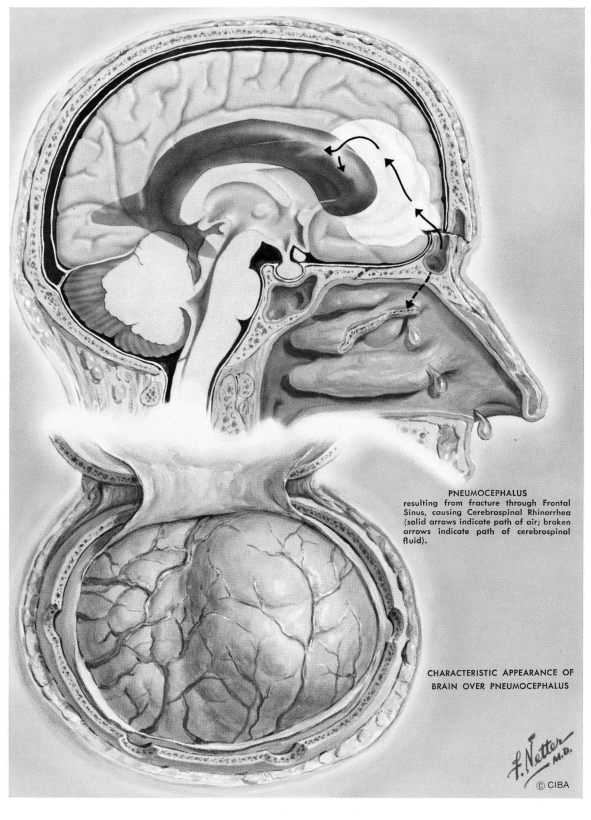

PNEUMOCEPHALUS
resulting from fracture through Frontal
Sinus, causing Cerebrospinal Rhinorrhea
(solid arrows indicate path of air; broken
arrows indicate path of cerebrospinal
fluid).

**CHARACTERISTIC APPEARANCE OF
BRAIN OVER PNEUMOCEPHALUS**

Traumatic pneumocephalus, though comparatively rare, must be recognized early and treated promptly to prevent serious complications and sequelae. This condition is almost invariably due to injury of one of the accessory nasal sinuses which permits air to enter the brain or the ventricular system.

In 1884, Chiari was the first to demonstrate postmortem that air entered the frontal lobe and ventricular system through a vent communicating with the ethmoidal cells. In 1913, Luckett first reported x-ray evidence of air in the ventricles of the brain following a skull fracture. Since then, many interesting reports of such cases have been published.

Although skull fracture is the most frequent cause of pneumocephalus, it should be remembered that it may occur after a severe sneezing spell in patients who have unusual prolongation of the arachnoid along the olfactory nerves.

The most frequent portal of entry of air is a fracture which involves the posterior walls of the frontal sinus or the cribriform plate of the ethmoid bone. Cases have been reported of fracture through the middle ear and mastoid bone which allows escape of the cerebrospinal fluid and entry of air into the cranium.

A bone fracture is usually accompanied by a tear of the dura, which may extend through the arachnoid into the cerebral tissue or the ventricle, thereby establishing a sinus through which fluid and air exchange. The air may be trapped in the subdural, subarachnoid, or ventricular space, or even within the brain substance. Not infrequently, the dural tear and sinus tract may be so small as to escape detection at operation.

It is estimated that two to five per cent of skull fractures develop cerebrospinal rhinorrhea. The complaints of severe headache accompanied by discharge of clear fluid from the nostril or the middle ear following a head injury should immediately raise the suspicion of pneumocephalus. X-ray films of the skull will readily show air

intracranially, if it is present.

Other more unusual causes of cerebrospinal rhinorrhea and pneumocephalus include intranasal manipulations, chronic infections in the region of the cribriform plate, erosion into the anterior cranial fossa by an orbito-ethmoidal osteoma, downward extension of a pituitary or other neoplasm into the sphenoidal sinus and craniotomy.

Meningitis is, of course, the greatly feared complication. With the availability of antibiotics, the outlook has become far more favorable today than it had been previously. The escaping cerebrospinal fluid should be studied for cells and cultured for organisms.

Nonoperative treatment includes rest in the sitting posture, avoidance of blowing the nose, and measures favoring the lowering of intracranial pressure.

Spontaneous healing usually occurs. However, if the rhinorrhea continues for two weeks or longer and fails to show any lessening in the quantity of escaping fluid, surgical repair of the cranial and dural defects should be carried out without any further delay.

PLATE 83

FRACTURES AND DISLOCATIONS OF THE SPINE

Experiences with spinal injuries during World War II, which included 2600 paraplegics, have completely changed our concepts about the care and treatment of these patients. With today's program of rehabilitation, eighty per cent of serious spine injuries can get on crutches, and seventy-five per cent of these with training can be gainfully employed or go to school.

Fractures and dislocations of the spine are due to trauma, which may be direct, indirect or both. Direct blows produce fractures of the spinous processes, transverse processes or laminae, but rarely involve articular facets or vertebral bodies. Indirect injuries, such as falling from a distance or diving into shallow water, may produce a fracture dislocation of the spine which reduces itself but the spinal cord damage may be complete and irreversible. If the injury results in articular displacement or a wedge-shaped vertebral fracture, the abnormal neurologic findings will be in keeping with the extent of the spinal cord pathology. This may vary from slight edema to extensive intraspinal hemorrhage. The higher the lesion, the worse the prognosis.

Important considerations of spinal injuries are:

1. Transportation. Unfortunately, unskillful moving or lifting of such patients may convert an insignificant injury into a complete transection of the spinal cord. Inability to move any extremity means the lesion is in the cervical region, requiring several persons to transport such a casualty. With the patient on his back, traction is applied to the head, countertraction to the legs and the body raised as one rigid piece and placed on the stretcher. If the legs are paralyzed, the lesion is in the thoracic or lumbar region. The patient should, therefore, be transported in face-down position in hyperextension.

2. History and Neurological Examination. The type of injury, site of pain, degree of motor and sensory impairment, and reflex status should be elicited rapidly and carefully. If repeated neurologic examinations show signs of increasing spinal cord compression, surgery is advisable.

3. Diagnosis. As a rule, a tentative working diagnosis can be made swiftly. Most fractures and dislocations at C1 and 2 are fatal. Fractures of the odontoid, with partial displacement, may cause only stiffness of the neck and the head to be held tilted away from the lesion. With complete dislocation at the atlanto-axial joint, tilting of the head is toward the lesion. Fractures and dislocations at C3, 4 and 5, involving the phrenic nerve, cause death by respiratory paralysis. With a transverse lesion at C4 and 5 segments, the forearms are flexed and rotated outward with the arms in abduction; while

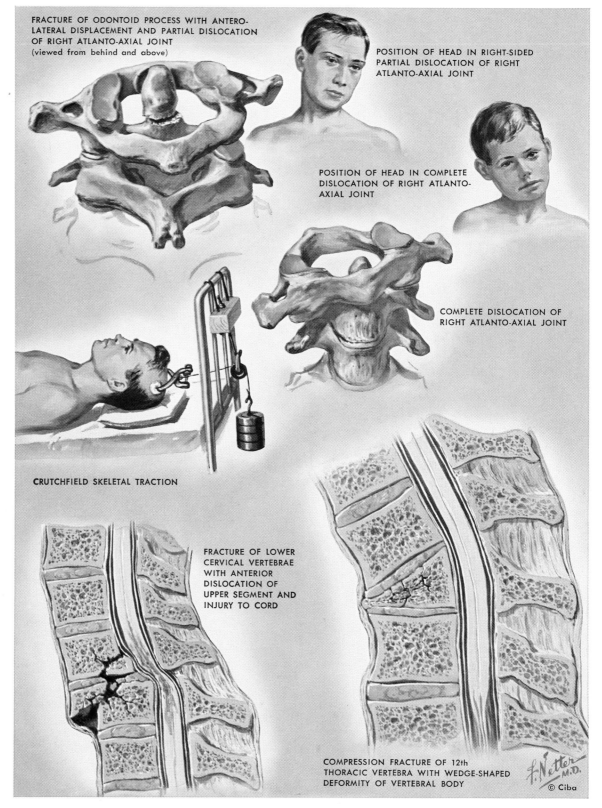

FRACTURE OF ODONTOID PROCESS WITH ANTERO-LATERAL DISPLACEMENT AND PARTIAL DISLOCATION OF RIGHT ATLANTO-AXIAL JOINT (viewed from behind and above)

POSITION OF HEAD IN RIGHT-SIDED PARTIAL DISLOCATION OF RIGHT ATLANTO-AXIAL JOINT

POSITION OF HEAD IN COMPLETE DISLOCATION OF RIGHT ATLANTO-AXIAL JOINT

COMPLETE DISLOCATION OF RIGHT ATLANTO-AXIAL JOINT

CRUTCHFIELD SKELETAL TRACTION

FRACTURE OF LOWER CERVICAL VERTEBRAE WITH ANTERIOR DISLOCATION OF UPPER SEGMENT AND INJURY TO CORD

COMPRESSION FRACTURE OF 12th THORACIC VERTEBRA WITH WEDGE-SHAPED DEFORMITY OF VERTEBRAL BODY

a transverse lesion at C6 and 7 causes a similar position of the arms except that the forearms lie on the chest. Lesions at thoracic segments spare the arms. The level of loss of sensation depends upon the location of the lesion. Paralysis of the legs is of the upper motor neuron type with urinary retention. Lesions at L1 vertebra or below produce signs of lower motor neuron involvement with sphincter disturbances.

4. X-ray. If films show compression of the spinal cord by bony fragments, prompt operation must be considered.

5. Operative Indication. Subarachnoid block by Queckenstedt test is no indication for operation because mild edema or intraspinal hemorrhage will promptly produce block. Fractures or compression of the cervical spine should have skeletal traction — Crutchfield tongs — which is much less hazardous than cervical laminectomy. Laminectomy in the thoracic or lumbar region is indicated if x-rays show impingement of bony fragments or there are signs of progressive spinal cord compression.

6. Nonoperative Treatment. Besides traction or hyper-

extension it is important to include the care of

(a) Skin. Meticulous cleanliness, prevention of pressure over bony prominences by the use of a foam mattress or Stryker frame, frequent turning, high protein balance and transfusions, are all necessary to prevent decubitus. The treatment of decubitus is débridement, control of infection and skin grafts.

(b) Sphincter. Munro tidal drainage prevents urinary infections and facilitates automatic bladder function. Early ambulation, positive protein balance and muscle building prevent bladder calculi. Rectal control by the clock is aided by mild catharsis and daily colonics.

(c) Skeletal development of arms and chest muscles by special exercises. High protein and vitamin diet lead to early ambulation.

(d) Psychic Rehabilitation. After pain is completely relieved, the patient must realize and accept his disability. With the encouragement of the surgeon, and by example of other patients, he can be inspired to learn a vocation and develop intellectual and social interests.

PLATE 84

HERNIATION OF LUMBAR INTERVERTEBRAL DISCS

The very common symptom, backache, is due to various causes which may be organic, psychosomatic, or purely psychogenic. Every patient with recurrent and disabling back pain should have a carefully taken history, a complete physical and neurologic examination and thorough laboratory and x-ray studies.

In 1911 Goldthwait first reported that "lumbago," "sciatica" or paraplegia may be the result of a herniated intervertebral disc. Mixter and Barr in 1934 emphasized that protrusion and extrusion of various portions of the intervertebral disc is one of the most frequent causes of low back pain.

With very rare exception, the etiology of intervertebral disc herniation is trauma. The trauma may be acute or chronic. The pathologic changes following trauma to the intervertebral disc begin with a tear in the posterior joint capsule — annulus fibrosus — and in the lateral portion of the posterior longitudinal ligament. A bulge or herniation appears at the weakest point of the joint capsule resulting in back pain and/or root irritation. With rest and conservative measures, the bulge may recede and the back pain subside.

Although the tear may heal, some progressive degeneration of the involved structure takes place. If the herniation fails to recede, nerve root irritation will continue and cause radiating leg pain, paresthesias, numbness, or so-called "sciatica."

With chronic trauma, the sequence of symptoms and pathologic changes is similar but slower. In the advanced stage, the intervertebral space is narrow with osteoarthritic changes at the vertebral margins and intervertebral foraminae.

There are four fluctuating phases of the clinical syndrome of herniated intervertebral discs. The size and position of the herniation at each phase determine the clinical picture.

1. Irritation. Back pain with or without sciatic radiation is the most outstanding symptom. The clinical findings include a diminution in lumbar curve, spasm of the spinae erecti muscles, a tilt of the trunk and partial disability. If no further protrusion takes place, bed rest with a board under the mattress, local heat, light massage and traction, will usually result in

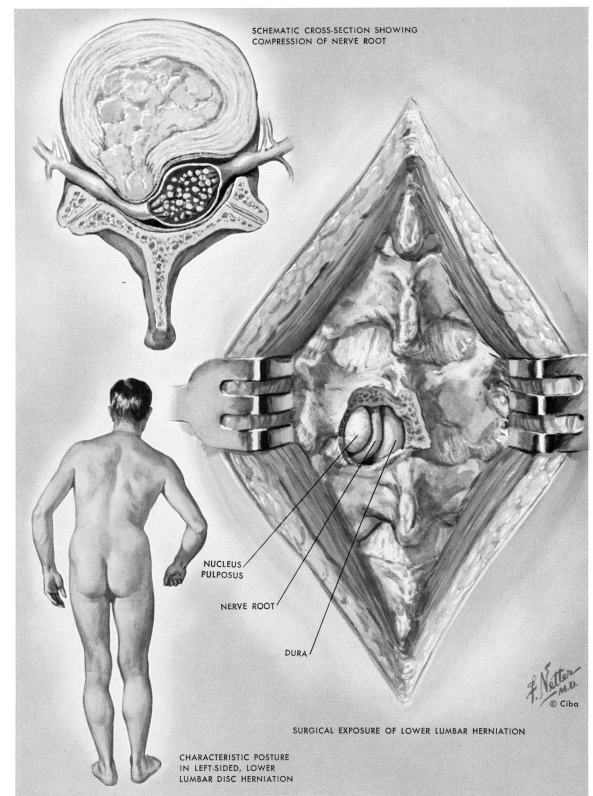

SCHEMATIC CROSS-SECTION SHOWING COMPRESSION OF NERVE ROOT

NUCLEUS PULPOSUS

NERVE ROOT

DURA

SURGICAL EXPOSURE OF LOWER LUMBAR HERNIATION

CHARACTERISTIC POSTURE IN LEFT-SIDED, LOWER LUMBAR DISC HERNIATION

subsidence of symptoms. Further herniation will produce

2. Compression. The herniated disc displaces and compresses the adjacent nerve root against the neighboring bony and ligamentous structures. The back pain may lessen but the "sciatic" pain may become intense and is usually aggravated by coughing, sneezing, or increased activity. Paresthesias in the outer aspect of the calf, foot or toes are frequent symptoms. The positive findings are loss of lumbar curve, spasm of lumbar muscles, tilt of the trunk, focal tenderness, limitation of straight leg raising and Lasègue's sign on the involved side, mild, indistinct hypalgesia over the outer calf and absent to diminished ankle jerk. Next is the phase of

3. Paresis. At this stage, root compression has intensified the pain so that the patient is almost totally disabled. The findings include weakness of the lower extremity, muscle atrophy, peroneal palsy, demonstrable sensory deficit, and diminished to absent knee or ankle jerk. Still further herniation of the joint contents may produce

4. Paralysis. The sequestrated disc may be so large

and so critically situated that it behaves like a neoplasm compressing the roots of the cauda equina, resulting in paralysis of the lower extremities, marked sensory loss and disturbance of function of bladder and bowel.

Not infrequently, laboratory aids are necessary to establish a positive diagnosis of a herniated intervertebral disc. X-rays of the spine as well as spinal fluid examinations are necessary to rule out congenital defects, inflammatory or neoplastic lesions. Myelography, using three to six cc. of Pantopaque® in the subarachnoid space, is the most reliable test for the accurate diagnosis and localization of a herniated intervertebral disc.

Treatment. When treatment is instituted, conservative measures consisting of bed rest, local heat, traction, and various supports should be tried for six weeks. In the event that the response to such treatment is inadequate and the patient is still disabled, Pantopaque myelography should be undertaken. If the myelogram shows evidence of disc herniation, then an interlaminar operation, as illustrated, is necessary.

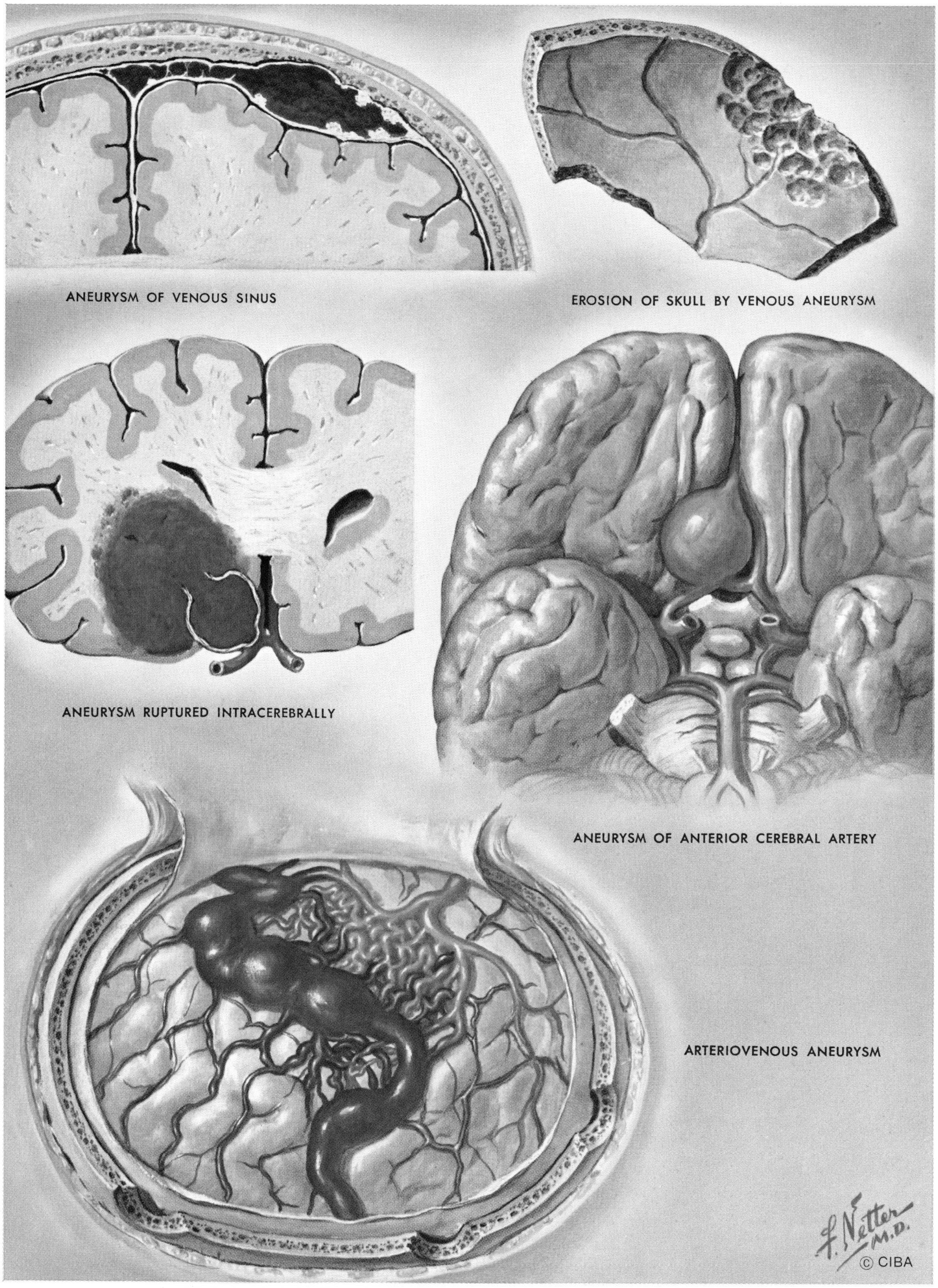

PLATE 85

ANEURYSM OF VENOUS SINUS

EROSION OF SKULL BY VENOUS ANEURYSM

ANEURYSM RUPTURED INTRACEREBRALLY

ANEURYSM OF ANTERIOR CEREBRAL ARTERY

ARTERIOVENOUS ANEURYSM

INTRACRANIAL ANEURYSMS

Intracranial aneurysms, next in frequency only to aortic aneurysms, are vascular dilatations resulting from localized defects in vascular elasticity. They are more frequent in men and occur at all ages, particularly during the second and third decades. They are found usually at the points of bifurcation of the Circle of Willis at the base of the brain. Although mainly due to congenital or developmental defects in the vessel wall these aneurysms may also be the result of hypertension, arteriosclerosis, emboli, or infections, very rarely of syphilis. Aneurysms may also be found within the cerebral substance, over the surface of the brain, within the cavernous sinus, or adjacent to large venous sinuses.

Intracranial aneurysms are frequently multiple, vary in size from a pea to a plum, and may remain symptomless during life. Rupture of an intracranial aneurysm is due to increase in intravascular tension brought on by extreme exertion or straining, very rarely from external trauma. Such a rupture is the most common cause of "spontaneous" subarachnoid hemorrhage. But there are other less frequent causes for subarachnoid bleeding such as vascular hypertension, infections, blood dyscrasias, and sometimes nephritis. Small leaks will produce mild meningeal signs but a large rupture is followed by explosive headache, vomiting, coma, stiff neck, Kernig's sign, fever and albuminuria.

Besides general signs of subarachnoid bleeding, a ruptured aneurysm will also show focal signs of pressure and hemorrhage. A frequent example is a rupture of the middle cerebral artery into the internal capsule spreading to the basal ganglia and speech areas producing hemiplegia and aphasia.

The diagnosis of ruptured aneurysm is made by the apoplectic onset of symptoms, signs of meningeal irritation, focal signs of cerebral damage, and uniformly bloody spinal fluid. The exact location and size of such aneurysms can be visualized by arteriography.

Treatment of subarachnoid bleeding consists of symptomatic relief and lumbar puncture to reduce intraspinal pressure and for the removal of bloody spinal fluid. The advisability of isolating and trapping aneurysms intracranially will depend upon the size and the location of the aneurysm. Ligation of the common or internal carotid artery is a less formidable task, and has fewer complications.

Prognosis. In a recent study of over 150 patients with ruptured intracranial aneurysms, forty per cent died during the first attack. Of the remaining patients, fifty per cent had a second attack within three weeks, and only forty per cent survived this attack.

There are other types of intracranial aneurysm which require consideration:

1. Arteriovenous aneurysms over the cerebral cortex are most frequently located at the Sylvian-Rolandic junction. They consist of tangled arterial loops communicating through a capillary bed with dilated and tortuous veins. They produce symptoms of mild recurrent seizures, jacksonian in type, with transient palsies which arouse the suspicion of "epilepsy." Arteriography demonstrates the size and location and ramifications of such an aneurysm. Surgical removal is frequently dangerous and most often it is unsatisfactory. Partial ligation of the arterial trunk may be beneficial.

2. Arteriovenous aneurysm of the cavernous sinus is due to trauma producing a fistulous communication between the internal carotid artery and the cavernous sinus. The signs are pulsating exophthalmos, chemosis of the conjunctiva, engorged retinal veins, ocular palsy and a bruit. After finger compression of the carotid artery has established adequate collateral circulation, partial or total ligation of the artery is advisable.

3. Aneurysms of the venous sinus involve the adjacent dura, erode the inner table of the skull, compress the brain and produce loculated arachnoidal cysts with focal brain atrophy. Recurrent headaches, focal or generalized seizures, may be the only symptoms. Diodrast® injection through the superior longitudinal sinus will demonstrate such a lesion. Treatment consists of excision of the aneurysm and involved dura without disturbing the circulation of the sinus.

PLATE 86

HYPERTENSIVE APOPLEXY

Hypertensive apoplexy is a sudden effusion of blood into the cerebral tissues as a result of vascular hypertension. It occurs at any age and beyond forty years is a common cause of death. Sudden increase in intravascular pressure following severe exertion, trauma or emotional tension may precipitate a cerebral hemorrhage, but it may also occur during sleep.

The etiology of vascular hypertension is still unknown. Inherited overactivity of the autonomic system, particularly the intracranial portion of the vegetative nervous system (ventral medial hypothalamic nuclei) is responsible for some forms of vascular hypertension. Psychomotor factors — anxieties, submerged drives, etc., also bear a relationship to intermittent elevations in blood pressure. About seventy per cent of patients with recurrent elevations in blood pressure eventually develop malignant vascular hypertension.

There are two forms of hypertensive apoplexy:

1. The benign form shows transient manifestations because the vascular spasms are mild and infrequent. Eventually the terminal arterioles become deficient in blood supply resulting in temporary local cerebral ischemia and minor hemorrhage. There follow encephalomalacia (cerebral softening) and cyst formation. Early complaints are transient faintness, dizziness, mild headache and forgetfulness; but in later stages, there are minor attacks of motor, sensory and speech disturbances. Restoration of function follows improved cerebral circulation. Glial scars of previous cerebral hemorrhages are found often in fatal cases of malignant hypertensive apoplexy.

2. Malignant hypertensive apoplexy may occur months or years after a benign cerebrovascular episode, and may even occur without previous warning. The vascular rupture and hemorrhage is explosively sudden, usually in an area of cerebral softening and frequently involving the middle cerebral artery or its branches (lenticulostriate artery — artery of hemorrhage). The hemorrhage displaces and destroys portions of the internal capsule and spreads to involve adjacent areas, but if it ruptures into the ventricles the outcome is promptly fatal. Primary hemorrhage in the pons is rare and as a rule rapidly fatal. Intracerebellar hemorrhage, very rare indeed, causes occipital and cervical pain, vomiting and ataxia and is fatal when it ruptures into the fourth ventricle.

The immediate signs of a hypertensive apoplexy are a sudden collapse, coma, dilated pupils, hemorrhages in the fundi, eyes deviated toward the lesion, respiratory difficulties (Cheyne-Stokes), with puffing of the cheek on the side of the paralysis, and loss of tendon and sphincter reflexes. The

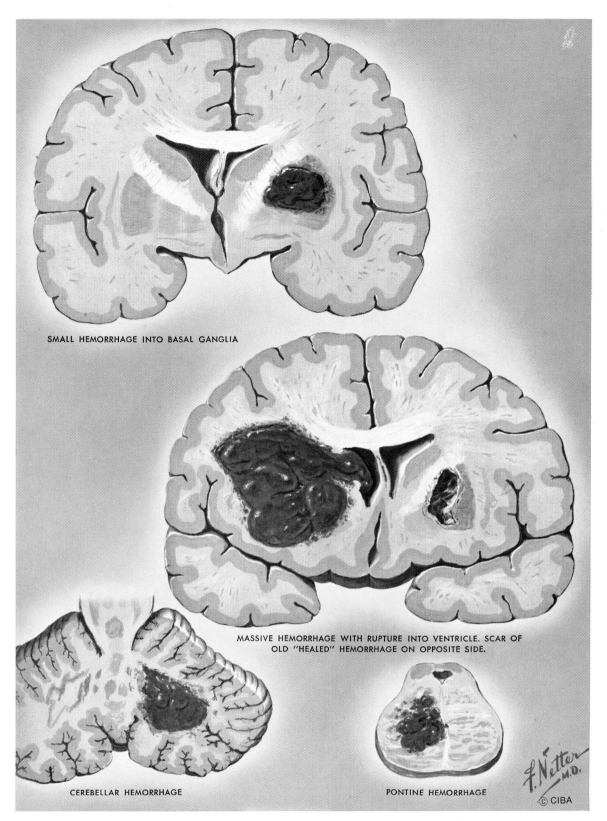

SMALL HEMORRHAGE INTO BASAL GANGLIA

MASSIVE HEMORRHAGE WITH RUPTURE INTO VENTRICLE. SCAR OF OLD "HEALED" HEMORRHAGE ON OPPOSITE SIDE.

CEREBELLAR HEMORRHAGE

PONTINE HEMORRHAGE

spinal fluid is usually uniformly xanthochromic or bloody.

If death does not supervene, recovery begins with return of consciousness which may appear within 24 to 36 hours. Abnormal neurological signs such as paralysis, facial weakness, aphasia, and pathological reflexes may point to the location of the hemorrhage. After six to eight weeks, signs of returning function appear first in the leg, then the arm, and lastly fine finger movements. Usually the gait is spastic in circumduction, the arm is inwardly rotated, the hand edematous, and the fingers clenched in the palm. Contractures and rigidities present serious problems of rehabilitation. Aphasia may be permanent but when speech returns it is slow and very seldom complete. Mental symptoms, emotional instability, and thalamic pains are distressing sequelae.

The prognosis is unfavorable if coma persists or is increasing during the first 48 hours, if hyperpyrexia continues, or if there are signs of cardiorespiratory-renal failure.

Treatment should begin long before the onset of cerebral vascular symptoms. The patient must realize what influence his work, environment, and emotions have upon his vascular hypertension. A change in philosophy may reduce the stress and strain upon his cerebral vessels. Reduction of weight, removal of infected foci, bowel regulation, habits of rest and relaxation, and special diet (Kempner rice diet and low salt) influence vascular tension favorably. The incidence of apoplexy can be decreased by fifty per cent with bilateral sympathectomy and splanchnic denervation in properly selected patients.

In the acute phase of apoplexy the head should be slightly elevated, respiratory passages cleared, oxygen given liberally and it may be necessary to carry out nasal tube feeding. Special and skillful nursing care is essential. Procaine injections into the stellate ganglion are helpful in only one-third of the patients. Recently, injections of Priscoline® into the carotid artery have been favorably mentioned.

Surgical evacuation of the intracerebral clot is seldom beneficial.

PLATE 87

Venous Anomalies

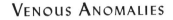

Venous anomalies of the brain, dural sinuses and spinal cord are numerous and variable. They vary considerably in size, location, distribution and configuration and are frequently accompanied by degenerative cerebral and spinal malformations. The clinical behavior of these venous anomalies is unpredictable. At times, a comparatively small venous malformation may produce alarming symptoms, and then again massive clusters of venous channels in critical areas may be quiescent for years.

The venous anomalies of the brain are frequently situated at the Sylvian-Rolandic junction and may present such a tangled collection of veins that an angiomatous neoplasm is suspected. However, the venous character of the lesion can be established by the absence of pulsation, the venous blood content, and by the gradual decrease in the vessel caliber from the point of origin. Displacement of the rolandic vein either anteriorly or posteriorly from its usual position is not infrequent, and with this shift there are associated difficulties in exact cerebral localization.

The symptoms of cerebral venous abnormalities are few indeed but when these malformations are accompanied by cerebral dysfunction or degeneration, they burst forth at irregular intervals with jacksonian or generalized convulsive seizures. With repeated seizures there may be transient motor weakness and subsequent mental deterioration.

The interior of the brain is also affected by venous anomalies which take the form of a cavernoma often communicating with venous dilatations over the cerebral cortex or with large dural sinuses. The vein of Galen may stray from its usual midline position and on some occasions has been found to enter the superior longitudinal sinus instead of the straight sinus. Excision or ligation of the main tributaries leading to these cerebral malformations has been followed by amelioration of symptoms.

The dural sinuses have their share of venous anomalies. Recent investigations have shown that the caliber of either transverse sinus varies considerably, that the transverse sinus on either side may be very small or entirely absent and that the right or left transverse sinus predominates in venous drainage from the superior longitudinal

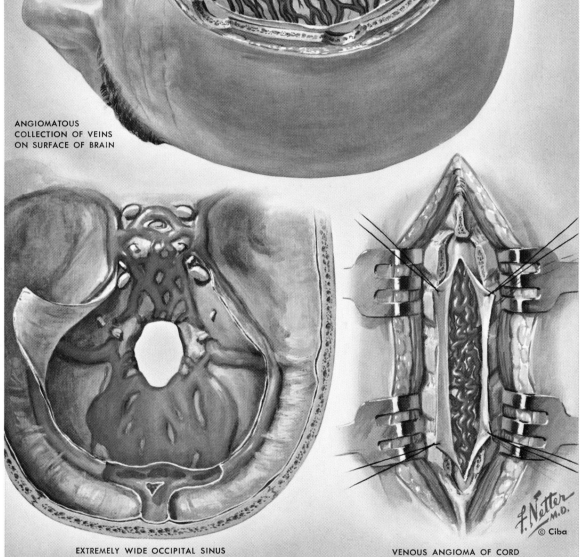

ANGIOMATOUS COLLECTION OF VEINS ON SURFACE OF BRAIN

EXTREMELY WIDE OCCIPITAL SINUS

VENOUS ANGIOMA OF CORD

sinus with equal frequency. The occipital sinus, known to have the greatest variability in size and position, may be totally absent, eccentrically placed or be so wide as to form a "lake" involving half of the cerebellar dura and presenting serious difficulties for surgical exposure of this region. The petrosal and cavernous sinuses have their share in these venous anomalies and may even be totally absent on one side without clinical signs.

There are three methods for diagnostic visualization of these venous anomalies. First, they may appear during the venous phase of angiography; second, they may be demonstrated by direct injection of Diodrast through a catheter in the superior longitudinal sinus; and third, some venous anomalies can be demonstrated by retrograde injection of Diodrast through a catheter inserted in the basilic vein which has been guided to the jugular bulb.

Venous anomalies of the vertebral system and the spinal cord are being recognized with increasing frequency, particularly since the introduction of Pantopaque myelography. Indentations and deformities of the dura and displacement of the nerve roots by extradural varicosities have been visualized with Pantopaque studies and have been demonstrated at operation. Such varicosities produce symptoms chiefly of nerve root irritation and pressure. Partial laminectomy with decompression and coagulation of varicosities has proved beneficial.

Varicose veins of the spinal cord most frequently found in the thoracic region arise mainly from the posterior spinal veins. These varicosities which are two to five times the normal caliber of spinal veins extend over two to three segments of the spinal cord and give the appearance of an elongated tangle of worms. They cause the clinical symptoms and signs of progressive spinal cord compression with periods of remission. Pain due to nerve root irritation is an outstanding symptom. Myelographic studies with Pantopaque show partial to complete subarachnoid block with tortuous defects outlining the corresponding venous malformations. Decompression by laminectomy, ligation of some of the main venous trunks and subsequent x-ray therapy have been followed by clinical improvement.

PLATE 88

CEREBRAL ARTERIOSCLEROSIS

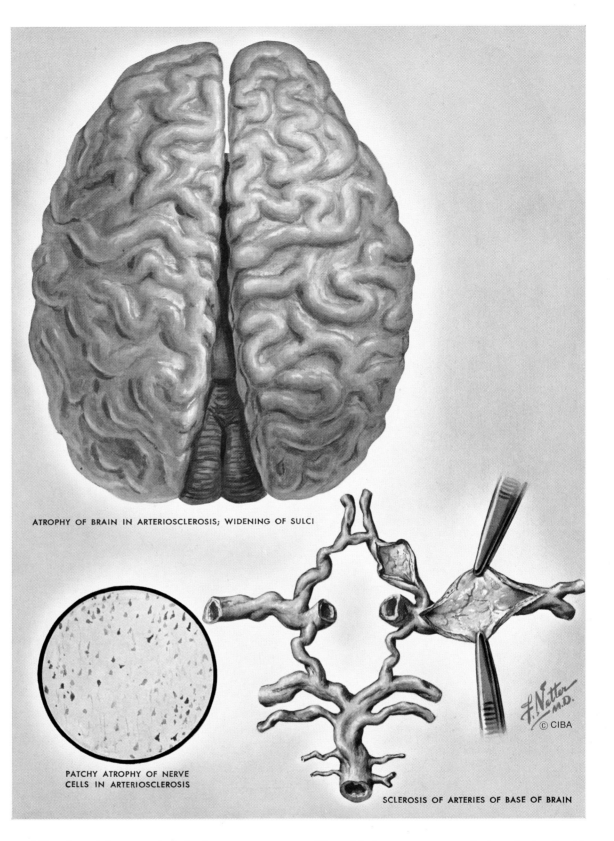

ATROPHY OF BRAIN IN ARTERIOSCLEROSIS; WIDENING OF SULCI

PATCHY ATROPHY OF NERVE CELLS IN ARTERIOSCLEROSIS

SCLEROSIS OF ARTERIES OF BASE OF BRAIN

Cerebral arteriosclerosis is a progressive obliterative process of the cerebral vessels which is responsible for circulatory disturbances in various parts of the brain. In many it is the result of nature's wear and tear, "a man is as old as his arteries," but there are other factors which hasten these vascular changes, such as heredity, metabolic disturbances, strenuous physical work, toxic and infectious conditions, particularly those due to alcohol, lead and syphilis. Cerebral arteriosclerosis may exist alone or be part of a generalized arteriosclerosis. However, there are many with cerebral arteriosclerosis who reach advanced age and retain remarkable physical and mental vigor.

The brain of cerebral arteriosclerosis shows a mottled appearance with generalized atrophy and thickened opalescent leptomeninges which are slightly adherent to the cerebral cortex. The convolutions are irregularly prominent because of the widening of the deep sulci. These pathological changes are most striking in the frontal lobes. The vessels at the base of the brain are hard, thickened and tortuous with plaques scattered throughout. Upon section of the brain there is atrophy of the gray matter, more so in the upper layers, with little change in the white matter. The ventricular system is symmetrically dilated — ex-vacuo. Scattered throughout the cortex are minute areas of softening with cyst and scar formation, and in the subcortical layers the process at times has a particular affinity for the basal ganglia. Early microscopic examination of the small arteries shows narrowing due to proliferation of the intima with endothelial granulations. These are later replaced and organized by fibroblasts as a result of necrosis and thrombosis. The adventitia is seldom involved. The cortical nerve cells show patchy atrophy and evidence of degeneration. In only fifty per cent of patients with cerebral arteriosclerosis are there comparable sclerotic changes in the retinal vessels.

In spite of advanced cerebral arteriosclerosis the patient may show no abnormal signs or symptoms and his mentality may be surprisingly acute and reflect great wisdom. The early abnormal cerebral symptoms begin with a slowing up of mental acuity, slight changes in personality, emotional instability, forgetfulness, particularly for recent events, poor judgment, difficulty in concentration, and intellectual deterioration. The personal appearance may become slovenly and there may be spells of crying and laughing without appropriate stimulus. Acts of jealousy, infidelity, sexual perversions and other asocial behavior are not unusual. With advancing cerebral pathology, there are symptoms of mild headache, dizziness, syncopal attacks, occasional nausea and vomiting, fleeting aphasia, transitory paralysis, parkinsonian features, and in late stages signs of mild delirium, senile dementia and psychosis.

There are several forms of presenile psychosis which must be differentiated from the true senile psychosis:

1. Pick's disease is chiefly found in women over sixty years and results from progressive atrophy and degeneration of the upper cortical layers. Arteriosclerosis of the cerebral vessels is slight or absent. Poor judgment, impaired intellect and transient aphasia are the outstanding symptoms. The disease may continue from five to ten years.

2. Alzheimer's disease first appears about the age of fifty and is due to premature cerebral arteriosclerosis with glial changes. It is characterized by rapid deterioration of memory, poor judgment, deficient intellect and loss of moral values. Occasionally there are focal signs of aphasia and apraxia.

3. Biswanger's dementia presenilis has its onset between forty and fifty years of age and is characterized chiefly by poor memory, lack of insight, euphoria, grandiose ideas, failing judgment and indifference and deterioration in moral standards. Occasionally there are convulsive attacks. The Wassermann test is negative.

The treatment of cerebral arteriosclerosis is chiefly symptomatic and should be in keeping with the patient's physical and mental capacities. Most helpful are a well-balanced daily program of rest, relaxation and activity, regulation of bowels, sufficient sleep, and social interests. There is no need for dietary restrictions. Institutional or custodial care may be necessary. Medication should be kept at a minimum and limited to small doses of iodides, barbiturates and aspirin.

PLATE 89

PURULENT MENINGITIS

Only those who witnessed, over a decade ago, the tragedies of purulent meningitis and its complications will fully appreciate the miracle wrought by the antibacterial drugs. It is hoped that the time is not too distant when purulent meningitis will become a pathologic curiosity.

Meningitis, an inflammation of the meninges, is most often bacterial in origin. The subarachnoid space is secondarily involved and reflects only the reaction to the inflammation.

The primary bacterial causes of meningitis are meningococcus, pneumococcus, Streptococcus haemolyticus, Hemophilus influenzae, Staphylococcus aureus, Streptococcus viridans, and others. These organisms gain entry into the central nervous system usually through the upper respiratory tract, but may enter by direct extension from infections of the accessory nasal sinuses, dural sinuses, osteomyelitis of the skull, penetrating wounds of the meninges, or by blood metastases from distant infectious foci such as occur in pneumonia, endocarditis, osteomyelitis, and septicemia. Predisposing factors to meningitis are undernourishment, physical exhaustion, debility, crowded living conditions, and the like.

The initial meningeal response to the invading organisms is meningeal congestion, edema, and minute hemorrhages. The inflammatory response of the pia-arachnoid and choroid plexus is first lymphocytic, then it promptly and rapidly shifts to an increase of polynuclear leukocytes. The cellular and chemical reaction in the cerebrospinal fluid varies with the progress or the recession of the infection showing first a turbid or cloudy appearance, then becoming increasingly thick, yellowish, or greenish, and finally changing to a plastic exudate. This exudate, a mixture of leukocytes, fibrin, and red blood cells, spreads over the surface of the brain, fills the basilar cisternae, envelops cranial nerves, and extends over the posterior aspect of the thoracic and lumbar spinal cord and roots. The infection also extends to involve the brain, resulting in meningo-encephalitis, and into the ventricles, producing ependymitis.

Any patient, particularly a child, with fever, malaise, and headache should, without fail, be tested for neck resistance and Kernig's sign. It is far better to be suspicious of meningitis and analyze the spinal fluid than to wait for the full-blown clinical signs of unmistakable meningitis.

The onset of meningitis may be abrupt and severe with high fever, chills, arthralgia,

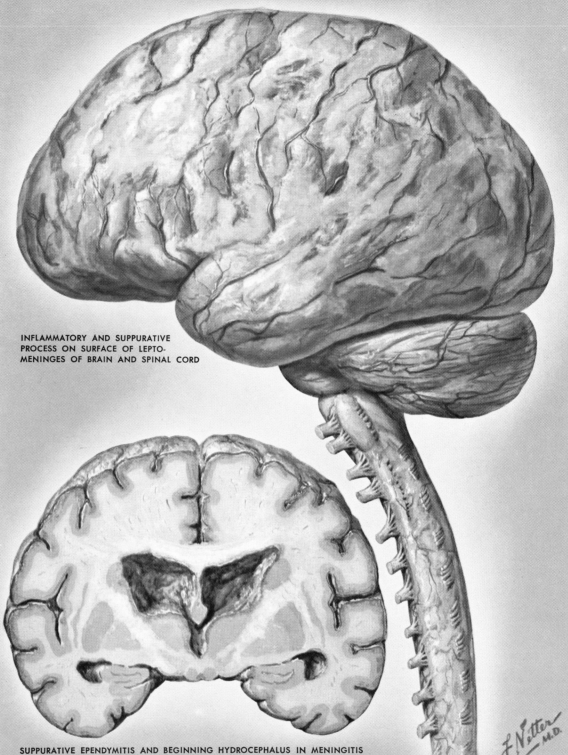

INFLAMMATORY AND SUPPURATIVE PROCESS ON SURFACE OF LEPTO-MENINGES OF BRAIN AND SPINAL CORD

SUPPURATIVE EPENDYMITIS AND BEGINNING HYDROCEPHALUS IN MENINGITIS

and somnolence progressing to convulsions and delirium. Hyperpyrexia, toxemia, bradycardia, and herpes are evident. The neck is stiff, Kernig's and Brudzinski's signs are positive. The deep reflexes are hyperactive, the cranial nerves are frequently involved, and Babinski's sign is positive. The skin often shows red, splotchy, elevated petechiae of meningococcemia, rarely gangrenous skin blebs, and most unusual, gangrene of the toes. Spinal fluid leukocytes vary in number from 15 to 15,000 with ninety to ninety-five per cent being polynuclears. Cultures from the spinal fluid, blood, and skin lesions frequently show intracellular and extracellular organisms. The diagnosis depends mainly on spinal fluid studies. Most important is evidence of an increase in spinal pressure, cell count, and globulin, as well as the presence of organisms on smear and culture growths, and a reduction of spinal fluid sugar content.

In advanced meningitis there is increased intracranial pressure due to subarachnoid block resulting in deepening coma, marked head retraction, papilledema, cranial nerve

palsies, and Biot's or Cheyne-Stokes respirations. Atypical or relapsing forms of meningitis are not unusual. Late complications of meningitis such as cranial nerve palsies, neuritis, deafness, and subarachnoid block are more easily prevented than treated.

The treatment of meningitis should begin before the onset of the disease. Prophylactic treatment of upper respiratory and other infections with antibacterial drugs has undoubtedly prevented countless cases of meningitis. The complete removal of infected foci is essential to treatment. Early treatment with massive doses of "cross-fire" antibacterial drugs should be started simultaneously with the diligent hunt for the organism in the blood and spinal fluid. Antibacterial treatment should be determined by the type of organism present and its tested sensitivity to the drug. Treatment should continue for at least five to ten days after spinal fluid, blood studies, and temperature are normal. Fluid intake should be adequate, and alkalosis prevented by the administration of 1/6 molar lactate solution.

PLATE 90

TUBERCULOSIS OF THE BRAIN AND SPINE

Tuberculosis of the brain and spine is secondary to tuberculosis elsewhere in the body. Bodily resistance rendered low from intercurrent disease or malnutrition causes the tubercle bacilli to become activated. The body responds chiefly with increased epithelioid and lymphocytic cell formation which tends to wall off the spread of infection by forming reticular fibers and connective tissue. The giant cell response is in inverse ratio to the virulence of the bacilli. As the tubercle bacilli multiply, their toxins and the resulting impairment of the blood supply lead to degeneration, necrosis, and caseation. When the infection is brought under control, encapsulation, sclerosis, and calcification follow. Unfortunately, when the defensive mechanisms break down the infection becomes disseminated and frequently enters the central nervous system.

Tuberculoma

The tuberculoma is found near the Sylvian fissure, in the cerebellum or pons, or less frequently, near the longitudinal sinus. It starts as a minute tubercle near a blood vessel in the meninges. After embedding itself in the brain substance, it gradually increases to the size of a pea or walnut and shows a calcified periphery and a softer grayish-yellow center. When a tuberculoma compresses cerebral blood vessels, softening follows, but it may produce the symptoms and signs of an intracranial neoplasm by obstructing the cerebrospinal fluid circulation.

Tuberculous Meningitis

This type of meningitis is most common between the ages of two and five but may occur at any age. The involved pale meninges show a tenacious fibrinopurulent exudate about the Sylvian fissure, the base of the brain, and the cranial nerves. Over the cerebral surface one may detect minute whitish granular specks — tubercles — of varying size and number. Subarachnoid block which causes the ventricles to dilate with an accompanying ependymitis is not unusual. In addition, lymphocytes infiltrate the cerebral perivascular spaces producing a meningoencephalitis.

The symptoms of tuberculous meningitis are insidious and often follow such debilitating diseases as measles or whooping cough. The earliest, apparently innocent, manifestations are failing health, loss of appetite and weight, mild headaches, restlessness, and low grade fever. If these symptoms continue for more than several days, tuberculous meningitis should be suspected and the spinal fluid analyzed. As the disease advances, headache, vomiting, and fever become more pronounced, there is a decrease in the pulse rate and night cries are noticed.

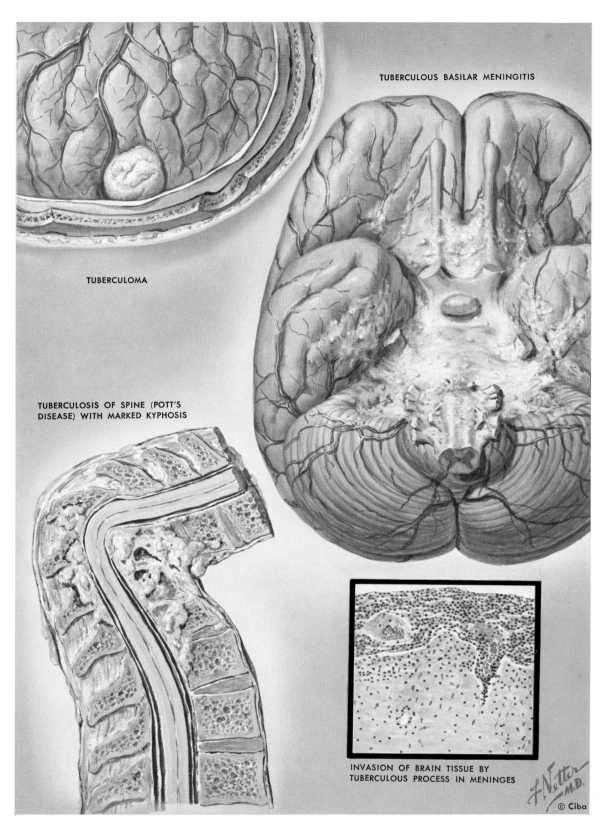

TUBERCULOMA

TUBERCULOUS BASILAR MENINGITIS

TUBERCULOSIS OF SPINE (POTT'S DISEASE) WITH MARKED KYPHOSIS

INVASION OF BRAIN TISSUE BY TUBERCULOUS PROCESS IN MENINGES

In later stages the neck becomes stiff and retracted; somnolence, convulsions, delirium, paresis, and cranial nerve involvement supervene. In the terminal stages the patient becomes more toxic and dehydrated, hyperpyrexia continues, and convulsions become more frequent. The neurologic findings are mainly stiff neck, positive Kernig's and Brudzinski's signs, papilledema, occasionally a retinal tubercle, ocular palsies, facial weakness, aphasia, and hemiplegia. Most important for early diagnosis is analysis of the spinal fluid which at first shows mild turbidity, few lymphocytes, increasing globulin, and reduction of sugar and chloride content. The spinal fluid after standing 12 to 24 hours forms a pellicle often harboring the tubercle bacilli.

Pott's Disease

Tuberculosis of the spine, which begins during childhood, involves the bodies of one or more vertebrae and at times the adjacent joints. Over seventy-five per cent of patients with this disease are under ten years of age. From the primary focus in the lungs or retropharyngeal space, the infection spreads to the vertebral bodies producing caseation, softening, and eventually collapse and deformity. The thoracic and lumbar vertebrae are most frequently involved, and there may be an accompanying pleural or psoas abscess. The pathologic process may be hastened by trauma. As the tuberculous mass extends into the spinal canal, there is a resulting pachymeningitis externa, root irritation, and spinal cord compression, but rarely dural penetration. Early and repeated x-ray studies of the spine indicating soft tissue changes, narrowing of intervertebral spaces, and bony destruction lead to prompt and accurate diagnosis.

In advanced stages x-rays demonstrate vertebral destruction, angulation, and gibbous formation. The early symptoms of Pott's disease are slow and insidious, beginning with mild back pains and tenderness, root irritation, and occasionally areas of hyperesthesia and herpes zoster. When there is evidence of spinal deformity, root irritation and cord compression, the disease is already advanced and progressing rapidly.

PLATE 91

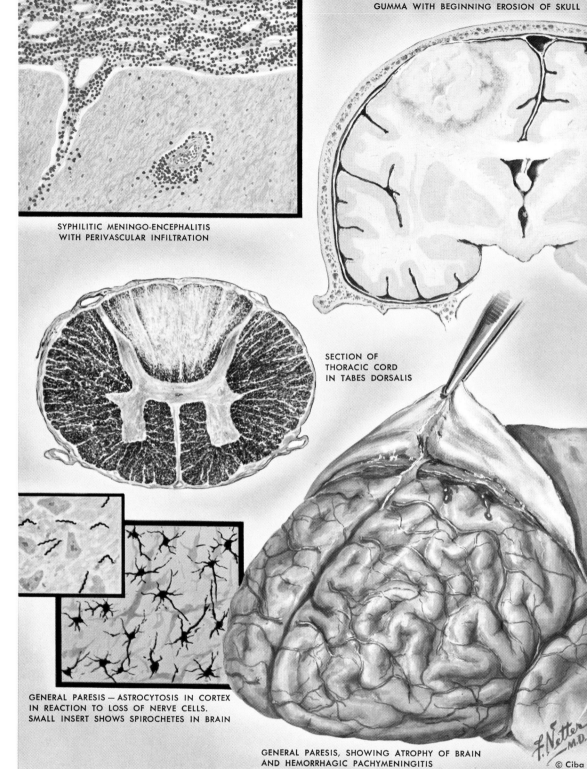

SYPHILITIC MENINGO-ENCEPHALITIS
WITH PERIVASCULAR INFILTRATION

GUMMA WITH BEGINNING EROSION OF SKULL

SECTION OF
THORACIC CORD
IN TABES DORSALIS

GENERAL PARESIS — ASTROCYTOSIS IN CORTEX
IN REACTION TO LOSS OF NERVE CELLS.
SMALL INSERT SHOWS SPIROCHETES IN BRAIN

GENERAL PARESIS, SHOWING ATROPHY OF BRAIN
AND HEMORRHAGIC PACHYMENINGITIS

NEUROSYPHILIS

Within five momentous years the cause, laboratory diagnosis, and treatment of syphilis were tremendously advanced. In 1905 Schaudinn demonstrated the organism causing syphilis — Treponema pallidum (*Spirochaeta pallida*); Wassermann (1908) described the agglutination test; and Ehrlich brought forth specific therapy for the disease — salvarsan.

The Treponema pallidum is a delicate, spiral parasite whose size, shape, and activity are best appreciated in a darkfield preparation from a primary venereal lesion. Syphilis of the nervous system occurs in less than twenty per cent of those patients primarily infected and takes several forms. The meninges, brain, and spinal cord response to the spirochetal parasite is evidenced by a chronic, inflammatory process of cellular and interstitial tissues which produces mainly small lymphocytic cells, epithelioid, and giant cells. Eventually the granulomatous process leads to endarteritis, degenerative and gummatous lesions.

The diagnosis of neurosyphilis can be established early, even before symptoms appear. Neurosyphilis is indicated by a spinal fluid cell count of more than 12 lymphocytes, an increased total protein, a positive complement fixation, and Lange's colloidal gold test.

The most frequent forms of neurosyphilis are:

1. Syphilitic meningitis usually occurs within two years following the primary infection with symptoms of nocturnal headache, malaise, stiff neck, fever, and cranial nerve palsies. The spinal fluid studies reveal an increase in lymphocytes, an elevated total protein, and a positive Wassermann reaction.

2. Meningovascular syphilis occurs about two years after the primary lesion, producing cranial nerve palsies, cerebrovascular accidents, and not infrequently convulsions. The positive findings are Argyll Robertson pupils, an increase in lymphocytes and total protein in the spinal fluid, and a positive Wassermann reaction.

3. Tabes dorsalis predominates in males, usually occurring between 25 to 45 years of age and has its onset 5 to 15 years after the primary infection. During these years the smoldering parasite produces a chronic infection leading to degenerative and sclerotic changes in the posterior nerve root fibers of the spinal cord, spinal ganglia cells, long fibers of the posterior column of the spinal cord, optic nerves, and ocular motor nuclei. The symptoms of lightning root pains, gastric crisis, spastic gait, failing vision, as well as urinary and sexual disturbances vary in their order of appearance and intensity. The optic nerves show progressive primary atrophy, the pupils are small, irregular, fail to react to light, but do react to accommodation (Argyll Robertson). Vibration sense is impaired. Romberg's sign is positive and ataxia is present. The knee and ankle jerks are absent. Only fifty per cent of these patients show a positive Wassermann reaction in the blood and spinal fluid.

4. Dementia paralytica, also called general paresis, predominates in males and usually occurs between the ages of 40 and 45. It is due to a diffuse, chronic, inflammatory process producing degenerative and sclerotic changes in the dura, meninges, and brain resulting in thickening of the dura, pachymeningitis hemorrhagica, atrophy of cortical cells giving a worm-eaten appearance, and proliferation of astrocytes. This process has a particular affinity for the frontal lobes. Noguchi, in 1913, with special stains and preparations, demonstrated the Treponema pallidum in the brain of paretics. The disease is insidious, the main symptoms are headaches, insomnia, personality change, delusions of grandeur, impaired judgment, disturbed emotional responses, slurring speech, tremors, and sexual indiscretions, all progressing to dementia. A generalized convulsion may be the first sign of the disease. Argyll Robertson pupils, described above, are characteristic of this condition. Blood and spinal fluid Wassermanns are positive in ninety to ninety-eight per cent of the cases.

5. Gumma of the brain or spinal cord is rare indeed, presenting the symptoms and signs of an expanding lesion in the central nervous system. Surgical removal of the gumma, supplemented with penicillin therapy, gives excellent results.

PLATE 92

ABSCESS OF BRAIN AND SPINE

The triumph of antibacterial drugs over most types of infection has greatly reduced the incidence of brain abscess. Whether acute or chronic, cerebral abscess is secondary to an extracerebral focus of infection, such as the middle ear, the ethmoid, or the frontal sinus. Abscess may develop following infections about the face, osteomyelitis of the skull, or a foreign body penetrating the brain. The intracranial infection may reach the brain through dehiscence, diseased bone cells, or more frequently by propagating thrombophlebitis of intercommunicating veins from mucous membranes to the meninges and intracerebral vessels.

Thrombophlebitis may spread along the diploe, often eroding the inner table of the skull, producing a "collar button" extradural abscess. Penetration of the dura leads to a subdural or more commonly to intracerebral abscess. The location of the focus and the direction of spread determine the localization of the abscess, be it temporal, cerebellar, frontal, or occipital.

Less frequently, a cerebral abscess develops from embolic metastases from distant sources, such as a lung abscess, bronchiectasis, osteomyelitis, endocarditis, or infections of the liver or urinary tract. About one-half of metastatic brain abscesses are multiple, compared to the solitary abscess caused by direct extension. They vary considerably in size, location, and degree of encapsulation.

A brain abscess begins with the multiplication of bacteria within the cerebral white matter. This produces ischemia, thrombosis, and acute cerebritis. There follow central softening, necrosis, and disintegration of brain tissue which is surrounded by a zone of hyperemia. The infection is usually limited by capsule formation, which consists mainly of proliferating endothelial cells, capillaries, astrocytes, and gitter cells. The central zone goes on to pus formation, from which it may be impossible to demonstrate organisms either on smear or culture. Unsatisfactory encapsulation will lead to meningitis, suppurative encephalitis, or rupture into a ventricle. The most frequent causative organisms of brain abscess are staphylococci, pneumococci, streptococci or mixed types. Rarer forms, chiefly from metastatic foci, are actinomyces, coccidioides, or monilia.

Diagnosis of brain abscess is frequently difficult. Early symptoms consist of malaise, nocturnal headache, fever, slight stiffness of the neck, vomiting, and bradycardia. Headache is the most constant symptom, and often is of the congestive type intensified by stooping, straining, or coughing. With increasing intracranial pressure there is increasing headache, papilledema, drowsiness, and eventually coma. Focal signs depend on the location and size of the abscess. Temporal lobe abscess produces contralateral facial weakness, hemiparesis, third and sixth nerve palsy, homonymous hemianopsia, aphasia, and abnormal reflexes. Localizing signs of a cerebellar abscess are tilting

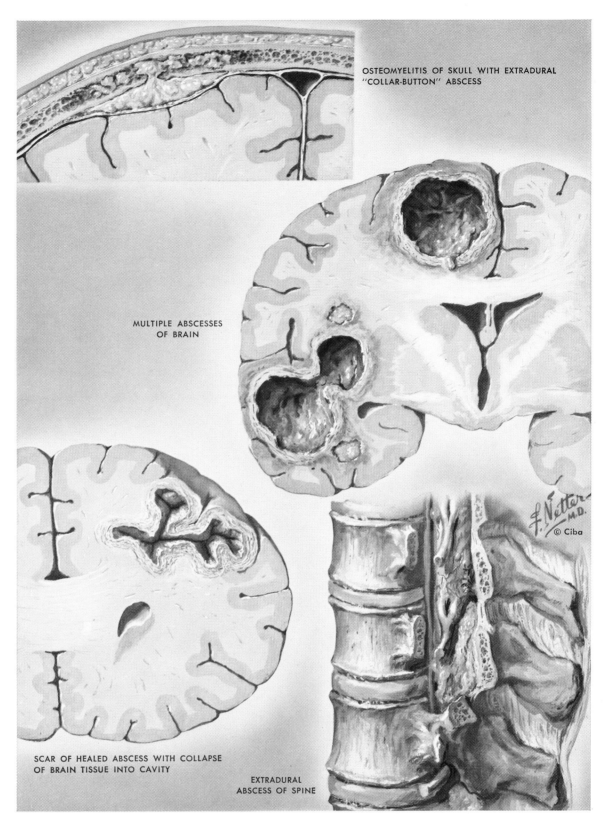

OSTEOMYELITIS OF SKULL WITH EXTRADURAL "COLLAR-BUTTON" ABSCESS

MULTIPLE ABSCESSES OF BRAIN

SCAR OF HEALED ABSCESS WITH COLLAPSE OF BRAIN TISSUE INTO CAVITY

EXTRADURAL ABSCESS OF SPINE

of the head and nystagmus toward the side of the lesion, recurrent vomiting, thickness of speech, ataxia, and dysdiadochokinesia. Frontal lobe abscess betrays few signs; mainly mental changes, inequality of pupils, convulsions, and incontinence.

Electro-encephalography, cerebral arteriography, or ventriculography may be necessary for exact localization of single, recurrent, or multiple abscesses. Early spinal fluid studies usually show increased pressure and total protein; polynuclear cells are increased. Following encapsulation, cell count and total protein diminish and lymphocytes predominate. Persistence or reappearance of polynuclears in the spinal fluid indicates poor encapsulation.

Acute Epidural Spinal Abscess

This condition is a surgical emergency. It can and should be recognized before the onset of neurologic signs. The infection reaches the epidural spinal space either by direct extension from a vertebra or by a septic embolus from a remote focus. The pathologic changes consist of

thrombophlebitis of the extradural venous plexus with subsequent pus formation, which produces compression of the spinal cord. Extension of the septic thrombosis to the veins within the spinal cord leads to secondary myelomalacia. This process advances with hourly rapidity and may readily produce irreversible damage.

Acute epidural spinal abscess should be suspected with a history of antecedent local infection which is followed within a week or two by acute fever, chills, and excruciating back pains. Mild stiffness of the neck and exquisite spinal tenderness are the most significant signs. Massive doses of antibacterial drugs are not curative. One should not wait for localizing signs to become evident. Spinal fluid examination will reveal subarachnoid block, xanthochromia, and increased total protein.

Myelography using Pantopaque will localize the pathologic condition. Laminectomy must follow immediately to save life and to prevent paralysis, loss of bladder and rectal control, decubitus ulcer, ascending urinary infection, and a drawn-out death from renal failure.

PLATE 93

ANTERIOR POLIOMYELITIS

(Polioencephalitis)

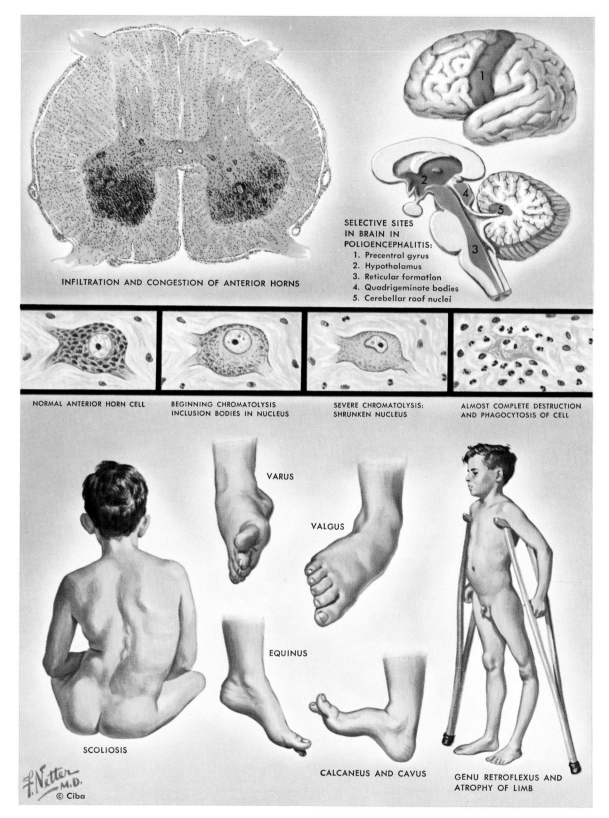

INFILTRATION AND CONGESTION OF ANTERIOR HORNS

SELECTIVE SITES IN BRAIN IN POLIOENCEPHALITIS:
1. Precentral gyrus
2. Hypothalamus
3. Reticular formation
4. Quadrigeminate bodies
5. Cerebellar roof nuclei

NORMAL ANTERIOR HORN CELL

BEGINNING CHROMATOLYSIS INCLUSION BODIES IN NUCLEUS

SEVERE CHROMATOLYSIS: SHRUNKEN NUCLEUS

ALMOST COMPLETE DESTRUCTION AND PHAGOCYTOSIS OF CELL

VARUS

VALGUS

EQUINUS

SCOLIOSIS

CALCANEUS AND CAVUS

GENU RETROFLEXUS AND ATROPHY OF LIMB

Anterior poliomyelitis (polioencephalitis) is an acute infectious viral disease affecting various parts of the central nervous system. Classical lesions involve the motor cells in the anterior horn of the spinal cord. Poliomyelitis is found all over the world. It often occurs in an epidemic form, though it may be sporadic. The disease is seen most frequently during the summer and early autumn. Tonsillectomies performed during these months increase the risk of contracting the bulbar form of poliomyelitis. In most recent epidemics, fifty per cent of the cases were under seven years of age, the peak being between three and six years, but recently more young adults have become victims of this disease. From fifty to eighty per cent of all cases escape permanent paralysis.

In 1909, Landsteiner and Popper recovered the filtrable virus and reproduced the disease in monkeys by intraperitoneal injections of a suspension made from the spinal cord of fatal cases. It is believed that poliomyelitis is transmitted by contact mainly through the upper respiratory tract along the olfactory nerves or the retropharyngeal space. However, some investigators believe the portal of entry to be the gastrointestinal tract.

There are several types of viruses causing human poliomyelitis, and these vary considerably in virulence. Once in the body, the virus shows affinity for certain areas of the central nervous system.

Pathologic changes within the spinal cord and brain consist mainly of hyperemia and edema of the pia, minute capillary hemorrhages, and perivascular infiltration of lymphocytes which choke off the small blood vessels. Pressure exerted on the anterior horn cells and interstitial tissue is most striking in the lumbar and cervical enlargements of the cord. Anterior horn cells show dissolution of mitochondria, progressive chromatolysis, shrinkage of nuclei, and finally degeneration of cells extending to the axons. The anterior horn cells disappear and

are replaced by sclerotic, interstitial (gitter) cells. Completely degenerated anterior horn cells cannot be restored. Therefore, with necrosis of the motor cells, paralysis of muscles innervated by them follows.

Various forms of the disease are:

1. Preparalytic or Abortive. As a rule, the onset is sudden and may be manifested by coryza, anorexia, cough, malaise, and gastrointestinal complaints. These symptoms are followed by irritability and restlessness, or somnolence, a suggestive Kernig's sign, and stiffness of the neck. Spinal fluid is clear, but may have an increase in cell count. Symptoms may last only several hours or a few days and then be followed by complete recovery, or the patient may enter the paralytic stage of the disease.

2. Paralytic. This stage usually presents an acutely ill patient with severe headache, toxemia, stiff neck, pain and tenderness of muscles, hyperpyrexia, and enlargement of the spleen and lymph nodes. Immediate paralysis is rare, but it usually appears within a few days after the initial symptoms. It is asymmetrical, involving mainly

the lower extremities; less often the arms; rarely the intercostal muscles or sphincters.

The blood count often reveals moderate leukocytosis with an increase in polymorphonuclears. The spinal fluid remains clear. However, the cells are increased. At first they are mainly polymorphonuclear, but then shift to lymphocytes. Paralysis is less likely with fewer than 100 cells but more likely with 500 or more cells.

3. Bulbar-Spinal. This type has a fatality rate from six to twenty-three per cent in various epidemics or in various localities. Pathologic changes, previously described, are found in the precentral gyrus, corpus striatum, hypothalamus, reticular formation, quadrigeminal plate, and cerebellar nuclei. Clinical signs are those of meningeal irritation, ocular and facial palsies, speech disturbances, and difficulty in swallowing. Paresis of the diaphragm, neck, intercostal muscles, and occasionally the abdominal muscles, when it occurs, causes respiratory paralysis. Spinal fluid findings are similar to those found in the paralytic stage.

PLATE 94

EPIDEMIC ENCEPHALITIS AND RABIES

Epidemic Encephalitis (von Economo's Disease, Encephalitis Lethargica)

This is an acute infectious disease producing diffuse inflammatory and progressive degenerative changes in the brain and spinal cord. It is believed that the disease is caused by a filtrable virus, although none has been identified as yet, which enters the nervous system through the nasopharynx. It occurs most commonly in the winter and spring, affecting both sexes equally and all ages. Those between 10 and 40 are more prone to contract it. The disease was pandemic during World War I, reaching the United States in 1918. Only sporadic cases have been reported since 1925.

Macroscopically, the nervous system shows engorged vessels on the surface of the brain and areas of hyperemia in the meninges. On section, disseminated pinpoint hemorrhages are often associated with hyperemia in the basal ganglia, midbrain, and pons. Microscopically, lesions are found in the gray matter and are either degenerative or inflammatory and infiltrative. In the former, necrosis of neurons is associated with neuronophagia, while the latter are characterized by perivascular infiltration of monocytes and plasma cells and marked glial proliferation.

The disease is protean in its manifestations and may simulate any neurologic syndrome depending on the dominant area of pathology. The onset may be abrupt or insidious with such symptoms as malaise, headache, fever, lethargy, and transient diplopia. Patients whose recovery is apparently complete may show signs of chronic encephalitis years later.

In some patients the main symptoms are fever, stiff neck, somnolence, lethargy, reversal of sleep pattern, diplopia, pupillary and ocular signs, mental disturbances, delirium, and paresis of the extremities.

In another type the dominant features are motor hyperirritability, myoclonic contractions of muscles affected singly or as a group, rigidities, spasticities, hyperactive reflexes, and pathologic toe signs. In addition, choreiform, athetoid or other irregular or rhythmic movements occur, which may be unilateral or generalized.

There are other types in which mental disturbances are most prominent. These include memory defects, confusion, disorientation, bursts of manic-depressive behavior, alternating delirium, somnolence, stupor, and emotional upheavals. The disease may be brief or persist for months.

The spinal fluid is usually clear, containing from 10 to 20 cells, the majority of which are monocytes. Rarely are there more than 100 cells. Globulin and sugar are only slightly, if at all, elevated. The Wassermann reaction is negative although the colloidal gold curve is luetic in type.

Postencephalitic sequelae may appear months or even years later. These include the parkinsonian syndrome with or without tremor, mask-like facies, abnormal jaw movements, drooling, oculogyric crises, nystagmus, tremors of face and tongue, ataxia, disturbances in sleep mechanism and excessive salivation and sweating. Mental and emotional deficiencies are observed particularly in children.

The disease must be differentiated from almost every type of neurologic disturbance. These include encephalitis from other in-

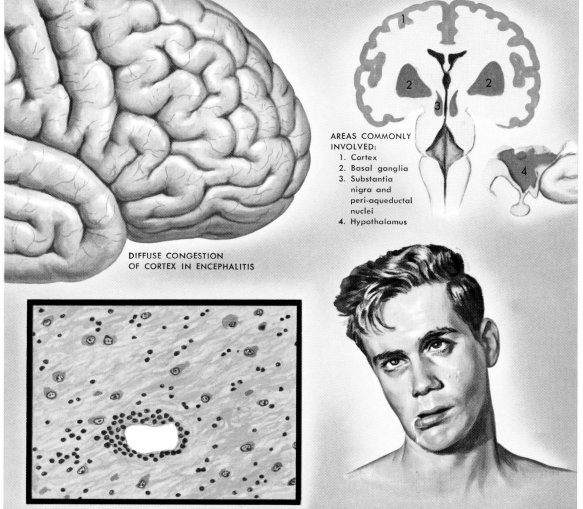

DIFFUSE CONGESTION OF CORTEX IN ENCEPHALITIS

AREAS COMMONLY INVOLVED:
1. Cortex
2. Basal ganglia
3. Substantia nigra and peri-aqueductal nuclei
4. Hypothalamus

PERIVASCULAR INFILTRATION WITH MONONUCLEAR CELLS

POST-ENCEPHALITIC FACIES. ABNORMAL JAW MOVEMENTS, DROOLING, EXPRESSIONLESS, MASK-LIKE

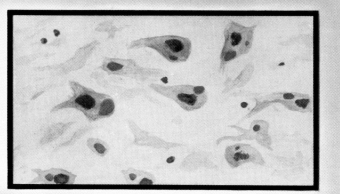

RABIES — NEGRI INCLUSION BODIES IN NERVE CELLS OF BRAIN

fections, toxic or traumatic in origin, from tuberculous meningitis, lymphocytic meningitis, syphilis of the nervous system, and brain tumor.

Mortality of epidemic encephalitis has been as high as twenty to thirty per cent. Recovery is usually rapid but may be delayed from six months to two years.

There is no known specific treatment.

Rabies (Hydrophobia)

This is an acute infectious viral disease transmitted to man through a wound contaminated by the saliva of a rabid animal. In the Scandinavian countries, this disease has been easily and completely eradicated by muzzling all dogs. In 1881, Pasteur demonstrated the virus in the brain of a rabid animal and three years later effected a method for protection against the disease.

The most characteristic pathologic findings are meningeal congestion and Negri inclusion bodies in the cells of the cerebral cortex, Ammon's horn, cerebellum, and pons. However, inability to demonstrate Negri bodies

does not rule out rabies. In addition, there is perivascular infiltration with small lymphocytes.

The incubation period of rabies varies from 10 to 60 days. It is shorter with extensive or multiple wounds, particularly when they occur about the face or head. The effects of the virus are greatly lessened if the skin has not been penetrated or if the bite has been through clothing.

In man, the premonitory symptoms are malaise, headache, anxiety, depression, insomnia, restlessness, delusions, hypersensitivity of the skin, and excessive salivation. During this stage there are alternating periods of rage and calmness. Convulsions may be brought on by so slight a stimulus as breath exhaled on the back of the neck. In the paralytic stage, which may start 24 to 48 hours after onset of symptoms, there are spasms of the larynx and pharynx; the patient's thirst increases, yet any attempt at drinking causes clenching of the jaws (hydrophobia). The entire body is seized with tonic contractions. Finally, convulsions become more intense, and death results from respiratory paralysis.

PLATE 95

TORULOSIS, TOXOPLASMOSIS, TRYPANOSOMIASIS

1. Torula histolytica (Cryptococcus neo-formans) is a yeast-like, nonspore-forming fungus producing a widespread chronic inflammation. The brain and spinal cord are involved in eighty per cent of cases. However, this fungus also affects the lungs, liver, spleen, kidney, and bone. The disease is being recognized with increasing frequency and, to date, there are about 225 reported cases, mostly in the United States.

When the fungus invades the nervous system, the pathological response consists of lymphocytes, epithelioid cells, and giant cells. These collect in the perivascular spaces, basilar meninges, cerebral gray matter, basal ganglia, thalamus, and cerebellar nuclei. The fungus produces a gelatinous type of spotty meningitis, a widespread meningo-encephalitis, or a localized granuloma resembling a gumma. Within the giant cells are spheroid bodies (torula) with large, round, vacuolated cells having a hyaline capsule with a dark-staining central nucleus. The fungus reproduces by budding, often producing cyst-like structures giving the brain a "soap bubble" appearance. The torula reaches the central nervous system through the blood.

The illness may begin acutely with chills and fever which subside, and are followed by prolonged and persistent symptoms of recurrent headache, mild stiffness of the neck, evidences of meningeal irritation, increased intracranial pressure, or spinal cord compression. Clinical findings are, mainly, ocular palsies, stiff neck, papilledema, and pathological reflexes, including positive Kernig's and Brudzinski's signs. This picture may simulate tuberculous meningitis, encephalitis, or tumor of brain or spinal cord.

The diagnosis is established by the findings of turbid or xanthochromic spinal fluid with elevated total protein, diminished sugar and chlorides, and most important, identification of the organism which resembles an encapsulated lymphocyte. Occasionally budding forms may be seen. Smears of the cells with India ink demonstrate the halo, the capsule formation, and the budding. Spinal fluid cultures on Sabouraud's medium will invariably show the torula. There is no definitive therapy for this disease although sulfonamides may be of value. Most patients die within two to four months from the onset of the illness; very few survive more than one year.

2. Toxoplasmosis is a congenital or acquired sporozoan infection, which chiefly involves the brain but may also produce lesions in the lungs, heart, liver and spleen. This organism is found in household pets and laboratory animals. Its mode of transmission to humans is still unknown.

The toxoplasmic organisms infiltrate along the blood vessels of the brain, producing a lymphocytic and granulomatous response with subsequent areas of necrosis, cystic cavities, and ventricular dilatation. In addition, there is bilateral focal chorioretinitis in the fundi. The onset is frequently at an early age with petit mal, convulsions,

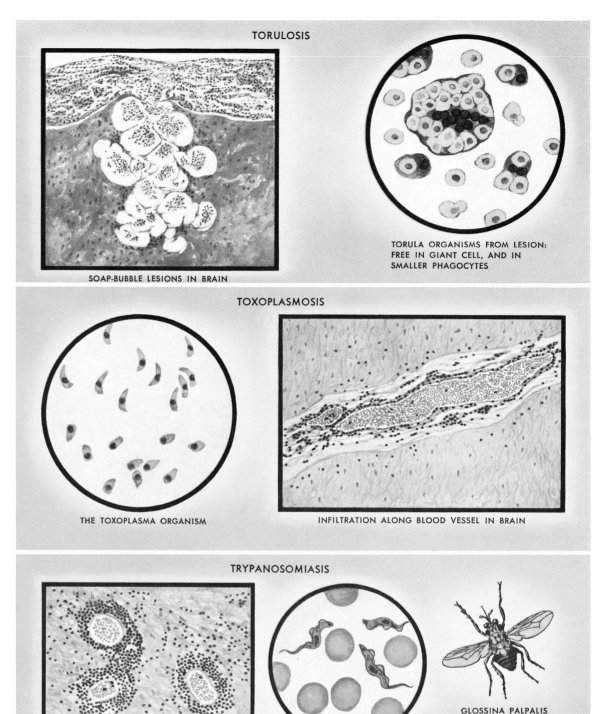

TORULOSIS

SOAP-BUBBLE LESIONS IN BRAIN

TORULA ORGANISMS FROM LESION: FREE IN GIANT CELL, AND IN SMALLER PHAGOCYTES

TOXOPLASMOSIS

THE TOXOPLASMA ORGANISM

INFILTRATION ALONG BLOOD VESSEL IN BRAIN

TRYPANOSOMIASIS

PERIVASCULAR ROUND-CELL INFILTRATION IN BRAIN TISSUE

TRYPANOSOMA GAMBIENSE IN BLOOD

GLOSSINA PALPALIS (specie of tsetse fly)

nystagmus, mental retardation, and poor vision due to vitreous opacities and large, irregular, overlapping chorioretinitis and retinal angiomatosis. Skull films show symmetrically scattered, rounded, or triangular flaky areas of calcification throughout the frontal and parietal areas and in the dentate nuclei. Electro-encephalograms reveal high voltage with slow wave activity. Spinal fluid in the encephalomyelitic form shows xanthochromic fluid, increased protein, normal or decreased sugar, up to 2000 leukocytes per cubic millimeter, most of which are lymphocytes and red blood cells. Demonstration of the organism or complement fixation test for toxoplasmosis establishes the diagnosis. There is no known treatment.

3. Trypanosomiasis (sleeping sickness) is due to infectious, fusiform, mobile parasites. In Central Africa the disease is usually caused by T. gambiense, although other trypanosomes may infect man. It enters the blood of humans following the bite by Glossina palpalis, a species of tsetse fly, breeding along the banks and forest swamps of West Africa. Within the body of the fly, the trypano-

somes undergo a series of changes over a period of 18 to 34 days before becoming infectious to man. In Brazil, where the disease is caused by T. cruzi and transmitted by one of the species belonging to Reduviidae, it is called Chagas' disease.

The trypanosomes circulate in the blood for a very brief interval and have a special affinity for the central nervous system where they produce packs of round cells in the perivascular spaces. The resulting pressure and ischemia are most striking at the base of the brain and medulla. There is associated cervical lymphadenopathy and splenic enlargement.

The disease is insidious in onset, with mild fever, rapid pulse, dull mentality, followed by slow, shuffling gait, tremors, thick speech, then progressing to prolonged and deepening lethargy, finally ending in death from meningitis or exhaustion.

The diagnosis is established by identification of trypanosomes in the blood, cerebrospinal fluid, or in gland puncture specimens.

PLATE 96

GLIOMATA

The cardinal signs of brain tumor — headache, vomiting, and papilledema — are due to increased intracranial pressure; the focal signs, however, are due to disturbed specific brain function. The clinical variables of brain tumors depend on their character, rate of growth, and critical position. A familiarity with the life history and clinical behavior of various intracranial tumors will, at times, permit accurate anatomic or even histologic diagnosis.

Gliomata originate from the supporting structures of the brain and comprise forty-two to fifty per cent of all intracranial neoplasms. They vary in size, location, clinical behavior, and histologic structure. The more embryonic the neoplastic cells, the more malignant the glioma, the more responsive is the tumor to x-ray and radium therapy. On the other hand, a histologically benign glioma may be malignant because of its proximity to vital brain centers. Some gliomata are infiltrative and destructive; others only displace normal structures. There are approximately ten types of glioma, but only the four most frequent ones will be described here. They are:

1. Astrocytoma, comprising forty per cent of all gliomata, is a slow-growing, well-demarcated neoplasm found most frequently in the lateral cerebellar lobes of children or in the temporal or frontal lobes of adults. These tumors are solid, but may also be cystic, containing xanthochromic or dark brown, oily fluid. The entire cyst wall may be neoplastic, or a "mural nodule" — the gliogenous tumor — may project from the cyst wall. When the nodule is totally removed, a permanent cure follows. Microscopically, the cells are round to oval with scant cytoplasm and dark-staining nuclei, which rarely show mitotic figures. With Cajal's gold sublimate or other differential stains, these cells show wiry or plump fibers in star-like radiation from the cell body. Areas of calcification are rare and show up as fine, flaky specks by x-ray.

The symptoms of recurrent increased intracranial pressure may extend over six to nine months before focal cerebellar, frontal, or temporal lobe signs appear. Ventriculograms, electro-encephalograms, or arteriograms will aid in early diagnosis. Survival following complete surgical extirpation may be from ten to twenty years or longer.

2. Oligodendroglioma comprise about four per cent of the glioma group. They are slow-growing, often well-demarcated neoplasms occurring in the cerebral hemispheres of adults. They originate in the white matter near the basal ganglia and extend along myelinated fibers. Grossly, oligodendroglioma appear firm, reddish, and solid, although rarely there may be associated cysts. Microscopically, they present a mosaic of irregular cells with uniformly spherical or rounded nuclei surrounded by a halo of cytoplasm. Mitotic figures are rare. Special stains show scant fibrillae. Areas of calcification are not unusual, and these readily show up as granular specks by x-ray. Clinically, the symptoms are insidious and slowly progressive and extend over a period of six months to a year before giving convincing evidence of an expanding intracranial neoplasm. Complete surgical removal is followed by long survival periods.

3. Ependymoma comprises about three per cent of gliomata and arises in the proximity of the lining of the lateral ventricles

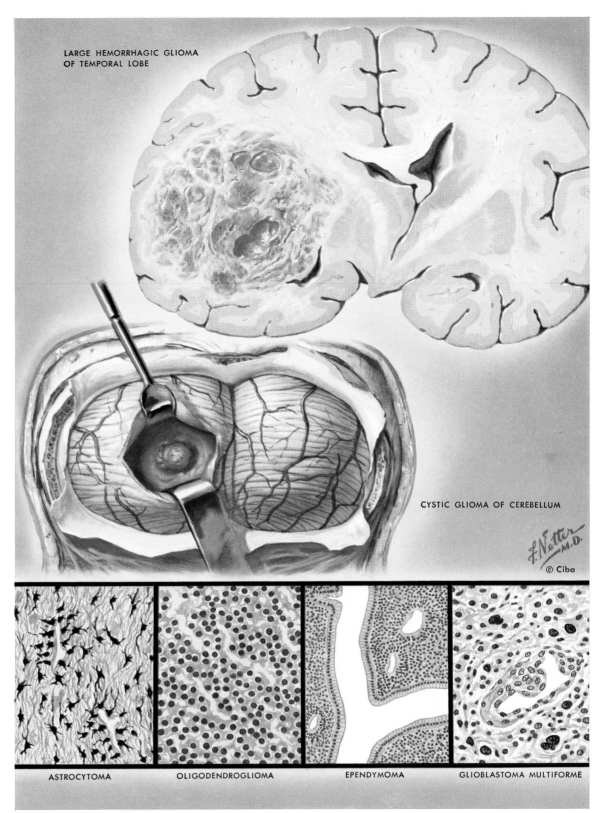

LARGE HEMORRHAGIC GLIOMA OF TEMPORAL LOBE

CYSTIC GLIOMA OF CEREBELLUM

ASTROCYTOMA   OLIGODENDROGLIOMA   EPENDYMOMA   GLIOBLASTOMA MULTIFORME

or the roof of the fourth ventricle. Ependymomas, when located in the region of the vermis, are firm and large and project through the foramen magnum; when found in the proximity of or attached to the lining of the lateral ventricles, they attain very large size and are often partly cystic. Microscopically, these tumors consist of large, polygonal cells arranged in pseudo-rosettes around blood vessels with intervening vacuolated areas. Special stains show blepharoplastin in the cytoplasm. Mitotic figures are occasionally seen in these tumors. Clinically, these tumors progress insidiously and unless critically situated give inconclusive signs and symptoms until the neoplasm has reached considerable size. X-rays of the skull often show fine specks of calcification and are most helpful in establishing the diagnosis. Ependymomas can be completely extirpated with excellent results.

4. Glioblastoma (Spongioblastoma) Multiforme is the most malignant type of glioma, occurring exclusively in the cerebral hemispheres. It occurs most often between 40 to 55 years of age and constitutes about thirty-five to forty per cent of all gliogenous neoplasms. Originating in the cerebral white matter, the cells multiply rapidly and irregularly. They advance without any semblance of demarcation until reaching the cortical surface, where the gyri and sulci are flattened and large surface vessels are displaced from their usual position. Glioblastomas spread along the long tracts crossing the midline to produce a "butterfly" pattern. Rapid growth produces cerebral edema, areas of degeneration, cystic formation, and scattered hemorrhages. This type of neoplasm may be multiple. Microscopically, there are areas of cellular disorganization, cystic necrosis, hemorrhage, endothelial proliferation with hyalinization, active bizarre mitotic figures and multinucleated giant cells. The clinical picture rapidly progresses with increased intracranial pressure, sudden convulsions, mental and intellectual impairment, paralysis and coma, with a high degree of papilledema. Radical surgical extirpation may be followed by a brief respite of from six to nine months, followed by recurrence. X-ray therapy has been temporarily beneficial.

PLATE 97

MENINGIOMATA

Meningiomata comprise thirteen to twenty-five per cent of all intracranial neoplasms. They also occur in the spinal canal. With few exceptions they are benign, well encapsulated, enucleable growths often attached to and involving the dura. Their rate of growth is unusually slow, frequently extending over many years, even a decade or more. Trauma, in some instances, bears a relationship to the site of the neoplasm. Meningiomas are very rare in youth and most frequent between the ages of 30 and 50. In a real sense, most meningiomas are extracerebral, for they do not infiltrate the brain but rather slowly displace brain tissue, forming a smooth bed. These tumors have favorite sites of origin, usually at the folds of dura adjacent to dural sinuses or in the vicinity of rich venous channels over the cerebral cortex or base of the skull.

Meningiomas vary considerably in size, location, and rate of growth. Grossly, they are well demarcated, firm, nodular, and at times lobulated with a thin, shiny, fibrous capsule. They may be as small as a pea or attain the proportions of a large potato. Not infrequently they are multiple.

On section the reddish-gray and granular tumor may be fibrous or soft. Rarely, cystic areas are present. Microscopically, there are several types of meningiomata and a single tumor may show considerable cellular variation. Most typical sections exhibit crowded clusters of fibroblastic cells containing round or oval nuclei and abundant cytoplasm. These cells are frequently arranged in whorl formation with scattered, dark-staining psammoma bodies and larger areas of calcification. Other types may show angioblastic elements, mitotic figures, or even sarcomatous changes.

Clinically, these tumors may be symptomless for many years, being situated in areas where they remain silent. Others may produce but few and transient complaints. Mild headaches, convulsions (focal or gen-

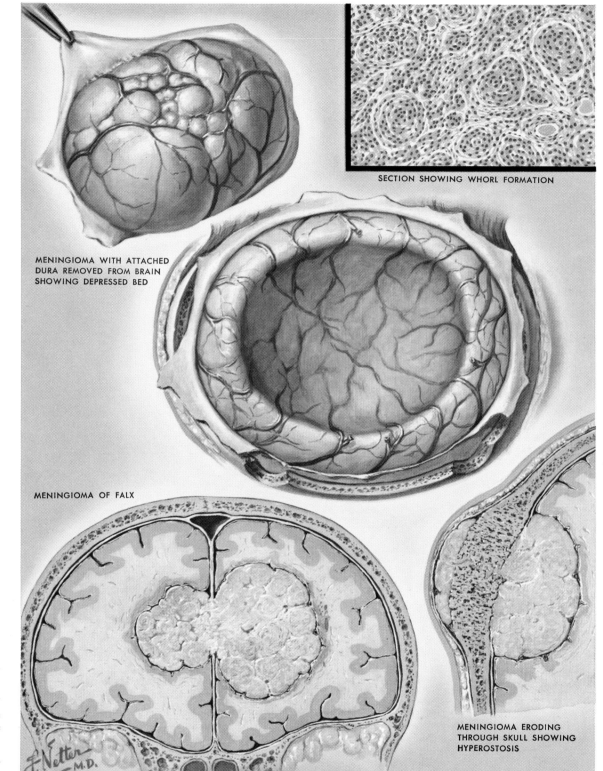

MENINGIOMA WITH ATTACHED DURA REMOVED FROM BRAIN SHOWING DEPRESSED BED

SECTION SHOWING WHORL FORMATION

MENINGIOMA OF FALX

MENINGIOMA ERODING THROUGH SKULL SHOWING HYPEROSTOSIS

eralized), and mental or personality changes may progress slowly for years without giving serious concern. When these tumors reach considerable size in relation to their point of origin, symptoms become disabling and at times alarming.

Symptoms and signs depend upon the location of origin. For example, tumors along the longitudinal sinus often start with jacksonian seizures, followed by hemiparesis and sensory disturbances which involve the leg more than the arm. Those in the olfactory groove cause anosmia and often mental symptoms. Meningiomas crossing the falx in a dumbbell-shaped arrangement may produce bilateral spasticity with sensory signs, raising the possibility of a spinal cord neoplasm. Others in the region of the anterior clinoids and wings of the sphenoid bone frequently produce primary optic atrophy, contralateral papilledema and uncinate phenomena. Meningiomas in the occipital lobe or posterior fossa produce hemianopsia or cerebellar signs.

X-rays of the skull are most helpful, for they show increased skull vascularity with deepening channels of the inner table and also punched-out areas of skull erosion over the site of the lesion. Subsequently, as the tumor cells infiltrate along the diploe and haversian canals, they produce bony reaction with resultant expansion of the inner and outer tables of the skull, giving x-ray evidence of hyperostosis and characteristic radiating bony spicules which are perpendicular to the thickness of the skull. Such a bony prominence can readily be felt underneath the scalp. In some types of meningiomas, x-rays show only dense areas of calcification or circular erosions of the inner tables of the skull.

Complete surgical enucleation is the only treatment. Because of their enormous size, critical location, and vascularity, these tumors often tax the skill, patience, courage, and judgment of even the most experienced neurosurgeon. At times, it may be necessary to complete removal of the tumor in more than one stage. In many instances, life and function depend primarily on skillful hemostasis.

PLATE 98

Acoustic Tumors

(Cerebellopontile)

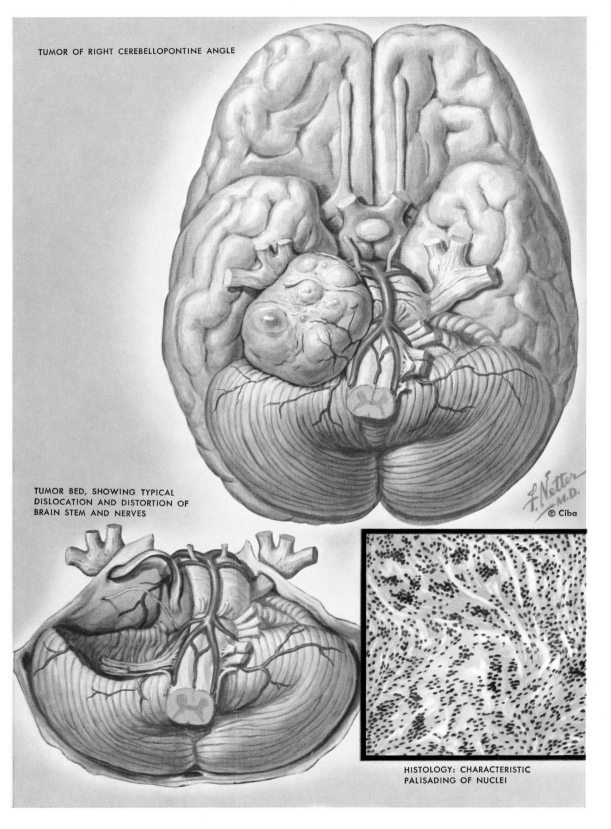

TUMOR OF RIGHT CEREBELLOPONTINE ANGLE

TUMOR BED, SHOWING TYPICAL DISLOCATION AND DISTORTION OF BRAIN STEM AND NERVES

HISTOLOGY: CHARACTERISTIC PALISADING OF NUCLEI

Acoustic tumors comprise eight to ten per cent of all intracranial neoplasms. They arise from the sheath of the eighth cranial nerve (vestibular portion) at the porus acusticus, probably from an embryonal rest. These encapsulated neoplasms, situated between the pons and cerebellum, gradually increase in size and begin to produce symptoms in adult life, frequently between the ages of 30 and 45. They are pale gray and irregularly nodular with a shiny capsule. At times they reach the size of a chestnut, usually weighing from fifteen to forty-five grams. Occasionally, there is an associated overlying arachnoidal cyst which may obscure the presence of the neoplasm.

On cross section these tumors are fibrous with yellowish-gray or reddish centers. Occasionally they are partly cystic. Most unusual are the findings of bilateral acoustic tumors associated with multiple meningiomata (von Recklinghausen).

Microscopically, these tumors consist mainly of two types of cells: (1) a fibroblastic type consisting of elongated, ovoid, spindle-shaped cells with dark-staining nuclei and fine wavy fibrils arranged in palisade formation and (2) a reticular type made up of homogenous collections of small, dark, rounded nuclei with loose, foamy cytoplasm. These tumors also show small areas of lipoid degeneration.

The symptoms produced by such tumors follow a fairly consistent pattern. At first there are symptoms of intermittent irritation, then compression of the structures occupying the cerebellopontile angle. In the late stages, because of obstruction of the aqueduct and fourth ventricle, signs of increasing intracranial pressure develop. Because acoustic tumors grow so slowly, the symptoms exist over a period of years. The earliest symptom consists of tinnitus, which is likened to the whistling of a peanut stand, associated with progressive unilateral deafness. When the deafness is complete, the tinnitus disappears. Repeated caloric tests will show progressive diminution in vestibular responses. Then follow unilateral transient numbness of the face, associated with diminished or absent corneal reflex, and at times trigeminal irritation simulating tic douloureux. Diplopia, external rectus palsy, facial asymmetry, slight drooling, and inability to tightly close the eyelids are early evidences of sixth and seventh cranial nerve involvement. When the tumor encroaches upon the cerebellum and pons and begins to obstruct the aqueduct, there appear such symptoms as periodic staggering gait, clumsiness of the hands, ataxia, nystagmus, thickness of speech, positive Romberg, dysdiadochokinesia, contralateral hemiparesis and hemihypalgesia. Somewhat later suboccipitofrontal headaches, vomiting, and papilledema appear.

Skull x-rays may show a dilated internal acoustic meatus and, in Towne's position, erosion of the petrous apex. Spinal fluid characteristically shows a very high total protein.

Among the less frequent tumors in the cerebellopontile angle which must be differentiated from acoustic tumors are papillomas, meningiomas, gliomas, and cholesteatomas. These tumors produce similar symptoms but are of different chronology and duration.

Surgical treatment of acoustic tumors is usually through a unilateral suboccipital craniotomy in the sitting position, with partial resection of the outer third of the cerebellum. Total extirpation of the tumor, which is attended by a high initial operative mortality, is complicated by complete facial paralysis. Some surgeons are content with an intracapsular tumor enucleation, which has a lower initial mortality, preserves the facial nerve, but is attended by a higher incidence of recurrence.

PLATE 99

SPINAL CORD TUMORS

The term spinal cord tumor is used to include any new growth within the vertebral canal. Such tumors may be completely extradural, they may be intradural-extramedullary (within the dura but not involving the substance of the cord), or they may be intramedullary, arising in the cord itself but occasionally invading it from without. They comprise 0.5 to 1 per cent of all tumors and occur at all ages; but seldom are they seen before the age of ten. They occur about one-tenth as frequently as intracranial neoplasms.

About 30 per cent of spinal cord tumors occur in the cervical region, 50 per cent in the thoracic region, and 20 per cent in the lumbar region. These tumors may be:

1. Primary (60-75 per cent), arising from epidural vessels or fat, dura, spinal nerves and arachnoid, or glial elements of the spinal cord.

2. Secondary (5-10 per cent), due to intraspinal extension from periosteal or osteal neoplasms in the spinal column (osteosarcoma of the vertebrae), or the intraspinal invasion by tumors arising in the neck, thorax, or abdomen.

3. Metastatic (20-25 per cent), from primary growths in the breast, thyroid, prostate, lung, kidney, or gastrointestinal tract.

About 60 or 70 per cent of all spinal cord neoplasms are found dorsal or dorsolateral to the spinal cord. However, they may be located ventrally or in various intermediate positions. With very few exceptions, such tumors are well encapsulated, clearly demarcated, and irregularly elongated. At times, they become cystic, and often they extend for two or more spinal segments. Cord tumors may lie above or beneath one or more spinal nerve roots, causing tension upon them. They may also be attached to, or intimately involve, the nerve root or the adjacent dura. The spinal cord, by slow compression, may be reduced to ribbon thinness and yet be capable of complete functional restoration.

The most frequent types of spinal cord neoplasms are neurofibromas (26-29 per cent), meningiomas (23-25 per cent), gliomas, including ependymomas (10-13 per cent), and hemangiomas (3 per cent). Of lesser frequency are lipomas, chordomas, cholesteatomas, dermoid cysts, and varicosities of the cord. Very rarely are such neoplasms multiple (neurofibromatosis). Secondary and metastatic lesions, however, are frequently multiple within the spinal canal, and invariably they involve the vertebrae. The histology of the most frequent of these primary tumors has been previously described in Plates 96, 97, and 98.

Spinal cord tumors produce symptoms and signs mainly by their mechanical effects, such as irritation and compression of the spinal nerve roots, compression and displacement of the spinal cord, and by obstruction of vascular supply. These mechanical alterations result in the symptoms and signs of progressive spinal cord compression, common to all spinal cord tumors, as well as focal or localizing neurological signs which depend upon the size, relative position and

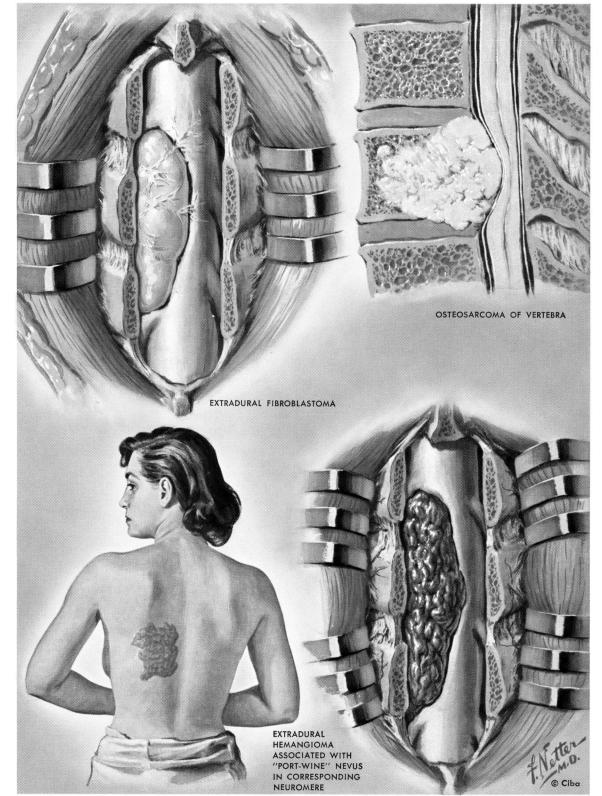

OSTEOSARCOMA OF VERTEBRA

EXTRADURAL FIBROBLASTOMA

EXTRADURAL HEMANGIOMA ASSOCIATED WITH "PORT-WINE" NEVUS IN CORRESPONDING NEUROMERE

level of the neoplasm. These focal signs are not infallible. Occasionally the sensory level may be indistinct, may shift, or even be misleading. This is particularly true if the tumor is anteriorly situated. Metastatic neoplasms to the spine may also produce bizarre findings. Because afferent sensory fibers require at least two cord segments before completely crossing to the opposite side of the spinal cord, the compressing lesion is usually found two to three dermatomes above the level of altered sensation. It is rather surprising that, on the average, spinal cord symptoms continue for 17 to 27 months before operative intervention.

General Symptoms and Signs of Spinal Neoplasms

1. Pain in the back is frequent and may, for a long time, be the only symptom of a spinal cord tumor. Yet it may be completely absent. The pain is due to nerve root or periosteal irritation or compression becoming increasingly severe and constant, but there may also be surprising periods of remission. Radicular and girdle-like pains are particularly frequent with intradural neoplasms, often simulating intercostal neuralgia, angina, and herpes zoster. On occasion, they even mimic an acute abdominal condition. The pain is characteristically made worse by activity, coughing, and straining. Lying down, which puts the spinal root on a stretch, often intensifies the pain, so that the patient is forced to sleep in a sitting position.

2. Sensory impairment may advance rapidly within several hours or days due to acute compression from a malignant tumor or hemorrhage within a benign neoplasm. However, as a rule, coldness, numbness, and tingling sensations begin in one extremity and progress slowly from below upwards until they reach the level of the lesion. Often the level of such sensory alterations has above it a narrow zone of hyperesthesia which marks the location of the tumor. Impaired sensation of pain, temperature, and light touch may precede any deficit in vibration and position sense. Sensory loss may go on to complete anesthesia, reaching a distinct dermatome level. *(Continued on following page)*

PLATE 100

SPINAL CORD TUMORS
(continued)

3. Motor weakness accompanies and keeps pace with sensory disturbances and consists chiefly of slowly increasing clumsiness, weakness, and spasticity, often starting in one extremity and spreading to the homolateral or contralateral extremity. Tumors situated anterolaterally produce homolateral weakness, diminution of touch and vibration below the level of the lesion, and impaired pain and temperature sensibility on the contralateral side (Brown-Séquard syndrome).

4. Sphincter disturbances in the early stages are marked by urgency, difficulty in starting urination and, gradually, urinary retention and overflow incontinence. Poor rectal sphincter control is a late symptom.

Spinal cord tumors also have special characteristics which depend upon their position relative to the dura and spinal nerve roots and also upon the spinal cord segment involved.

Extradural neoplasm arising from epidural structures, most often on the dorsolateral aspect, comprises about thirty to thirty-five per cent of all primary spinal cord tumors. The neurofibroma (fibroblastoma), meningioma, and hemangioma are the most frequent types, the latter at times showing a "port wine" nevus in the corresponding neuromere. Osteosarcomas, lymphosarcomas, Hodgkin's disease, cholesteatomas, dermoid cysts, and chordomas are also encountered extradurally. The clinical progress of extradural tumors is usually more rapid, showing early motor signs and delayed, indistinct sensory abnormalities. Following the withdrawal of spinal fluid by lumbar puncture, the sensory level frequently becomes more distinct. Metastatic carcinomas to the spine have preference for the extradural space and are rarely found intradurally. Tumors in this location are most likely to produce x-ray changes in the spine.

Intradural-extramedullary neoplasms comprise a little over fifty per cent of primary spinal cord tumors. The meningiomas, which are found most frequently in women over 40 between the second and eleventh thoracic vertebrae, usually adhere to and involve the undersurface of the dura. This type of tumor frequently makes a bed for itself by displacing and depressing the spinal cord.

The neurofibromas are distributed equally throughout the spinal canal and are often intimately attached to the spinal nerve roots. These tumors at times penetrate the dura and extradurally follow the nerve through the spinal foramen, forming a dumbbell-shaped neoplasm.

Lipomas have a predilection for the cervical and lumbar regions, while varicosities of the cord are more often found in thoracic segments. Xanthochromia is most frequent in tumors in this location. Tumors of the cauda equina and filum terminale are usually intradural-extramedullary. Their symptomatology is described on page 130.

Intramedullary neoplasms comprise ten to fifteen per cent of primary spinal cord tumors. They are elongated and fusiform and extend longitudinally within the spinal cord, having preference for the cervical and lumbar regions. The ependymomas and gliomas are the most frequent histologic types,

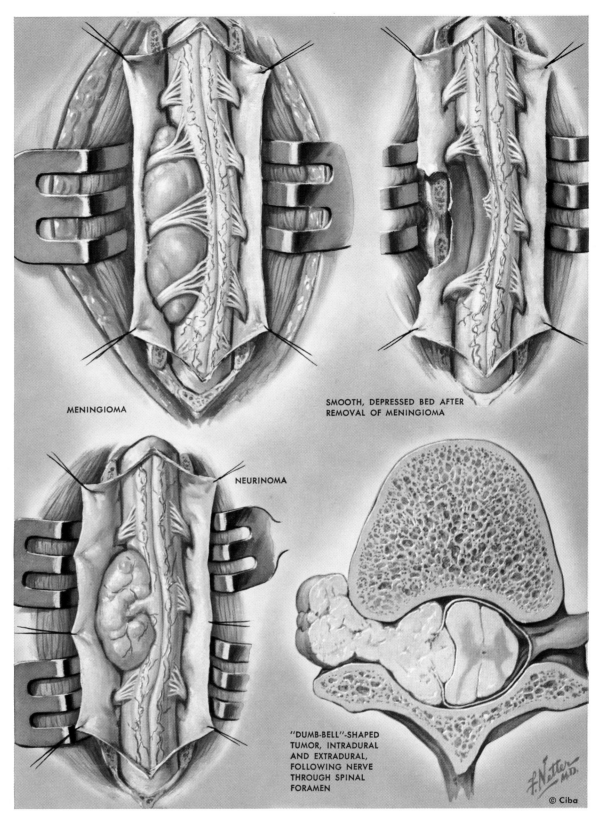

MENINGIOMA

SMOOTH, DEPRESSED BED AFTER REMOVAL OF MENINGIOMA

NEURINOMA

"DUMB-BELL"-SHAPED TUMOR, INTRADURAL AND EXTRADURAL, FOLLOWING NERVE THROUGH SPINAL FORAMEN

© Ciba

but angiomas, lipomas and dermoids may also be found within the spinal cord. These neoplasms enlarge slowly, showing bilateral impairment of pain and temperature sensibility, while tactile and position sense remain intact. Atrophy, spasticity, and fibrillations are frequent, and in many ways the symptoms clinically simulate syringomyelia. These neoplasms on occasion have been successfully and completely removed through an incision in the posterior columns of the spinal cord.

Special Localizing Neurological Signs at Different Vertebral Levels:

1. Cervical Region. Tumors in this area produce pain in the back of the neck and suboccipital region, particularly on motion. Clumsiness, weakness, and spasticity beginning in one upper extremity gradually spread to involve other extremities, finally producing a tetraplegia. If the tumor extends into the posterior cranial fossa, signs of intracranial obstruction may follow. Atrophy of the muscles about the shoulder girdle, arms, and intrinsic

hand muscles may be associated with hyperactive deep reflexes throughout, with bilateral Babinski and ankle clonus. A Horner syndrome may be present when the eighth cervical segment is involved. Focal percussion tenderness is frequently found over the spinous processes of the involved vertebrae. Sphincter disturbances are late or absent.

2. Thoracic Region. In this area abdominal and cremasteric reflexes disappear early. A band of hyperesthesia is frequently found just above the level of impaired sensation. Lower motor neuron signs of spastic paresis of the lower extremities with corresponding pathological toe signs and sphincter disturbances are typical findings. Percussion tenderness over any thoracic spine has important localizing value. Compression at the tenth thoracic segment will cause paralysis of the lower parts of the recti abdominalis. This can be demonstrated by having the patient raise his head. Unantagonized contraction of the upper rectus muscles will cause the umbilicus to move cephalad (Beevor's sign). (*Concluded on following page*)

PLATE 101

SPINAL CORD TUMORS
(concluded)

3. Cauda equina and filum terminale. Tumors of the conus and cauda equina begin with severe low back pain radiating first down one leg, then down the other — "bilateral sciatica." The sensory deficit may at first involve only one nerve root, but gradually spreads asymmetrically over the saddle area. Weakness usually starts with foot drop and dragging of one leg, slowly progressing to involve the entire leg, and then spreading to the other extremity. Sphincter disturbances and impaired sexual powers are early manifestations, particularly when the filum terminale interna is the primary seat of the tumor. Knee jerks and ankle jerks gradually diminish, finally disappearing. Cystometric tests will invariably show evidence of a neurogenic bladder. Decubitus ulcers over the sacrum, as well as ulcers on the heels and ankles, are frequently seen with neoplasms in this region. On the other hand, large neoplasms within the cauda equina have been removed in the absence of any abnormal neurologic sign. Giant herniated intervertebral discs in the lumbar region can readily reproduce the symptomatology of a cauda equina neoplasm.

Diagnosis. Patients with the history of progressive weakness and spasticity of the extremities, having disturbed sphincter function and showing a clear-cut sensory level, abnormal reflexes, and focal spinal tenderness, present no great difficulty in diagnosis. But if the neoplasm is small, producing only a few symptoms and equivocal neurological signs, the diagnosis is difficult and can be accurately established only with the aid of laboratory facilities, especially studies of spinal fluid and x-ray (flat plates and after use of a radio-opaque medium).

Spinal fluid studies consist mainly of manometric tests and spinal fluid analysis. The manometric test determines the patency of the subarachnoid space above the point of lumbar puncture. It should be done in the lateral recumbent position, and the excursions of the spinal fluid in the manometer during normal respiration, coughing, straining and jugular compression should be charted to rule out a partial or complete subarachnoid block. The manometric test by no means rules out a deforming or destructive lesion below the point of lumbar puncture. In addition, partial subarachnoid block can easily be missed. After withdrawal of spinal fluid for analysis, there may be sudden increase in symptoms with a more distinct sensory level. Subarachnoid block may also be due to inflammatory subarachnoid adhesions, pachymeningitis, extradural

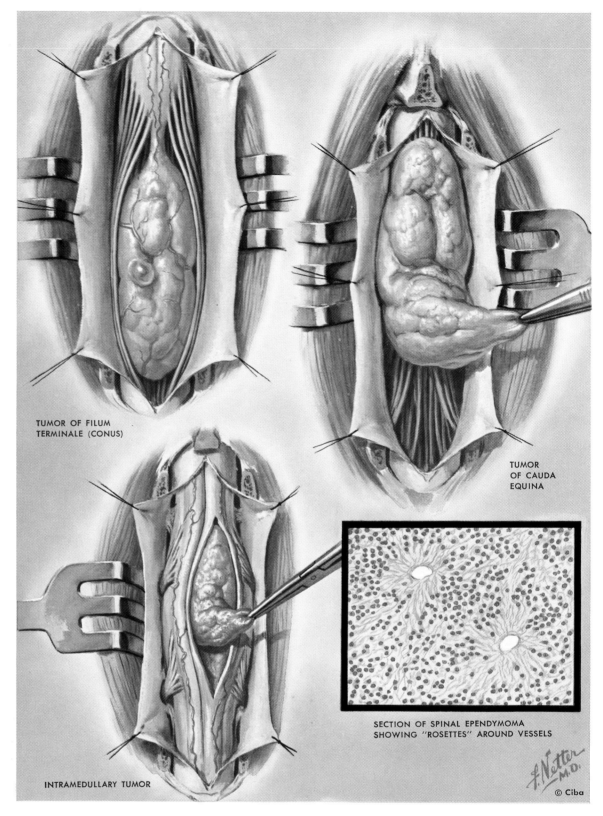

TUMOR OF FILUM
TERMINALE (CONUS)

TUMOR
OF CAUDA
EQUINA

INTRAMEDULLARY TUMOR

SECTION OF SPINAL EPENDYMOMA
SHOWING "ROSETTES" AROUND VESSELS

abscess, congenital and osseous deformities, and fracture dislocations of the spine.

About fifty per cent of obstructing neoplasms of the spinal cord show yellow (xanthochromic) spinal fluid. This is more likely the more caudad the neoplasm. Froin's syndrome, a condition of the spinal fluid found when blockage has occurred, is characterized by xanthochromia, high total protein, rapid coagulation, and increase of lymphocytes. This syndrome is not unusual in spinal cord neoplasms; it may also occur in giant herniated intervertebral discs. Spinal fluid total protein may be normal (20-40 mg.) with neoplasms, but usually is over 100 mg. per cent.

X-ray studies of the spine may show localized bony erosion, calcification within the neoplasm, partial or complete absorption of one or more pedicles, scalloping of the posterior aspects of the vertebral bodies, widening of the interpediculate spaces, and enlargement of the spinal canal due to the expanding neoplasm.

A radio-opaque medium, such as Pantopaque, which is

heavier than spinal fluid, may be injected into the subarachnoid space. Under fluoroscopy on a tilt-table this contrast medium can be guided and observed for various delays, deformities and defects within the subarachnoid space, and spot films taken instantaneously. About 6 cc. is used, and this can be withdrawn after the studies are completed. To date this contrast medium serves as the most reliable means of differentiating neoplastic from various congenital, inflammatory and degenerative lesions of the spinal cord.

Treatment is surgical. Over eighty-five per cent of primary neoplasms of the spinal cord are benign and can be completely enucleated. Following laminectomy, over ninety per cent of these patients recover completely, though at times very slowly, and finally are able to resume their previous gainful activity. The operative mortality in most neurosurgical clinics is less than one per cent. There are few procedures in surgery that bring such dramatic, gratifying and satisfactory results as the removal of a benign spinal cord neoplasm.

PLATE 102

TUMORS METASTATIC TO BRAIN AND SPINE

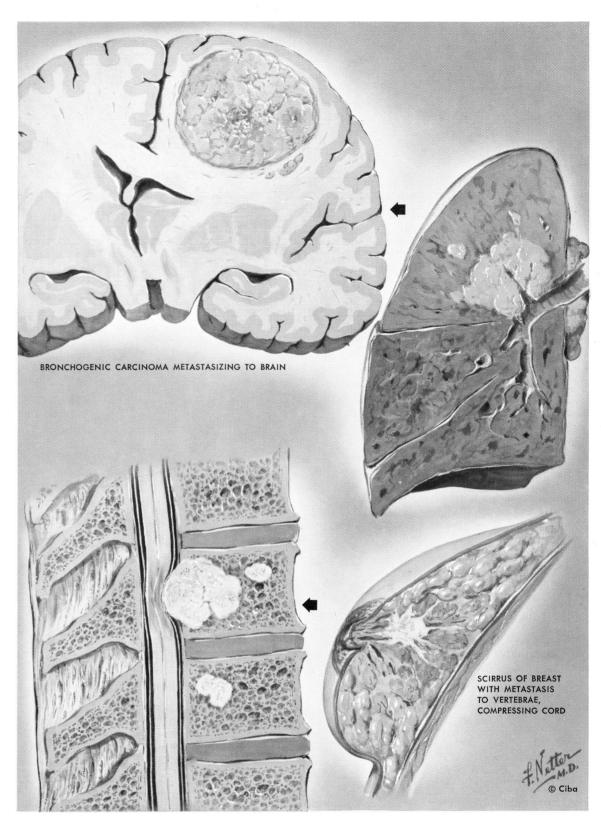

BRONCHOGENIC CARCINOMA METASTASIZING TO BRAIN

SCIRRUS OF BREAST WITH METASTASIS TO VERTEBRAE, COMPRESSING CORD

Neoplasms metastatic to the brain comprise three to five per cent of all brain tumors, and in over sixty per cent of the patients they are multiple, involving one or both cerebral hemispheres. Occasionally, they are limited to the posterior fossa. The primary extracranial neoplasm may be so small and inactive as to escape detection, and the intracranial metastases may be encountered unexpectedly at operation. In some patients a surprisingly long interval (5 to 15 years) may elapse from the removal of the primary growth to the onset of the intracranial symptoms. The most frequent sites of primary neoplasms which metastasize to the brain are the lung (thirty-five per cent, bronchogenic), the breast (twenty-five per cent), the kidney (seven per cent, hypernephroma), the thyroid, prostate, and gastrointestinal tract. Metastases to the skull and brain are chiefly from the breast, thyroid, prostate, and kidney. Metastatic melano- and lymphosarcoma are seldom found as solitary lesions.

Metastases to the brain vary considerably in size, shape, number, and location. Usually, they favor the cerebral cortex or lie just beneath it. The lesions appear well circumscribed with a wide margin of adjacent cerebral edema. Areas of cystic degeneration may also be encountered. The histology of the metastatic lesions, of course, resembles that of the primary growth.

The clinical course is usually rapid following the onset of intracranial symptoms and signs. Because the lesions are often multiple, the neurologic signs are frequently variable, widespread, and perplexing. A history of a pre-existing malignant growth or a chest film showing primary or metastatic lesions readily establishes the diagnosis. However, in some patients a thorough, systematic search may be necessary in order to ferret out the primary lesion.

Craniotomy and decompression with removal of the main metastatic mass may be followed by considerable palliative relief. This is particularly true with metastatic

hypernephroma. In most instances, however, postoperative prolongation of life is seldom over two months.

Metastatic tumors to the spine occur usually beyond the age of forty. The most frequent primary foci are the breast, thyroid, prostate, kidney, and gastrointestinal tract. The carcinomatous cells reach the spine by the blood stream or lymphatics and frequently lodge within the lateral aspects of the vertebral bodies or in the extradural space. Multiple myeloma, melano- and lymphosarcoma, and Hodgkin's disease also metastasize to the spinal column by way of the bloodstream and also by contiguity, having a special preference for the spinous processes and the vertebral arches. These extradural lesions involve the periosteum and compress the spinal nerve roots relatively early, producing severe and intractable back pain. As the malignant cells multiply, the vertebral bodies are subject to gradual destruction, compression, and finally sudden collapse. The histology of the metastatic lesions will depend upon the character of the primary growth.

Intense, intractable back pain is the most outstanding

and most persistent symptom of a metastatic neoplasm to the spine. For weeks or months such pain may be the only symptom. Usually, it is made worse by activity and fails to respond to all forms of medication, including morphine. Focal or percussion tenderness over one or several spinous processes or over the sacrum may be the only significant finding. X-rays of the spine or pelvis may be negative for a long time in spite of extensive pathologic bone infiltration. With the sudden collapse of the involved vertebral bodies and the accompanying impaired spinal cord circulation, there follows within hours or days acute and often complete spinal cord compression. The result is a flaccid paralysis of the extremities, sensory impairment which progresses upward to a distinct level of anesthesia, loss of sphincter control and absent deep reflexes. Spinal fluid studies may show xanthochromia, elevated total protein and, not infrequently, complete subarachnoid block. The exact level of the lesion can be verified by studies with a radio-opaque medium. Laminectomy for amelioration of symptoms has at times been surprisingly beneficial.

PLATE 103

SYRINGOMYELIA, HEMATOMYELIA AND HYDROMYELIA

Syringomyelia is a central cavitation of the spinal cord, most often affecting men (seventy per cent) during the second and third decades of life. It is found most frequently in the lower cervical and upper thoracic regions, but it also occurs in the medulla (syringobulbia) or brain stem (syringopontia). The cavity is near the central canal, is elongated and fusiform, and extends longitudinally for six to seven or more spinal segments.

Syringomyelia may result from (1) congenital maldevelopment (abiotrophy), (2) degenerative changes secondary to intraspinal hemorrhage or thrombosis, (3) dural and meningeal constrictions, or (4) atrophic gliosis secondary to an intramedullary neoplasm.

The fusiform bulging of the spinal cord is due to xanthochromic fluid within the syrinx, which is smoothly lined with glial and fibrous elements or ependymal cells. Degenerative changes start in the anterior commissure, involving the crossing pain and temperature fibers about the central canal, and steadily but slowly spread asymmetrically and longitudinally, forming a fusiform cyst with compression of the anterior horn cells and pyramidal tracts. This pathologic process may continue over a period of ten to twenty years or longer with periods of quiescence lasting for years. The process, however, may terminate acutely following a hemorrhage within the syrinx.

The earliest symptoms are awkwardness and weakness of the hands and fingers. The atrophic changes which follow eventually give the appearance of a "claw" hand and spread to involve the shoulder girdle. Spinal root pains are unusual and, if present, mild. Most characteristic is the dissociation of impaired pain and temperature sensibility with intact light touch and muscle sense. Vibration and position sense may be defective. Fibrillations of the involved muscles are frequent. Hyperactivity of deep reflexes and pyramidal tract signs are not unusual unless the lesion is in the lumbar region, where it produces a flaccid weakness of the lower extremities with diminished to absent deep reflexes. Vasomotor disturbances of the extremities, swelling of the hands, thickening of the skin, and arthropathies (Morvan's disease) may be encountered. When the cavitation involves the medulla or brain stem, we find, in addition, disturbances of the vagus, vestibular nuclei, trigeminal tract, and medial lemniscus. Spinal fluid studies

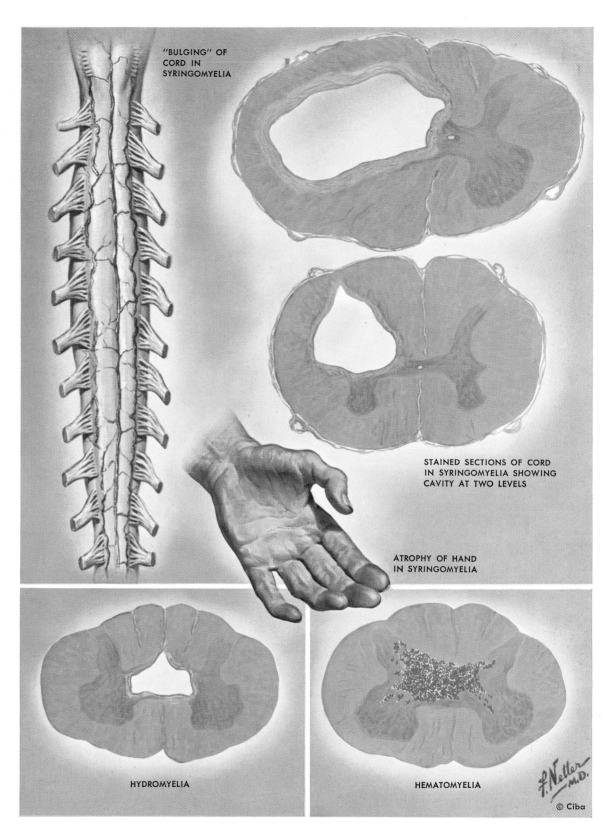

"BULGING" OF CORD IN SYRINGOMYELIA

STAINED SECTIONS OF CORD IN SYRINGOMYELIA SHOWING CAVITY AT TWO LEVELS

ATROPHY OF HAND IN SYRINGOMYELIA

HYDROMYELIA

HEMATOMYELIA

are within normal limits, but occasionally they show an elevated total protein and partial subarachnoid block.

Hematomyelia is due to hemorrhage within the spinal cord. It may result from (1) direct trauma — such as spinal fracture, stab or bullet wound, (2) transmitted injury to the spine — from fall on buttocks, severe strain, shell burst, or diving accident, or (3) intraspinal rupture of a miliary aneurysm, hemorrhage within a syrinx, blood dyscrasia, or caisson disease. Usually, the intraspinal hemorrhage follows immediately after the injury, but it may be delayed for several hours. In some instances where there is progressive myelomalacia, the hemorrhage may be delayed one or two weeks (delayed apoplexy).

The intraspinal hemorrhage may be petechial or massive, varying considerably in size and shape. It extends longitudinally for several segments to involve mainly the gray matter. The swollen and bluish spinal cord may also show traces of blood on the surface. Within the cord the hemorrhagic areas are arranged in perivascular cuffs with central thrombosis, edema, and disrupted architecture. In

massive hemorrhage, the involved spinal cord may be reduced to a pulp. Blood absorption, organization and repair may continue for many months and consist chiefly of phagocytosis by gitter cells, astrocytic and glial reaction, and changes in the anterior horn cells. Areas of softening remain with cystic cavities lined with glial and endothelial cells which have all the characteristics of syringomyelia. The symptoms and signs are in proportion to the extent of intraspinal hemorrhage and disorganization. If the hemorrhage is small, the abnormal neurological findings are correspondingly few and recovery surprisingly good, but seldom is it complete. If only one side of the cord is involved, a Brown-Séquard syndrome may result. If hemorrhage is massive, there follow a flaccid paralysis, a sensory level of anesthesia, loss of sphincter function, and absent reflexes.

Hydromyelia is a cystic dilatation of the central canal. It may be the result of congenital defects, trauma, central gliosis, or an early phase of syringomyelia. It may also be secondary to hematomyelia.

PLATE 104

MULTIPLE SCLEROSIS, AMYOTROPHIC LATERAL SCLEROSIS AND COMBINED SCLEROSIS

Multiple (Disseminated-Insular) Sclerosis

A demyelinizing degenerating disease affecting the brain and spinal cord. It is most common among young females (13 to 30 years) and is found more frequently in cold, moist and damp areas of the temperate zone. The etiology of multiple sclerosis is still unknown.

At first there is swelling and then demyelinization of the medullary sheath, which exposes nerve cylinders. This is followed by glial proliferation and organization. The well-demarcated sclerotic plaques which result are scattered irregularly throughout the white and gray matter of the brain and spinal cord. Most frequently, the involved areas are found in the cervical enlargement, the ventricles, pons, cerebellum, basal ganglia, and medulla. Very rarely are spinal roots involved.

The disease is variable and unpredictable with great fluctuation in neurologic symptoms and signs. There are three main types: (1) the acute form with a survival period of 10 to 20 months, (2) the chronic progressive form, which has a slow downhill course for many years (20 to 30), and (3) the remittent form, which has a fair prognosis for any one period of exacerbation.

The cardinal signs of intention tremor, nystagmus and scanning speech are found only in patients with fairly advanced lesions. The earliest symptoms are fleeting, deceptive, and fluctuating. Such symptoms as diplopia, blurred vision, urinary incontinence, spasticity and ataxia of the extremities, and euphoria are transient and may disappear for no obvious reason. Hysteria is often suspected. Absence of abdominal and cremasteric reflexes persists. A remission may last several months or even years. An exacerbation of signs may include optic pallor (temporal) going on to optic atrophy, scanning speech, horizontal nystagmus, intention tremors, ataxic and spastic gait, Romberg's sign, absent abdominal and cremasteric reflexes, and pathologic toe signs. Sensory defects are inconstant. In late stages there is deterioration of mind and personality. Spinal fluid shows a few cells, slight elevation in total protein, and paretic gold curve (fifty per cent) but negative Wassermann.

Amyotrophic Lateral Sclerosis

First described by Charcot in 1865, it is a slowly progressive disease of unknown etiology which begins in adult life and involves the anterior horn cells as well as the pyramidal tracts. In later stages, the motor nuclei of the medulla and pons become involved.

Atrophy of the anterior horn cells and ventral roots is most frequently found in the cervical enlargement. Degenerative changes of the pyramidal tracts show decreasing medullation of nerve fibers with neuroglial proliferation. These have been traced to motor cells in the cerebral cortex.

Symptoms start insidiously during middle life with fatigue, obscure pains, and awkwardness of fine finger movements.

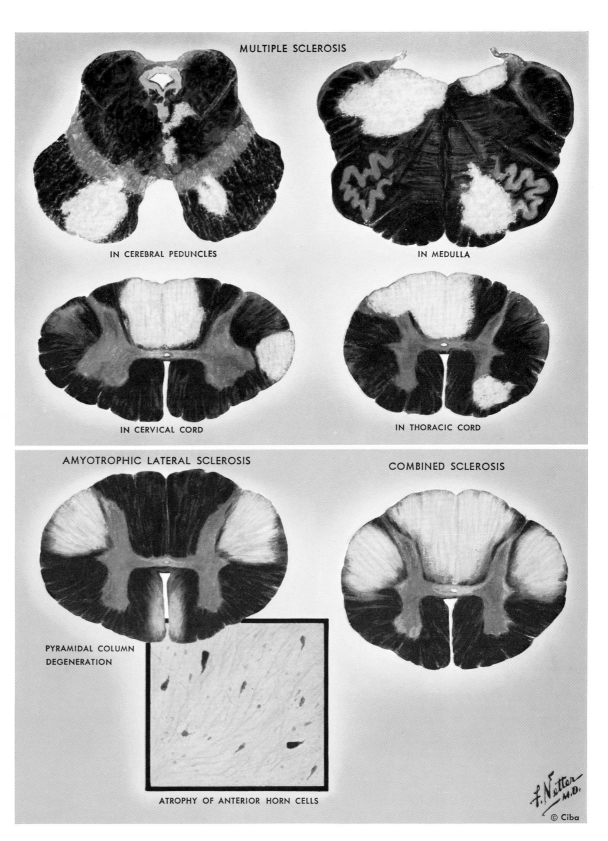

MULTIPLE SCLEROSIS

IN CEREBRAL PEDUNCLES

IN MEDULLA

IN CERVICAL CORD

IN THORACIC CORD

AMYOTROPHIC LATERAL SCLEROSIS

COMBINED SCLEROSIS

PYRAMIDAL COLUMN DEGENERATION

ATROPHY OF ANTERIOR HORN CELLS

F. Netter, M.D.

© Ciba

There is wasting of the small muscles of the hands with relative increase of spasticity of the flexor muscles over the extensors. Electrical tests show partial or complete nerve degeneration. Following involvement of the hands, atrophy of the arms, shoulder girdle, and trapezius occurs. One side may be more involved than the other. Muscle fibrillations are common. When nerve involvement spreads to the medulla and brain stem, we find tongue fibrillations, jaw clonus, dysarthria, and dysphagia. Involvement of the lower extremities is accompanied by a spastic gait, hyperactive deep reflexes, and pathologic toe signs. Sensation is unaffected and sphincters are almost never disturbed. Spinal fluid is normal. The course is downhill; survival is seldom more than three years.

Combined Sclerosis (Subacute)

A progressive, degenerative disease involving the posterior and lateral columns of the spinal cord. It frequently starts without known cause but may precede, coexist with, or follow pernicious anemia. It has also been found associated with chronic debilitating, cachectic and deficiency states. Axis cylinder and medullary sheath degeneration is most frequent in the mid-thoracic region, involving posterior columns, direct and indirect pyramidal tracts, and direct cerebellar tracts.

Onset is insidious with generalized weakness and vague gastrointestinal discomforts. Most characteristic is a sensation of "pins and needles" in toes and finger tips, which is symmetrical. Atrophy of the arms is more striking than that of the legs. Touch, vibration, position, deep pain, and muscle sensibility are steadily impaired, and the Romberg test becomes positive. Pain is uncommon, but there are sensations of girdle constriction. The lower extremities fatigue easily; the gait becomes spastic and ataxic with hyperactive deep reflexes and pathologic toe signs. The sphincters are seldom affected. In the terminal stages flaccid paraplegia, loss of reflexes, and mental changes appear. Occasionally, short remissions occur, but the disease is ultimately fatal, lasting 2 to 6 years. Spinal fluid studies are normal.

SUBJECT INDEX

(Numerals refer to pages, *not* plates)

THE CIBA COLLECTION OF MEDICAL ILLUSTRATIONS

SUPPLEMENT TO VOLUME I

NERVOUS SYSTEM

A Compilation of Paintings on the
Anatomy and Functional Relations of the

HYPOTHALAMUS

Prepared by

FRANK H. NETTER, M. D.

In collaboration with

W. R. INGRAM, PH.D.

Edited by

ERNST OPPENHEIMER, M.D.

Commissioned and published by

CIBA

CONTENTS

INTRODUCTION

Scientific interest in the hypothalamus began a little over 50 years ago. During the intervening years, there has been a gradual widening of knowledge with slowly progressive clarification of hypothalamic function. This has been accomplished despite the great technical difficulties imposed by the relative inaccessibility of the hypothalamus and its close physical relationship with other vital structures.

Much of the early work was devoted to the relationship between the hypothalamus and the pituitary. However, the impressive results of experiments on the visceral effects of destructive and irritative lesions of the hypothalamus led to the belief that here are located the controlling mechanisms of autonomic function. Indeed, some authorities have perhaps logically extended this concept to include the view that the hypothalamus is a center for the control of emotion. These ideas may have resulted from a somewhat excessive narrowness of viewpoint concerning localization of cerebral function.

The hypothalamus is unquestionably of great significance both phylogenetically and anthropologically. It plays striking rôles in many aspects of mammalian physiology. It undoubtedly contains integrative mechanisms which, in addition to their effect on behavior patterns, also aid in regulating the basic life functions of the organism. However, this integration is apparently carried out through its relationships with other parts of the nervous system, including the so-called higher levels, as well as through the endocrine system. It is in this field of interrelationship that some of the most pressing problems lie. It must be appreciated that while this interesting region of the brain is only part of a system of complex circuits, it is a very important link in these circuits and is so strategically placed that its derangement may have profound effects.

Space limitation has made it impossible to mention everything that is to be found in the literature on this subject. In some areas we may be guilty of oversimplification; this is inevitable in the present stage of our knowledge. However, the experimental evidence upon which the following material is based does at present appear to be both sound and reliable.

W. R. INGRAM, PH.D.
Professor and Head of the Department of Anatomy,
State University of Iowa, Iowa City, Iowa

PRINTED IN U.S.A.

ORIGINAL PRINTING BY COLORPRESS, NEW YORK, N.Y.
COLOR ENGRAVINGS BY EMBASSY PHOTO ENGRAVING CO., INC., NEW YORK, N.Y.
OFFSET CONVERSION BY THE CASE-HOYT CORP., ROCHESTER, N.Y.
THIS PRINTING BY THE CASE-HOYT CORP., ROCHESTER, N.Y.

PLATE I

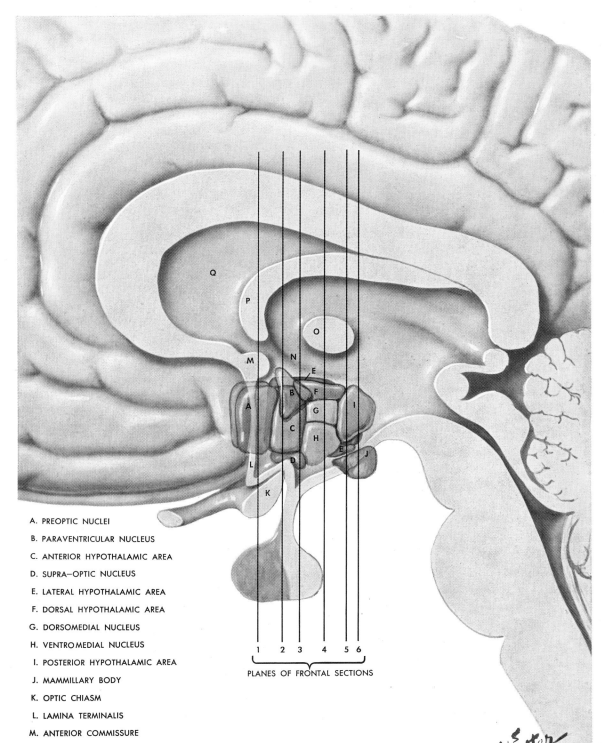

GENERAL TOPOGRAPHY
Planes of Frontal Sections

A. PREOPTIC NUCLEI

B. PARAVENTRICULAR NUCLEUS

C. ANTERIOR HYPOTHALAMIC AREA

D. SUPRA–OPTIC NUCLEUS

E. LATERAL HYPOTHALAMIC AREA

F. DORSAL HYPOTHALAMIC AREA

G. DORSOMEDIAL NUCLEUS

H. VENTROMEDIAL NUCLEUS

I. POSTERIOR HYPOTHALAMIC AREA

J. MAMMILLARY BODY

K. OPTIC CHIASM

L. LAMINA TERMINALIS

M. ANTERIOR COMMISSURE

N. HYPOTHALAMIC SULCUS

O. INTERMEDIATE MASS OF THALAMUS

P. FORNIX

Q. SEPTUM PELLUCIDUM

PLANES OF FRONTAL SECTIONS

The hypothalamus, a part of the diencephalon, is bordered anteriorly by the *lamina terminalis,* with the *anterior commissure* above and the *optic chiasm* below; posteriorly by the interpeduncular fossa; dorsally by the *hypothalamic sulcus,* marking the junction with the thalamus; and ventrally by the bulging tuber cinereum which tapers into the funnel-shaped infundibulum. Laterally, as seen in the subsequent frontal sections (see Plates 2, 3 and 4, pages 148-150), principal boundaries are provided by the substantia innominata, the internal capsule, the subthalamic nucleus and the basis pedunculi (see Plate 4, page 150). Mostly within these boundaries, but spilling over them in places are clustered a number of masses of cells which are referred to as the hypothalamic nuclei. Many of these groups of cells are well defined in some forms of lower animals. In man, however, they have become much less distinct and more diffuse, with a few exceptions, such as the *supra-optic* and *paraventricular nuclei*

and the mammillary complex. Many of these cell groups are, as a matter of fact, more distinct in the fetus than in adult man. One or two groups, however, are better developed in the human brain than in other species. This diffuseness is further complicated by the fact that many of these nuclei contain several histologically different types of neurons, and this intermingling of cell types, together with certain physiologic evidence, makes one wonder if many of these anatomic subdivisions have specific functional significance. Indeed, definite physiologic function has been unequivocally shown for only one or two pairs of these nuclei. Other localization of function thus far is, at best, regional.

The boundaries of these nuclei are not always based on concentrations of cells, but fiber bundles

and infiltrating fiber masses aid in setting up the topography of the region. Although specific allocation of function has as yet been largely lacking, the morphologic establishment of these entities can be valuable to the physiologist, pathologist and clinician in providing a means of descriptive communication. Observations based on precise localization of lesions, of points of stimulation or of the pickup of electrical phenomena or chemical change may some day fill out the many gaps in our knowledge of this small but complicated region.

The accompanying plate indicates the six planes of frontal sections upon which the subsequent three diagrammatic plates are based. These planes transect each of the principal nuclear groups of the hypothalamus.

PLATE 2

SECTIONS THROUGH HYPOTHALAMUS I

Planes 1 and 2

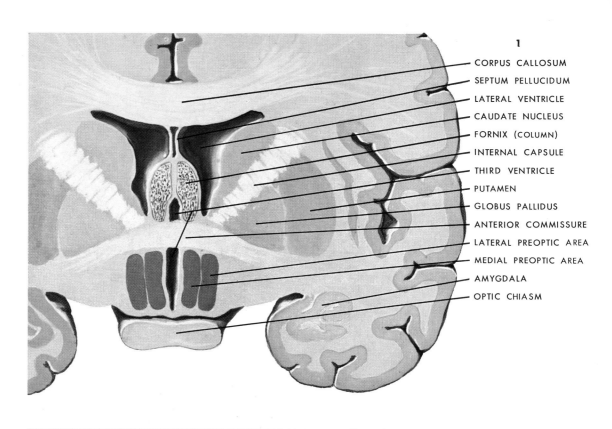

1

- CORPUS CALLOSUM
- SEPTUM PELLUCIDUM
- LATERAL VENTRICLE
- CAUDATE NUCLEUS
- FORNIX (COLUMN)
- INTERNAL CAPSULE
- THIRD VENTRICLE
- PUTAMEN
- GLOBUS PALLIDUS
- ANTERIOR COMMISSURE
- LATERAL PREOPTIC AREA
- MEDIAL PREOPTIC AREA
- AMYGDALA
- OPTIC CHIASM

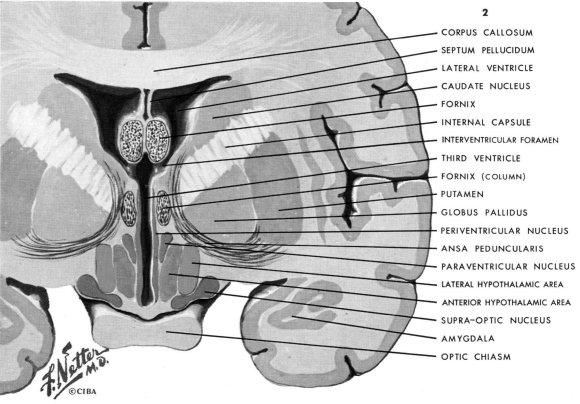

2

- CORPUS CALLOSUM
- SEPTUM PELLUCIDUM
- LATERAL VENTRICLE
- CAUDATE NUCLEUS
- FORNIX
- INTERNAL CAPSULE
- INTERVENTRICULAR FORAMEN
- THIRD VENTRICLE
- FORNIX (COLUMN)
- PUTAMEN
- GLOBUS PALLIDUS
- PERIVENTRICULAR NUCLEUS
- ANSA PEDUNCULARIS
- PARAVENTRICULAR NUCLEUS
- LATERAL HYPOTHALAMIC AREA
- ANTERIOR HYPOTHALAMIC AREA
- SUPRA-OPTIC NUCLEUS
- AMYGDALA
- OPTIC CHIASM

The *preoptic areas* are often grouped with the hypothalamic nuclei, although it is said that they are more properly part of the telencephalon than of the diencephalon. Although they extend forward beyond the *optic chiasm,* good evidence is available that they participate in temperature regulation (see Plate 14, page 160) and perhaps some other autonomic functions. They are closely related to the olfactory regions (see CIBA COLLECTION, Volume 1, *Nervous System,* page 62) laterally, and the medial forebrain bundle (see Plate 5, page 151) passes through the lateral one. This bundle forms connections between medial rhinencephalic structures, and possibly the anterior striatopallidal region and the hypothalamus and lower brain stem regions. Farther caudally (Plane 2), the *anterior* and *lateral hypothalamic areas* appear, the latter giving passage also to the medial forebrain bundle. The cell population of these areas at this level is

fairly uniform and consists of small neurons, except for a few large neurons scattered along a line between the paraventricular and supra-optic nuclei.

The latter two nuclei are the most conspicuous of the anterior and supra-optic regions. The *paraventricular nuclei* are slender wedge-shaped groups near the *third ventricle* ventromedial to the fornices. The *supra-optic nucleus* overlays the beginning of the optic tract, which separates it into two portions, a large anterolateral and a small posteromedial, which are united by a small layer of cells. The neurons of these two nuclei are large, with dark-staining Nissl substance condensed at the periphery, with relatively clear perinuclear regions. Both nuclei send fibers down the infundibular stem into the posterior lobe of the pituitary gland (see Plate 1, page 147 and Plate

10, page 156), although not all the cells of the paraventricular nuclei have this destination.

This portion of the hypothalamus is closely related topographically to the *ansa peduncularis* and the inferior thalamic peduncle, from which it receives some fibers which probably set up important connections with the insula, substantia innominata and thalamus. Connections with the *septum pellucidum* are also a feature of this region. It is a question, however, how many such connections are possessed by the supra-optic and paraventricular nuclei.

Several other smaller nuclei (not illustrated), including the nucleus suprachiasmaticus and nucleus supra-opticus diffusus, are also present in this region. Their significance is unknown, but they are related to the supra-optic commissures.

PLATE 3

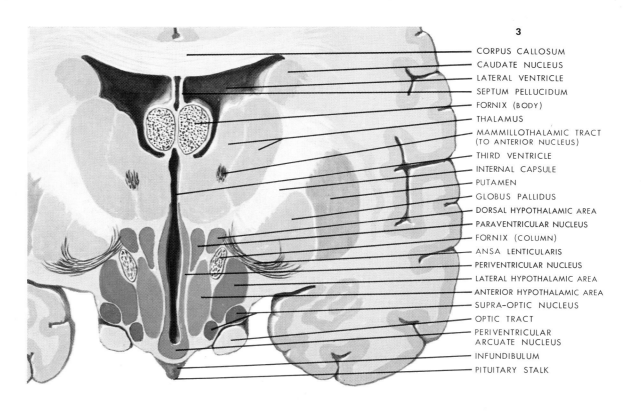

3

CORPUS CALLOSUM
CAUDATE NUCLEUS
LATERAL VENTRICLE
SEPTUM PELLUCIDUM
FORNIX (BODY)
THALAMUS
MAMMILLOTHALAMIC TRACT
(TO ANTERIOR NUCLEUS)
THIRD VENTRICLE
INTERNAL CAPSULE
PUTAMEN
GLOBUS PALLIDUS
DORSAL HYPOTHALAMIC AREA
PARAVENTRICULAR NUCLEUS
FORNIX (COLUMN)
ANSA LENTICULARIS
PERIVENTRICULAR NUCLEUS
LATERAL HYPOTHALAMIC AREA
ANTERIOR HYPOTHALAMIC AREA
SUPRA-OPTIC NUCLEUS
OPTIC TRACT
PERIVENTRICULAR
ARCUATE NUCLEUS
INFUNDIBULUM
PITUITARY STALK

SECTIONS THROUGH HYPOTHALAMUS II

Planes 3 and 4

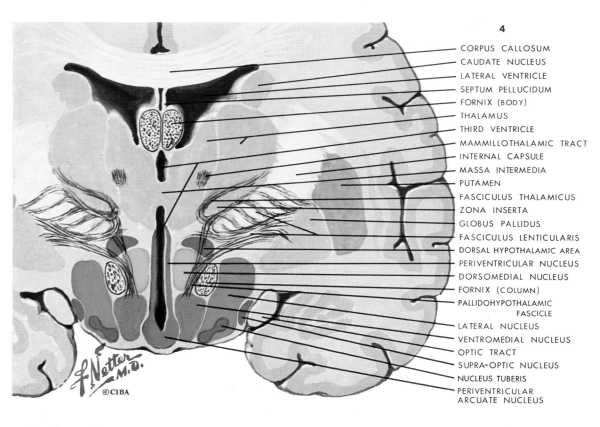

4

CORPUS CALLOSUM
CAUDATE NUCLEUS
LATERAL VENTRICLE
SEPTUM PELLUCIDUM
FORNIX (BODY)
THALAMUS
THIRD VENTRICLE
MAMMILLOTHALAMIC TRACT
INTERNAL CAPSULE
MASSA INTERMEDIA
PUTAMEN
FASCICULUS THALAMICUS
ZONA INSERTA
GLOBUS PALLIDUS
FASCICULUS LENTICULARIS
DORSAL HYPOTHALAMIC AREA
PERIVENTRICULAR NUCLEUS
DORSOMEDIAL NUCLEUS
FORNIX (COLUMN)
PALLIDOHYPOTHALAMIC
FASCICLE
LATERAL NUCLEUS
VENTROMEDIAL NUCLEUS
OPTIC TRACT
SUPRA-OPTIC NUCLEUS
NUCLEUS TUBERIS
PERIVENTRICULAR
ARCUATE NUCLEUS

In the tuberal portion of the hypothalamus (Plane 3), as the *optic tracts* diverge, some changes in configuration take place. A few cells of the *supra-optic nuclei* may remain, and the *lateral hypothalamic area* continues caudally in its characteristic position. The latter is now separated from the medial structures by the *fornix,* which passes caudoventrally through the tuber cinereum. In the medial region the small-celled *anterior nucleus* (or area) gives way to two good-sized nuclei, the *dorsomedial* and *ventromedial hypothalamic* groups (Plane 4). In adult man these are rather poorly defined, especially the former, which is more an area than a nucleus, consisting

of rather small cells. The ventromedial nucleus is well defined in lower animals and in the human fetus and can be seen in propitious adult material. Its neurons are more densely grouped than are those in the dorsomedial nucleus.

A rather conspicuous bundle of fibers, the *pallido-hypothalamic fascicle,* which seems to arise in the *globus pallidus,* enters the ventromedial nucleus, which also has been said to have important connections with the orbital portion of the frontal lobe and with the amygdaloid complex (see also Plate 6, page 152). The medial region of the hypothalamus also has rich connections with the thalamus, in part via the *periventricular nuclei.* The latter are thin sheets of small, moderately dark-staining neurons lining the lower part of the third ventricle, external to the

ependyma. At their lower end they expand into the *periventricular arcuate nuclei.* These structures appear to set up relays of unmyelinated fibers between the thalamus and hypothalamus.

Embedded in the lateral area some small irregular nuclei appear, the *nuclei tuberis.* The lateral nucleus itself, hitherto uniformly composed of small cells, at the level of the ventromedial nucleus begins to contain rather dense, irregularly grouped masses of large cells containing considerable Nissl substance. It is believed that these give rise to fairly large fibers which form part of the descending efferent pathways from the hypothalamus. Through these nuclei the fibers of the medial forebrain bundle (see Plate 5, page 151) continue to descend, many of them ending in the hypothalamus.

PLATE 4

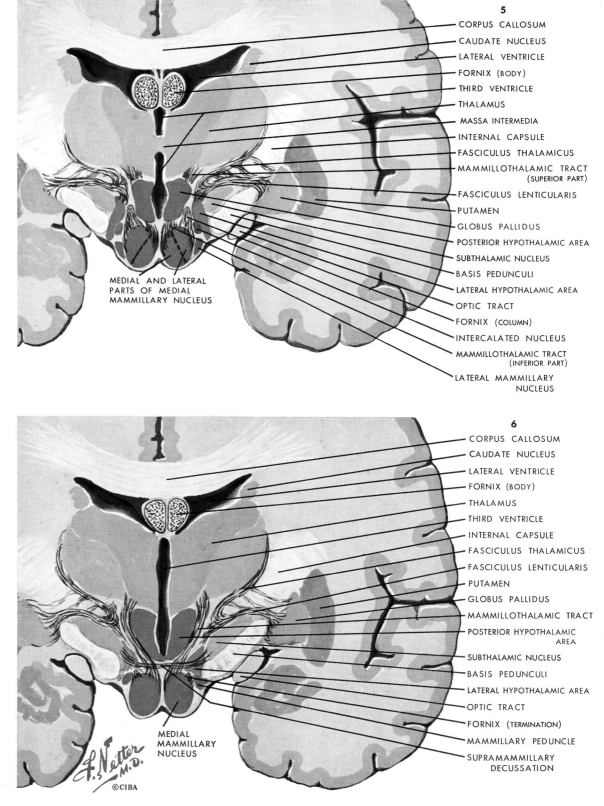

5

CORPUS CALLOSUM
CAUDATE NUCLEUS
LATERAL VENTRICLE
FORNIX (BODY)
THIRD VENTRICLE
THALAMUS
MASSA INTERMEDIA
INTERNAL CAPSULE
FASCICULUS THALAMICUS
MAMMILLOTHALAMIC TRACT (SUPERIOR PART)
FASCICULUS LENTICULARIS
PUTAMEN
GLOBUS PALLIDUS
POSTERIOR HYPOTHALAMIC AREA
SUBTHALAMIC NUCLEUS
BASIS PEDUNCULI
LATERAL HYPOTHALAMIC AREA
OPTIC TRACT
FORNIX (COLUMN)
INTERCALATED NUCLEUS
MAMMILLOTHALAMIC TRACT (INFERIOR PART)
LATERAL MAMMILLARY NUCLEUS

MEDIAL AND LATERAL PARTS OF MEDIAL MAMMILLARY NUCLEUS

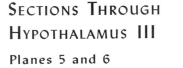

SECTIONS THROUGH HYPOTHALAMUS III

Planes 5 and 6

6

CORPUS CALLOSUM
CAUDATE NUCLEUS
LATERAL VENTRICLE
FORNIX (BODY)
THALAMUS
THIRD VENTRICLE
INTERNAL CAPSULE
FASCICULUS THALAMICUS
FASCICULUS LENTICULARIS
PUTAMEN
GLOBUS PALLIDUS
MAMMILLOTHALAMIC TRACT
POSTERIOR HYPOTHALAMIC AREA
SUBTHALAMIC NUCLEUS
BASIS PEDUNCULI
LATERAL HYPOTHALAMIC AREA
OPTIC TRACT
FORNIX (TERMINATION)
MAMMILLARY PEDUNCLE
SUPRAMAMMILLARY DECUSSATION

MEDIAL MAMMILLARY NUCLEUS

The mammillary region contains within a small area some very complex and enigmatic structures. This part of the hypothalamus is compressed by the ventromedial drift of the *internal capsules* which form the upper ends of the cerebral *peduncles,* and by the expansion of the so-called subthalamic area. This area is characterized by the formation of the *subthalamic nucleus* and by the intrusion of descending and ascending fibers from the lentiform nucleus (*fasciculus lenticularis,* putamen and globus pallidus, see Plate 3, page 149) and ascending fibers of the brachium conjunctivum and ascending sensory systems. The *lateral hypothalamic area* is reduced and condensed. It consists almost entirely of the large cells previously mentioned (see Plate 2, page 148), and the descending efferent fibers are now closely gathered, many of them unmyelinated.

A new cell mass, the *posterior nucleus* or *area,* appears between the third ventricle and the subthalamic areas. In its caudal extent it is bounded laterally by the *mammillothalamic tracts.* This nucleus contains both the small cell types characteristic of the anterior nuclei and agglomerations of larger neurons of the type found in the lateral nucleus. It is fairly well established that these neurons also give rise to the important descend-ing efferent pathways which pass down (1) through the central gray as the dorsal longitudinal fasciculus (see Plate 5, page 151) and (2) through the reticular formation of the brain stem.

The *mammillary formation,* so conspicuous on the ventral aspect of the brain and also obvious for the metaphoric significance of its name, is surprisingly complex. It consists of a *medial nucleus* which may be divided into at least two vague divisions; a *lateral nucleus* quite small in man and consisting of cells dense with chromidia; and several satellite nuclei, which include the premammillary area, the *nucleus intercalatus,* and the *supramammillary area.* The latter is related to the supra-optic commissure, which is composed largely of fibers from the subthalamic nuclei.

The *fornix* (see Plate 7, page 153), a massive bundle originating from the hippocampus, descends into the lateral part of the medial mammillary nucleus but appears to contribute fibers to all parts of the mammillary complex.

Some condensations of cells of the type found in the lateral hypothalamic region are, at times, found about the fornix, probably so arranged by mechanical displacement. They have been termed the nucleus perifornicalis, but these are not conspicuous in man. Stimulation of this region has produced spectacular autonomic effects; hence it is mentioned here.

The *mammillothalamic tract* connects the medial mammillary nucleus and the anterior thalamic nucleus, which connects with Area 24 of the gyrus cinguli. The mammillotegmental tract joins the descending hypothalamic connections. The *mammillary peduncle,* inconspicuous in man, arises in the mesencephalon and terminates in the lateral mammillary nucleus.

PLATE 5

SCHEMATIC RECONSTRUCTION OF HYPOTHALAMUS (THREE-DIMENSIONAL)

A three-dimensional reconstruction of the rather intricate internal structure of one lateral half of the hypothalamus is necessarily highly schematic. The diffuseness and poor differentiation of many of the cell masses in the human brain necessitate some rather arbitrary boundaries. Plate 5 also shows major fiber connections and the principal cell groups in their relationships one to another and to nearby regions. Rostrocaudally, the *preoptic nuclei* fade into the *lateral area* and the *anterior area* which, in turn, is more or less continuous with the *dorsomedial nucleus*. These structures, as mentioned in the texts to Plates 2, 3 and 4 (see pages 148-150), are made up of fairly uniform masses of rather small neurons, interspersed with fibers of passage as well as a local feltwork. Small cells merge with differently arranged cell groups and infiltrate between them so as to obscure some nuclear boundaries. In a sense, these neurons form a sort of matrix in which the more discrete nuclei might be said to be embedded. For this reason one may find in the literature such terms as "substantia grisea centralis", "nucleus tubero-mammillaris", "substance grise fondamentale", etc., applied to this pervading cellular system. The posterior part of the lateral area as well as the posterior nucleus distinguish themselves from this system because masses of large neurons accumulate in them (see page 150), which, as has been indicated, are the sources of part of the efferent fibers of the hypothalamus. Obviously, these nuclei must possess intricate connections with other hypothalamic regions, with the thalamus and striatal systems, with neopallial and rhinencephalic organizations, as well as, possibly, with the great afferent systems.

The *ventromedial nucleus* is another somewhat more distinct area which is said to receive important frontal, cortical and rhinencephalic, as well as thalamic and pallidal, connections. Disturbances in this region and in the nearby lateral area may lead to profound behavioral disorders (see Plates 15, 16 and 17, pages 161-163).

The *paraventricular* and *supra-optic nuclei* are very clear and distinctive, and their efferent connections are well estab-

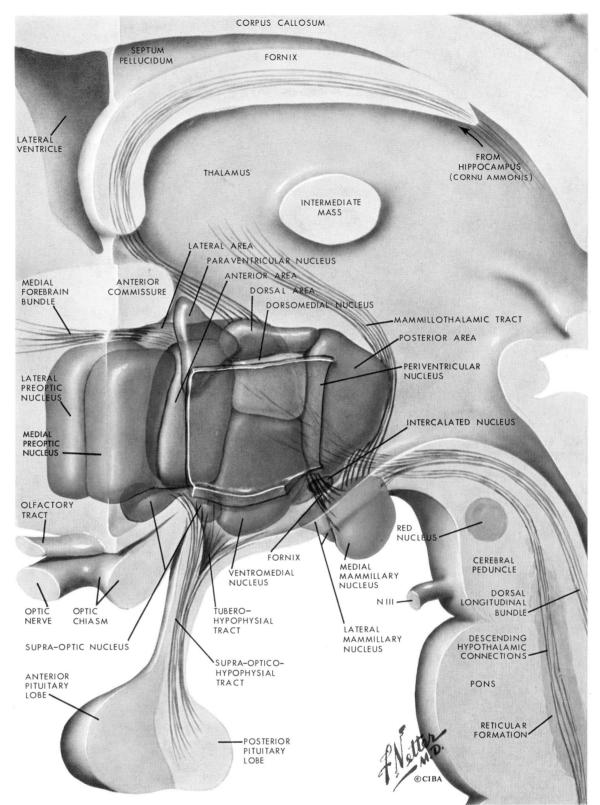

lished. They, especially the supra-optic, send fibers into the infundibular (*posterior*) *lobe* of the pituitary, where these fibers branch profusely and form much of the bulk of the lobe. It may be mentioned in passing that these neurons possess cytologic characteristics which have given some evidence of neurosecretory activity (see also Plate 10, page 156). Afferent neural connections are not clearly understood; that they exist is indicated by changes in activity of this system in response to noxious afferent stimuli and emotion-evoking situations. The relationship of the cells of these nuclei to capillaries and small blood vessels is peculiar, and the blood supply to these structures is very rich indeed (see Plate 8, page 154).

Nerve fibers from poorly defined regions in the tuberal and posterior portions of the hypothalamus also appear to enter the infundibular stem. It is very likely on physiologic grounds that many of these

fibers may possess neurosecretory characteristics.

The mammillary complex is clearly evident structurally, though its functions are physiologically obscure. Its massive connections through the *fornix, mammillothalamic tract,* mammillotegmental tract and *mammillary peduncle* have been mentioned (see page 150). The mammillotegmental tract (not illustrated) leaves the mammillothalamic tract to descend into the reticular formation of the brain stem to terminate in the dorsal and ventral tegmental nuclei. It is very probable that even more extensive connections exist.

Aside from the massive connections set up through the above-mentioned tracts and the medial forebrain bundle, it is not possible to demonstrate in a single figure the rich connections of the hypothalamus with other parts of the brain (see Plates 6 and 7, pages 152 and 153).

CEREBRAL REGIONS ASSOCIATED WITH HYPOTHALAMUS

Although the hypothalamus provides very important integrative mechanisms for autonomic activity and packs these neural circuits into small space, it is not the only site for such functions. Evidence has accumulated which justifies the postulate that the cerebral cortex can also influence the neural outflow, which we call autonomic. In the laboratory such effects can be produced experimentally by direct stimulation of the cortex of the frontal lobe and of the gyrus cinguli. These effects are less marked than those produced by stimulation of the hypothalamus but are nevertheless striking, and some of them do not depend upon the integrity of the hypothalamus. In the normal human subject many autonomic discharges are associated with subjective emotional experiences and also with behavioral patterns which an observer would class as emotional.

Behavior changes produced by cortical ablations are well known (see Plate 17, page 163). Also, changes in behavior, varying from mania and hyperphagia to apathy, aphagia (see Plate 15, page 161) and somnolence (see Plate 16, page 162), occur after certain hypothalamic lesions.

It is important, therefore, that the *hypothalamus* be regarded as part of a series of *complex neural circuits* involving brain stem, cerebral hemisphere and other parts of the diencephalon. These circuits are poorly understood, but evidence for rich connections with septal, subcallosal, preoptic and frontotemporal areas has been offered.

Some of these circuits and connections (see lower figure) may be direct, but many are probably indirect. It has been said that direct connections between the orbital portions of the *frontal lobes* and the hypothalamus exist, but they have not as yet been confirmed. Indirect connections with the *prefrontal areas* through the *medial thalamic nuclei* are well established. The hypothalamus is also connected with the *gyrus cinguli* by way of the *anterior thalamic nuclei* and with *rhinencephalic structures* via the fornix and stria terminalis. The nucleus amygdalae, or better, the amygdaloid complex (because it is composed of several nuclei), for the sake of brevity, "amygdala", is also said to send direct connections to the ventromedial hypothalamic nucleus. If this is confirmed, it will be very interesting in view of the fact that lesions of the latter in animals produce definitely different behavioral changes than do lesions of the amygdalae. After experimental destruction of the amygdalae, an animal is tame, unafraid and hypersexual, while after destruction of the ventromedial nuclei it is savage, often hyperphagic (see also Plate 15, page 161) and hyposexual.

The hypothalamus is undoubtedly influenced, probably indirectly, by the great sensory systems which have such

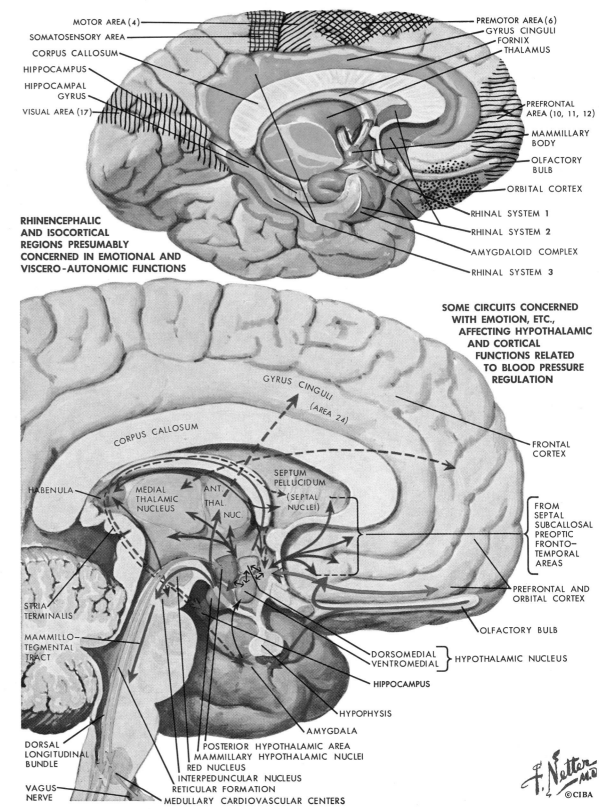

RHINENCEPHALIC AND ISOCORTICAL REGIONS PRESUMABLY CONCERNED IN EMOTIONAL AND VISCERO-AUTONOMIC FUNCTIONS

SOME CIRCUITS CONCERNED WITH EMOTION, ETC., AFFECTING HYPOTHALAMIC AND CORTICAL FUNCTIONS RELATED TO BLOOD PRESSURE REGULATION

rich thalamic connections, and the complex responses evolved through thalamic and cortical integration must have some behavioral and autonomic expression through the hypothalamic route. In recent years increasing evidence implicates rhinencephalic structures in emotional and visceral autonomic functions. Pribram,[1] on the basis of a careful survey of the accumulated evidence, proposes a classification of these structures into three rhinal systems, which are illustrated schematically in the upper figure of the accompanying picture. Reduced to simple terms, these may be described as follows: The *first rhinal system,* which is connected with the *olfactory bulb,* consists of the olfactory tubercle, diagonal band, prepiriform cortex and corticomedial nuclei of the amygdaloid complex. The *second rhinal system,* which is connected with the first, consists of portions of the subcallosal and frontotemporal cortex, the *sep-*

tal nuclei and the basolateral nuclei of the amygdalae. The *third rhinal system,* connected with the second system, consists of the *hippocampal structures* (see also Plate 7, page 153) and entorhinal and cingulate cortex. Only the first of these systems has direct olfactory connections, while the others, though still called rhinencephalic and though they have become very extensive even in a microsmatic animal such as man, have adapted to other functions. They appear to be related to emotional and visceral activities. In laboratory animals, stimulation of these structures has produced respiratory and vascular changes as well as gross movements.[2] The effects of ablations are mentioned later (see Plate 17, page 163). These areas also have direct and indirect connections with the hypothalamus and thalamus and are sometimes referred to as the "limbic lobe", a term introduced many years ago

(Continued on page 153)

(*Continued from page 152*)

by Broca. Some evidence (not yet completely established) suggests that drugs such as reserpine may produce part of their effects by their influence on these limbic systems.

Among the more obscure associations of the hypothalamus are the stria medullaris thalami, the stria terminalis, the medial forebrain bundle and the fornix. The stria medullaris connects the medial olfactory area, amygdala and preoptic area with the habenular nucleus. The *stria terminalis* arises chiefly in the amygdala and runs forward in the groove between the thalamus and caudate nucleus to contribute fibers to the anterior commissure (see Plate 2, page 148), preoptic area and hypothalamus. In man this system seems more sparse than in lower animals.

The medial forebrain bundle (see Plate 5, page 151) links the ventromedial olfactory areas with the preoptic areas, hypothalamus and mesencephalic tegmentum. The position of this tract in the hypothalamus corresponds with the lateral hypothalamic areas, shown in the sections of the hypothalamus (see Plates 3 and 4, pages 149 and 150).

The most conspicuous of these connections is the *fornix*. This massive, harp-shaped, bilateral structure is formed of fibers which arise for the most part from the pyramidal cells of the hippocampus. These fibers enter the fimbria of the hippocampus, which lies medial to the hippocampus in the floor of the inferior horn of the *lateral ventricle* of each side. They run posteriorly and curve dorsalward in a bundle called the *crus of the fornix,* which passes forward, becoming attached to the undersurface of the *corpus callosum,* and courses medially to become approximated with its fellow from the opposite side in the *body of the fornix.* Continuing forward, these bundles again diverge somewhat to form the *columns of the fornix,* which turn ventrally behind the anterior commissure and then posteriorly through the hypothalamus to terminate mainly in the mammillary bodies. Interconnection of the hippocampi is set up by fibers passing from one crus into the other through the *hippocampal commissure.* Fibers of the fornix end in both medial and lateral mammillary nuclei (see page 150). Some studies indicate that many fibers have terminations in the hypothalamus anterior to the mammillary region.[3] It is said, too, that a scattering of fibers passes caudally into the mesencephalon, and that some are contributing to the stria medullaris thalami. It is also possible that some fornix fibers end in the septum pellucidum, in the habenula and in the tuberal region. Some authorities offer evidence that fibers arising in the hypothalamus ascend in the fornix toward the hippocampus.

The *hippocampus* is part of the archipallium (rhinencephalon). It consists of a band of a very special type of cortex which has been rolled into the inferior horn of the lateral ventricle at the *hippocampal fissure.* This fissure marks the boundary between hippocampal complex and hippocampal gyrus. The *dentate fascia,* a serrated band of complex cortex,

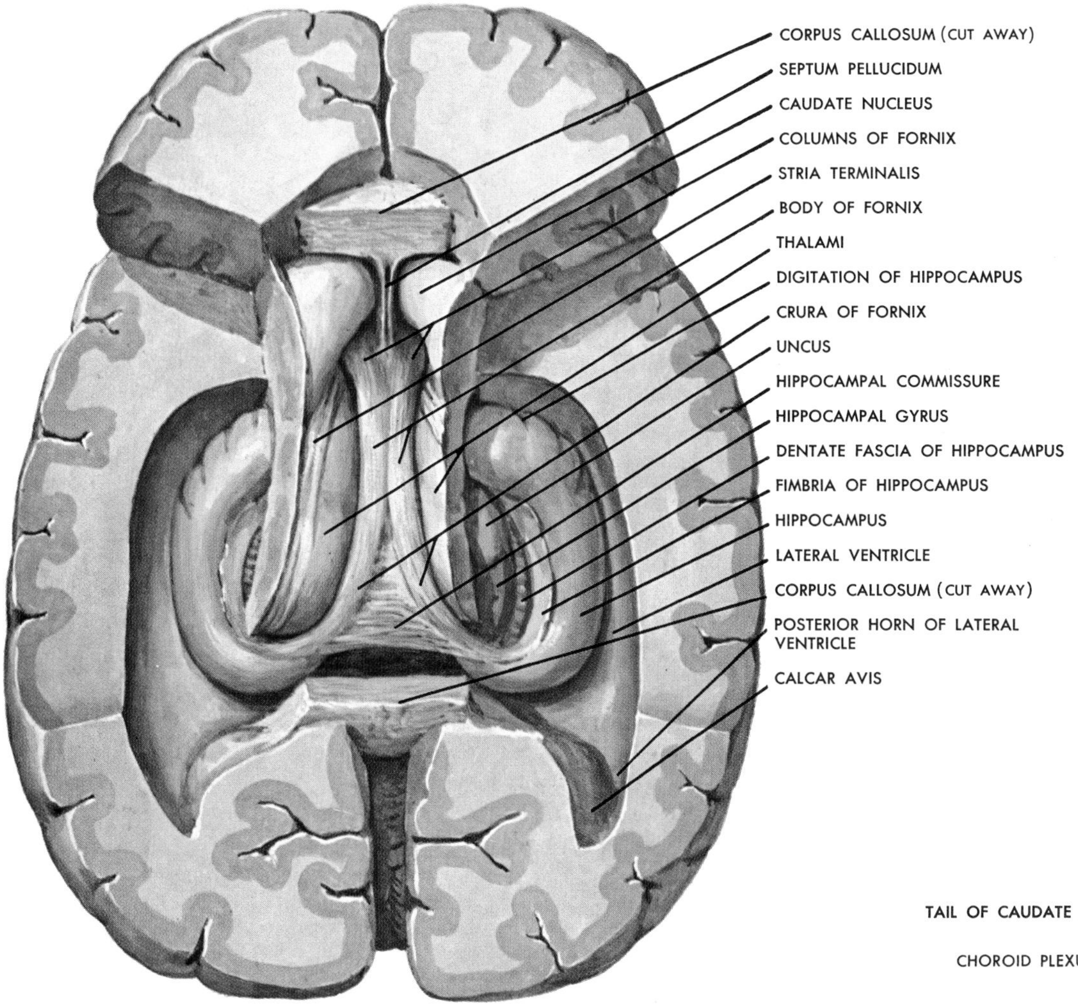
CORPUS CALLOSUM (CUT AWAY)
SEPTUM PELLUCIDUM
CAUDATE NUCLEUS
COLUMNS OF FORNIX
STRIA TERMINALIS
BODY OF FORNIX
THALAMI
DIGITATION OF HIPPOCAMPUS
CRURA OF FORNIX
UNCUS
HIPPOCAMPAL COMMISSURE
HIPPOCAMPAL GYRUS
DENTATE FASCIA OF HIPPOCAMPUS
FIMBRIA OF HIPPOCAMPUS
HIPPOCAMPUS
LATERAL VENTRICLE
CORPUS CALLOSUM (CUT AWAY)
POSTERIOR HORN OF LATERAL VENTRICLE
CALCAR AVIS

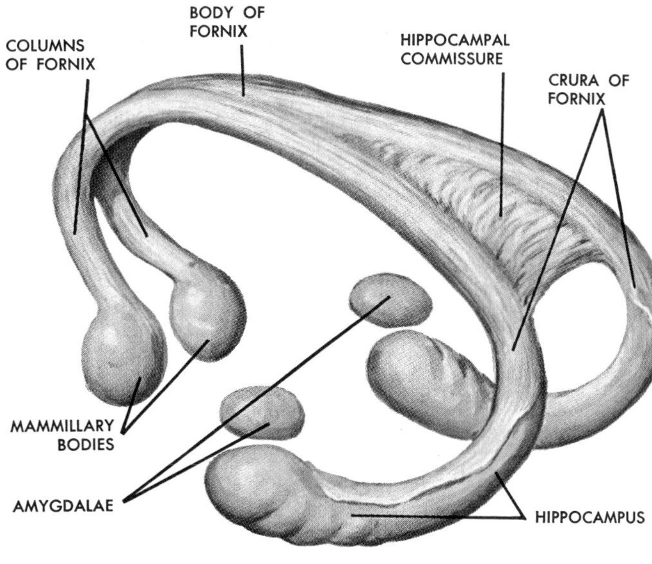
BODY OF FORNIX
COLUMNS OF FORNIX
HIPPOCAMPAL COMMISSURE
CRURA OF FORNIX
MAMMILLARY BODIES
AMYGDALAE
HIPPOCAMPUS

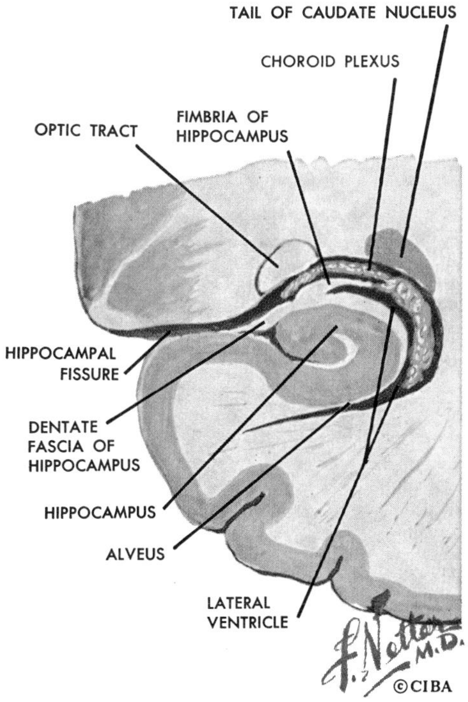
TAIL OF CAUDATE NUCLEUS
CHOROID PLEXUS
OPTIC TRACT
FIMBRIA OF HIPPOCAMPUS
HIPPOCAMPAL FISSURE
DENTATE FASCIA OF HIPPOCAMPUS
HIPPOCAMPUS
ALVEUS
LATERAL VENTRICLE
F. Netter M.D.
©CIBA

lies between the hippocampal fimbria and the fissure[4] and seems partially distinct from the hippocampus but is closely related to it structurally.

In lower animals the hippocampus extends posteriorly and dorsally to become attached to the splenium of the corpus callosum. In man this does not occur as far as the main hippocampus is concerned, but a thin layer of primitive hippocampal tissue covers the splenium of the corpus callosum and extends forward over it. Embedded in this so-called indusium griseum are two slender bundles of fibers, the medial and lateral longitudinal striae, sometimes called the fornix longa. It seems that the corpus callosum in its great growth has invaded and distorted the original hippocampal structures.

Although they belong to the rhinencephalon, the hippocampus and fornix do not seem to be related directly to the sense of smell. No deficiency of olfactory sense has been observed in cases of congenital absence of these structures in man. From the functional standpoint, Papez[5] included the fornix as part of a circuit which he suggested to be a mechanism of emotion. However, lesions of the fornix in monkeys have not produced very obvious emotional changes, while in cats the chief effects have been enhancement of pleasure reactions.

It is thus evident that the hypothalamus does not sit alone at the head of the autonomic table but shares this station with other forebrain systems, both neopallial and rhinencephalic, as well as with the great sensory integration mechanisms of the thalamus. Out of these relationships, of which our knowledge is still superficial indeed, come patterns of behavior which are modifiable by situations and which are accompanied by autonomic adjustments which adapt the individual to changes in both external and internal environment.

PLATE 8

BLOOD SUPPLY OF HYPOTHALAMUS

Vascular Relation to Hypophysis

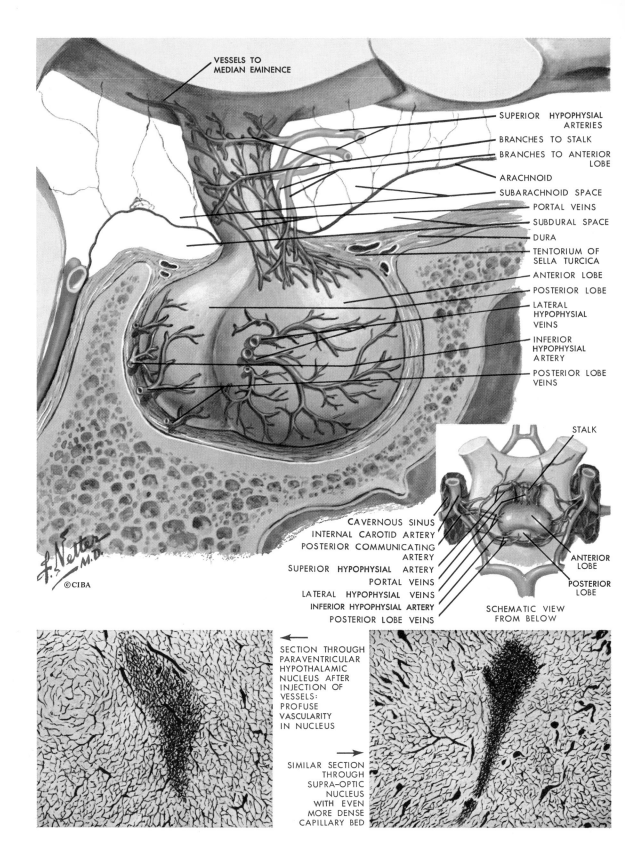

VESSELS TO MEDIAN EMINENCE

SUPERIOR HYPOPHYSIAL ARTERIES
BRANCHES TO STALK
BRANCHES TO ANTERIOR LOBE
ARACHNOID
SUBARACHNOID SPACE
PORTAL VEINS
SUBDURAL SPACE
DURA
TENTORIUM OF SELLA TURCICA
ANTERIOR LOBE
POSTERIOR LOBE
LATERAL HYPOPHYSIAL VEINS
INFERIOR HYPOPHYSIAL ARTERY
POSTERIOR LOBE VEINS

CAVERNOUS SINUS
INTERNAL CAROTID ARTERY
POSTERIOR COMMUNICATING ARTERY
SUPERIOR HYPOPHYSIAL ARTERY
PORTAL VEINS
LATERAL HYPOPHYSIAL VEINS
INFERIOR HYPOPHYSIAL ARTERY
POSTERIOR LOBE VEINS

STALK
ANTERIOR LOBE
POSTERIOR LOBE
SCHEMATIC VIEW FROM BELOW

SECTION THROUGH PARAVENTRICULAR HYPOTHALAMIC NUCLEUS AFTER INJECTION OF VESSELS: PROFUSE VASCULARITY IN NUCLEUS

SIMILAR SECTION THROUGH SUPRA-OPTIC NUCLEUS WITH EVEN MORE DENSE CAPILLARY BED

The hypothalamus receives its blood supply through small arteries which arise from the *circle of Willis*. Venous blood is drained into the cavernous sinus.

The *superior hypophysial arteries* spring from the posterior communicating arteries or from the internal carotid and supply the infundibular stem and the anterior lobe of the pituitary. These vessels, however, do not supply blood to the hypothalamus. The arterial supply and venous drainage of the hypothalamus are completely independent from those of the pituitary gland and stalk, according to Wislocki[6] and Green.[7]

The superior hypophysial arteries communicate within the substance of the stalk and *median eminence* (the anterior portion of the beginning of the stalk, which is less distinct in man than in carnivores, in which the stalk slants posteriorly) with an interesting group of so-called *hypophysial portal veins*. These vessels arise from a mass of capillary whorls and loops which spiral among the nerve fibers of the stalk and form a network on the surface of the stalk or within the pars tuberalis. Coursing downward, they enter the pars distalis within which they divide into the characteristic sinusoids of that lobe.

From these sinusoids blood passes into a group of *lateral hypophysial veins* which drain into the *cavernous sinus*. This system is of great importance for the neurohumoral theory of control of the anterior lobe, for, according to this concept, neurosecretion released by nerve fibers within the stalk is transmitted to the anterior lobe via the portal veins (see Plate 9, page 155). The cell bodies of these neurons are in the hypothalamus.

The posterior lobe of the hypophysis receives blood through one or more *inferior hypophysial arteries* (arising from the internal carotid arteries) which form arterioles and capillaries within the substance of the lobe. Venous drainage is into the cavernous sinus.

The hypothalamus receives a rich blood supply, and certain cell groups are especially endowed in this respect. The *supra-optic* and *paraventricular nuclei* are pervaded by the *most dense capillary networks* in the brain.[8] This is important since changes in the physicochemical status of the blood appear to modify the activities of these neurons.

PLATE 9

RELATIONS OF HYPOTHALAMUS TO ANTERIOR LOBE OF PITUITARY

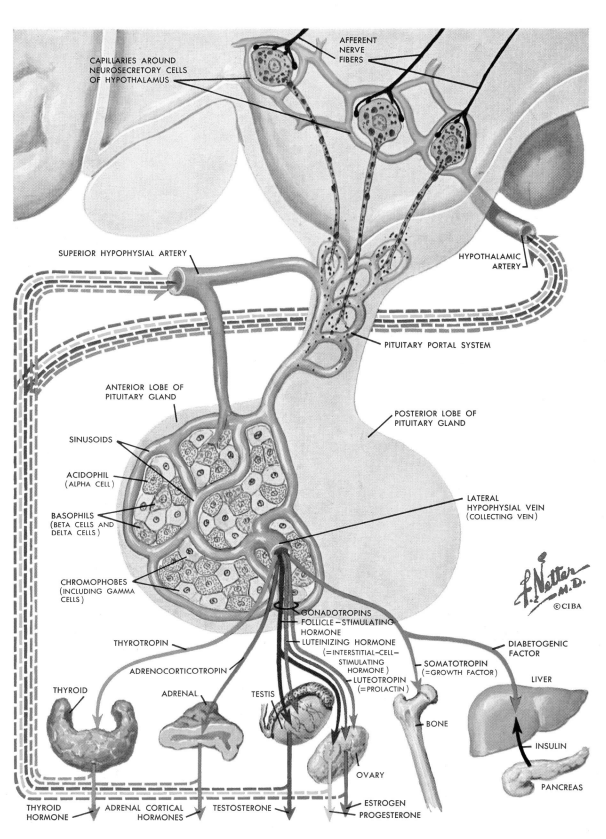

CAPILLARIES AROUND
NEUROSECRETORY CELLS
OF HYPOTHALAMUS

AFFERENT
NERVE
FIBERS

SUPERIOR HYPOPHYSIAL ARTERY

HYPOTHALAMIC
ARTERY

PITUITARY PORTAL SYSTEM

ANTERIOR LOBE OF
PITUITARY GLAND

POSTERIOR LOBE OF
PITUITARY GLAND

SINUSOIDS

ACIDOPHIL
(ALPHA CELL)

BASOPHILS
(BETA CELLS AND
DELTA CELLS)

LATERAL
HYPOPHYSIAL VEIN
(COLLECTING VEIN)

CHROMOPHOBES
(INCLUDING GAMMA
CELLS)

GONADOTROPINS
FOLLICLE—STIMULATING
HORMONE
LUTEINIZING HORMONE
(=INTERSTITIAL−CELL−
STIMULATING
HORMONE)
LUTEOTROPIN
(=PROLACTIN)

THYROTROPIN

ADRENOCORTICOTROPIN

SOMATOTROPIN
(=GROWTH FACTOR)

DIABETOGENIC
FACTOR

LIVER

THYROID

ADRENAL

TESTIS

BONE

INSULIN

OVARY

PANCREAS

THYROID
HORMONE

ADRENAL CORTICAL
HORMONES

TESTOSTERONE

ESTROGEN
PROGESTERONE

F. Netter M.D.
©CIBA

Some strong evidence has accumulated in recent years that the hypothalamus can influence the secretory activities of the anterior lobe of the pituitary. This does not mean that the latter is completely under hypothalamic control, because under the present state of our knowledge we must assume that a great number of anterior lobe functions are autonomous, in accordance with changes in the concentration of various hormones in the blood. Granted, however, that hypothalamic influence is important, for instance in the formation and release of the *luteinizing hormone* in response to copulatory stimuli in some animals,[9,10] the problem remains as to how that influence is brought to bear. In the opinion of the best authorities, the number of nerve fibers entering the lobe from the infundibular stem is too small to have any effect on the gland cells. Furthermore, no evidence has been disclosed that nerve fibers from the superior cervical ganglion have any but vascular connections. Hence, in the accompanying plate, the neurosecretory hypothesis has been resorted to (as also outlined in Plates 8 and 10, pages 154 and 156).

In accord with this theory, which is supported by a body of acceptable evidence, neurosecretions released into the *hypophysial portal system* regulate the secretory activity of the anterior lobe cells. Presumably, the release of neurosecretory materials varies according to the stimuli received by the hypothalamic neurons either through nervous connections or through changes in the composition of the blood. Thus, for example, in the nonspontaneously ovulating animals, the act of copulation stimulates hypothalamic neurons, which release a neurosecretion that, in turn, promotes release of luteinizing hormone from the anterior lobe.[11,12] The secretion of gonadotropic, adrenotropic or thyrotropic hormones is, as concluded from many experimental data, dependent upon the level of gonadal, adrenocortical or thyroidal hor-

mones, respectively, in the blood. It is widely assumed that the site of such regulating mechanism is the cells of the anterior lobe, which respond directly to the stimuli deriving from the changing blood levels. However, in the light of our present knowledge, it cannot be excluded that some neurosecretory mechanism is involved and that the receptors for these stimuli are located in the hypothalamus, whence they are passed on, in turn, to the anterior pituitary. Both possibilities are supported by experimental evidences, none of which permits, however, a final decision.

With this background Plate 9 is essentially self-explanatory, but it should be mentioned that not all relationships are as definitely settled as they appear in the schematic picture. For instance, the so-called diabetogenic hormone and the somatotropic factor might be identical. It might also be noted that the cellular sources of the various anterior lobe hormones

are not yet definitely settled, although evidence has been submitted that the *alpha cells* (eosinophilic) of the anterior lobe produce growth hormone, that the *beta cells* of the basophilic groups produce thyrotropin and that gonadotropin originates in the *delta cells*. The functions of the *chromophobes* and gamma cells are unknown.

It is easy to visualize how lesions of the hypothalamus might influence the production of anterior lobe hormones, and good experimental and clinical data support this assumption. It has also been verified that one type — the so-called cerebral type of precocious sexual development in children — is the manifestation of hypothalamic derangement, usually a tumor which need not be of hypothalamic origin. Some of these endocrine relationships are discussed in *Reproductive System*, Volume 2 of THE CIBA COLLECTION OF MEDICAL ILLUSTRATIONS, pages 4 to 6 and 80.

PLATE 10

CONTROL OF WATER EXCRETION
Antidiuretic Hormone

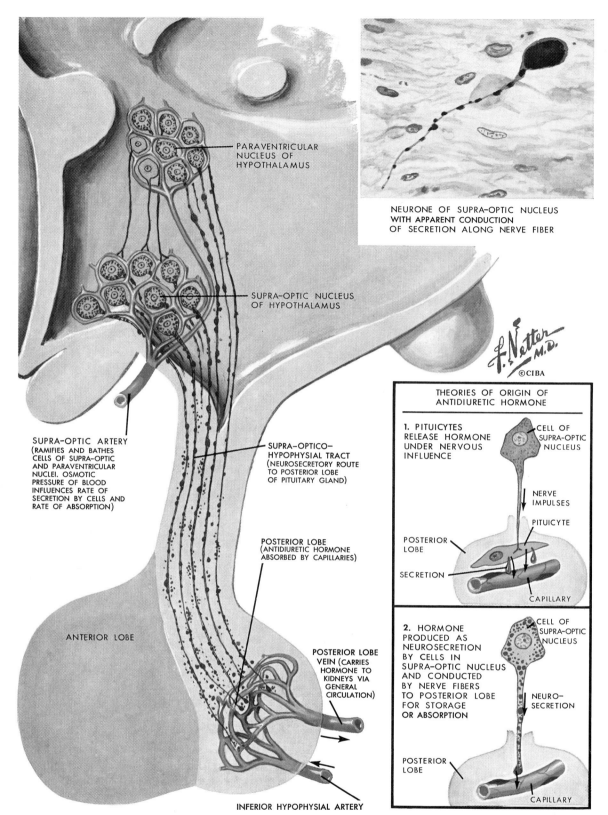

NEURONE OF SUPRA-OPTIC NUCLEUS
WITH APPARENT CONDUCTION
OF SECRETION ALONG NERVE FIBER

PARAVENTRICULAR
NUCLEUS OF
HYPOTHALAMUS

SUPRA-OPTIC NUCLEUS
OF HYPOTHALAMUS

SUPRA-OPTIC ARTERY
(RAMIFIES AND BATHES
CELLS OF SUPRA-OPTIC
AND PARAVENTRICULAR
NUCLEI. OSMOTIC
PRESSURE OF BLOOD
INFLUENCES RATE OF
SECRETION BY CELLS AND
RATE OF ABSORPTION)

SUPRA-OPTICO-
HYPOPHYSIAL TRACT
(NEUROSECRETORY ROUTE
TO POSTERIOR LOBE
OF PITUITARY GLAND)

POSTERIOR LOBE
(ANTIDIURETIC HORMONE
ABSORBED BY CAPILLARIES)

ANTERIOR LOBE

POSTERIOR LOBE
VEIN (CARRIES
HORMONE TO
KIDNEYS VIA
GENERAL
CIRCULATION)

INFERIOR HYPOPHYSIAL ARTERY

THEORIES OF ORIGIN OF
ANTIDIURETIC HORMONE

1. PITUICYTES
RELEASE HORMONE
UNDER NERVOUS
INFLUENCE

CELL OF
SUPRA-OPTIC
NUCLEUS

NERVE
IMPULSES

PITUICYTE

POSTERIOR
LOBE

SECRETION

CAPILLARY

2. HORMONE
PRODUCED AS
NEUROSECRETION
BY CELLS IN
SUPRA-OPTIC NUCLEUS
AND CONDUCTED
BY NERVE FIBERS
TO POSTERIOR LOBE
FOR STORAGE
OR ABSORPTION

CELL OF
SUPRA-OPTIC
NUCLEUS

NEURO-
SECRETION

POSTERIOR
LOBE

CAPILLARY

It has been known for a long time that the posterior lobe of the pituitary provides some powerful hormones. One of these is an oxytocic principle, or oxytocin, which causes contraction of uterine muscle. In some mammals this substance, a peptide hormone, which, incidentally, has recently been synthesized, plays an important rôle physiologically in parturition, but in man the intrinsically produced hormone seems not to be essential. Another principle found in the posterior lobe is the antidiuretic hormone (see also Plate 11, page 157), in the absence of which the clinical picture of diabetes insipidus develops. This hormone also has a mild pressor effect when it is administered in large doses of pituitary extracts. The latter effect, for which no physiologic rôle has been established, may be due to an accompanying substance present in the extract,

or it may represent the result of a toxic overdose of the antidiuretic principle. In any event, no other specific pressor substance has as yet been separated from the antidiuretic substance.

The latter substance, which is essential for keeping water excretion by the kidney within useful limits, is released into the capillaries of the infundibular stem and process. *Two theories* as to its formation have been offered. One suggests that the hormone is secreted by the glialike pituicytes of the posterior lobe, under control of the nerve fibers of the *supra-opticohypophysial tracts*. After a high section of these tracts, or destruction of the *supra-optic nuclei,* the antidiuretic hormone is no longer produced, but the pituicytes remain morphologically unchanged after section of the stalk. The cytologic evidence of secre-

tory activity by the pituicytes is poor. The other theory, elaborated in recent years by Scharrer,[13] Bargmann[14] and their associates, suggests that the antidiuretic hormone is a neurosecretion produced by the neurons of the *supra-optic nuclei*. This neurosecretion is said to migrate along the nerve fibers of the *supra-opticohypophysial tract* to be released into the capillaries of the posterior lobe. Changes in the amount of this substance released would depend upon the activity of the neurons responding to changes in the blood and tissue fluid which bathe them, and probably also to nervous influences. While final proof for this theory is still lacking, it is supported by some rather good cytologic and experimental evidence. Certainly it fits the well-established facts concerning diabetes insipidus and the control of water excretion.

PLATE II

REGULATION OF WATER BALANCE

The rôle of the hypothalamus in regulating water balance centers principally in the *supra-optic nucleus*. It is possible that some cells of the paraventricular nucleus (see Plate 10, page 156) also participate. The axons of these neurons pass down the infundibular stem and branch to form a dense meshwork among the pituicytes, or modified glial cells, of the posterior lobe (infundibular process) of the pituitary. The neurosecretory theory of posterior lobe function has been discussed on page 156.

The supra-optic nuclei receive an exceptionally rich blood supply (see Plate 8, page 154). This is important because changes in the activity of these neurons seem to be caused primarily by variations in the osmotic pressure of the blood. Thus, when the blood in the hypothalamic vessels becomes hyperosmotic, as may be the case in dehydration, the neurons of the supra-optic nuclei respond by increasing the production and/or release of antidiuretic hormone, leading to a rise in its titer in the plasma. When blood with a greater antidiuretic activity reaches the kidney, the hormone displays its action presumably in the *distal convoluted tubules*.

On the other hand, when hydration occurs, the effects are the reverse. If a normal person drinks a large quantity of water or other fluid, the resulting decrease in osmotic pressure of the blood, even though small, inhibits the secretory activity of the supra-optic neurons. Then, as the concentration of antidiuretic hormone in the blood falls, the distal tubule can no longer promote as much reabsorption of water, and the output of urine increases (water diuresis). Excess fluid is then excreted and normal osmotic blood pressure is restored.

Besides changes in the blood, other factors may affect the activities of the supra-optic neurons. Some of these may be emotional. Other evidence supports the notion that noxious peripheral stimulation and stressful situations alter the rate of production of antidiuretic hormone. While these factors are important, it is doubtful if they can contravene the effects of osmotic changes in the blood. It may be added that certain drugs, such as morphine, also seem to change the level of secretion of this substance.

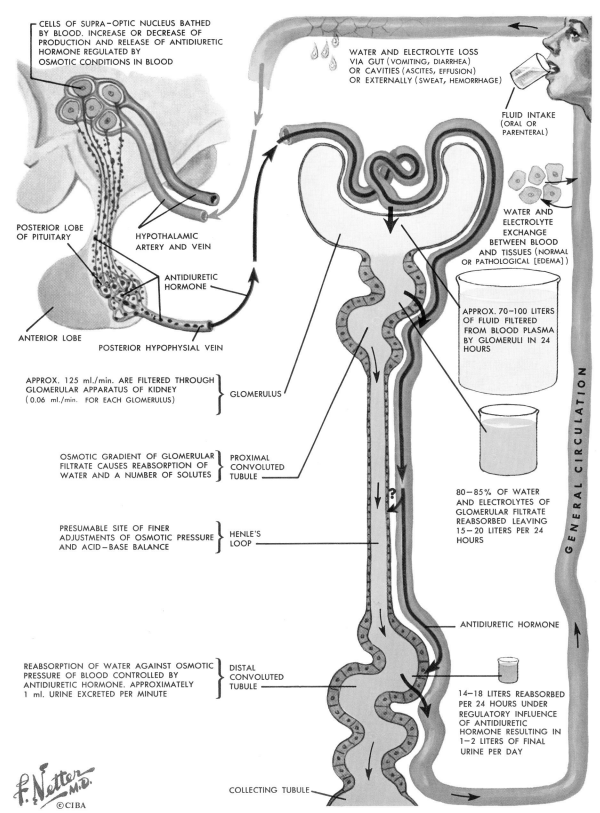

CELLS OF SUPRA-OPTIC NUCLEUS BATHED BY BLOOD. INCREASE OR DECREASE OF PRODUCTION AND RELEASE OF ANTIDIURETIC HORMONE REGULATED BY OSMOTIC CONDITIONS IN BLOOD

POSTERIOR LOBE OF PITUITARY

HYPOTHALAMIC ARTERY AND VEIN

ANTIDIURETIC HORMONE

ANTERIOR LOBE

POSTERIOR HYPOPHYSIAL VEIN

APPROX. 125 ml./min. ARE FILTERED THROUGH GLOMERULAR APPARATUS OF KIDNEY (0.06 ml./min. FOR EACH GLOMERULUS) — GLOMERULUS

OSMOTIC GRADIENT OF GLOMERULAR FILTRATE CAUSES REABSORPTION OF WATER AND A NUMBER OF SOLUTES — PROXIMAL CONVOLUTED TUBULE

PRESUMABLE SITE OF FINER ADJUSTMENTS OF OSMOTIC PRESSURE AND ACID–BASE BALANCE — HENLE'S LOOP

REABSORPTION OF WATER AGAINST OSMOTIC PRESSURE OF BLOOD CONTROLLED BY ANTIDIURETIC HORMONE. APPROXIMATELY 1 ml. URINE EXCRETED PER MINUTE — DISTAL CONVOLUTED TUBULE

COLLECTING TUBULE

WATER AND ELECTROLYTE LOSS VIA GUT (VOMITING, DIARRHEA) OR CAVITIES (ASCITES, EFFUSION) OR EXTERNALLY (SWEAT, HEMORRHAGE)

FLUID INTAKE (ORAL OR PARENTERAL)

WATER AND ELECTROLYTE EXCHANGE BETWEEN BLOOD AND TISSUES (NORMAL OR PATHOLOGICAL [EDEMA])

APPROX. 70–100 LITERS OF FLUID FILTERED FROM BLOOD PLASMA BY GLOMERULI IN 24 HOURS

80–85% OF WATER AND ELECTROLYTES OF GLOMERULAR FILTRATE REABSORBED LEAVING 15–20 LITERS PER 24 HOURS

ANTIDIURETIC HORMONE

14–18 LITERS REABSORBED PER 24 HOURS UNDER REGULATORY INFLUENCE OF ANTIDIURETIC HORMONE RESULTING IN 1–2 LITERS OF FINAL URINE PER DAY

GENERAL CIRCULATION

F. Netter M.D.
©CIBA

From the clinical standpoint, an understanding of these mechanisms is important in consideration of the ebb and flow of fluid in the normal as well as in the ailing organism. The total picture is, of course, tremendously complicated by the rôles of the liver, heart, adrenal, kidney, etc., especially as modified by pathologic conditions. For the individual who is normal with respect to these other organs, proper functioning of the hypothalamo-hypophysial system is essential for maintenance of fluid balance as well as for adaptability in conservation of fluid.

Lesions which destroy all or a large part of the supra-opticohypophysial system deprive the patient of all or part of his sources of antidiuretic hormone. When this occurs, the condition known as diabetes insipidus ensues, in which the patient excretes proportionately large amounts of urine of low specific gravity and, if able, ingests equivalent amounts of water. Such persons are susceptible to dangerous dehydration if deprived of access to water. They offer striking testimony for the importance of this mechanism in adaptation to restricted fluid intake, for while these patients can concentrate their urine to a limited extent, they cannot do so to a degree which makes existence adequately possible. However, the disease may be partially controlled by treatment with posterior lobe substance or extracts.

The causes of diabetes insipidus are varied; trauma, including basal skull fracture, tumors, infections, thrombosis or arteriosclerosis may be implicated. Usually in this disease the loss of neurons of the supra-optic nucleus and of their axons in the infundibulum and posterior lobe is almost complete. This attests the importance of these structures in maintaining a normal urine output consistent with good body economy.

MECHANISMS OF BLOOD-PRESSURE REGULATION

It has been known for many years that an animal can be deprived of its sympathetic nervous outflow and still live and maintain sufficient blood pressure for moderate normal activity (Cannon).[15] However, in situations demanding unusual effort or sustained activity above the normal, such operated animals cannot function adequately, because, among other things, the animals have lost the ability to increase cardiac activity and partially divert the flow of blood from the viscera to the muscles and nervous tissues. Therefore, it is to the advantage of the organism that it possess means for regulating blood flow and blood pressure in accordance with current body needs. Even in the absence of sympathetic outflow, some mechanisms for this regulation exist: (1) the *adrenal medulla* still secretes epinephrine, though its production is poorly regulated; (2) the contractions and relaxations of somatic muscles (in movement) help in forcing blood through the *peripheral vessels;* (3) under the influence of adrenal cortical hormones, sodium and water may possibly accumulate in the walls of blood vessels, thus reducing their caliber and increasing general pressure. However, nervous control is more efficient, since it provides both the rapid and the fine adjustments necessary for maintaining adequate general blood supply at all times and for protecting the heart from undue strain. Such regulation consists essentially in the capacity of the blood vascular compartment to change the caliber of its vessels and to alter the stroke volume and rate of the heart. Both the variable arterial caliber and the heart's output modify blood pressure and, according to regional changes in the vessels, may affect the blood supply to various systems or regions of the body.[16]

Local changes in blood flow may be due to local or segmental reflexes. Certain types of stimuli might effect spatially restricted *vasoconstriction* or *vasodilatation.* The latter might result in part

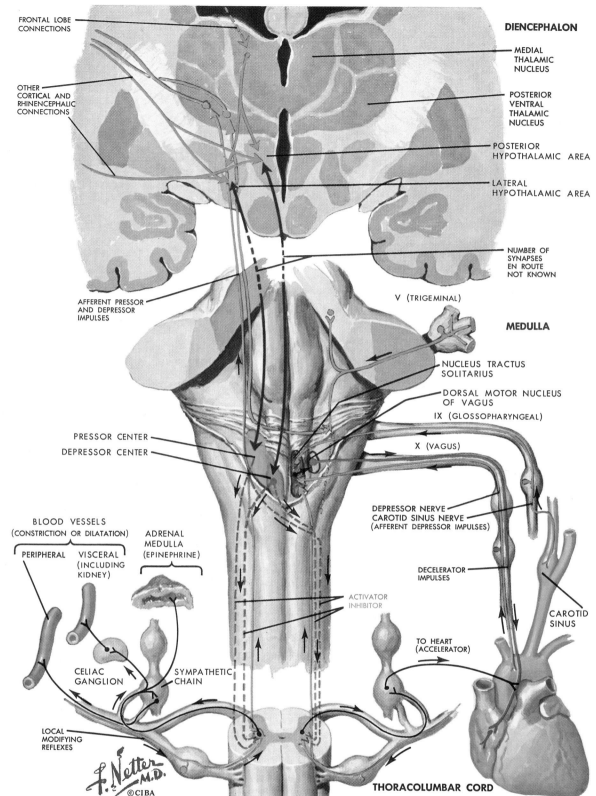

from axon reflexes or antidromic impulses. More generalized changes may occur in response to peripheral and visceral stimuli, principally noxious or libidinous, which activate ascending pathways and thus modify cardiovascular activity by their influence on regulatory mechanisms in the brain. Such afferent impulses may directly affect mechanisms in the *medulla oblongata,* or, more likely, *thalamic relays* which act through the hypothalamus and down again to the *bulbar and spinal outflow.* Also, through *cortical connections of the thalamus,* psychic elements may be brought in to modulate the responses. This type of effect is principally pressor, with increased cardiac activity and visceral and peripheral arteriolar constriction. The efferent limb of this long reflex arc travels mainly in *descending hypothalamic pathways,* and perhaps also pontile relays, to the vasomotor mechanisms (often and for historical reasons called "centers") in the bulb

and spinal cord, which, in turn, affect the blood vessels and the heart. The number of relays or synapses in this descending path is not known, and it is very likely that complex reverberating circuits are involved in this as in most neural activities.

The effects of situational circumstances on psychic activity and hence on vasomotor and cardiac regulation, according to the constitutional make-up of the individual, must be mentioned, because they are very important indirect modulators of autonomic activity in modern man (see also Plate 13, page 159).

Depressor effects are also part of the modulation system, *e.g.,* the moderator mechanisms which are set up through the *carotid sinus* and *aortic reflexes.* Situational modification of psychic activity may also act through hypothalamic and/or lower brain stem circuits to lower the blood pressure and depress the

(Continued on page 159)

(Continued from page 158)

heart. It is thus evident that *connections of the hypothalamus with both pressor and depressor systems* do exist. Their true course cannot be properly allocated and can be indicated only symbolically by arrows. The definite pressor and depressor regions in the hypothalamus are not clearly known, because in animal experiments a change in stimulus parameters, without altering the locus of stimulation, may reverse the response from elevation to depression of blood pressure.

It should be remembered that not all blood vessels of the body respond to a pressor situation by constriction. It is quite likely that, during neuroregulatory visceral and peripheral vasoconstriction, the vessels of the muscles, and perhaps of the heart, dilate. This is logical enough, since the most active tissues require the most blood, which is provided through dilated channels if the pressure elsewhere is high enough.

All this serves to illustrate the inadequacy of the term "center", as it has been used in the past and is still found from time to time in modern literature. The cardiovascular regulatory system extends from receptors to telencephalon and back to effectors, through various complicated circuits.

Efferent Pathways in Neurogenic and Humoral Hypertension (Plate 13)

Besides the reflex mechanisms concerned in the regulation of normal blood pressure, psychologic factors also participate, especially in persons who are susceptible to stresses and strains. Circumstances producing emotional reactions, internal conflicts and worry may so upset the normal regulatory machinery that excessive systolic and diastolic blood pressures result. Such effects are brought about through neural channels. The turmoil in the cerebral cortex of a worried individual is brought to focus, in a sense, upon the fundamental cardiovascular regulators at the lower level. This cortical activity, on theoretical grounds, especially concerns the frontal lobe and rhinencephalon, both of which have very close, direct and indirect *connections with the hypothalamus* (see Plate 6, page 152) and with the reticular formation of the lower brain stem. The hypothalamic neuron systems, brought to supernormal activity by the bombardment of cortical impulses, discharge down the brain stem and spinal cord by pathways involving unknown numbers of synapses and intercalated circuits. These impulses act upon the bulbar cardiovascular "centers", increasing the activity of the heart. Discharges to the spinal level activate the *thoracolumbar portion of the autonomic system* through which arteriolar constriction is brought about, especially in the great visceral vascular bed. The *adrenal medulla* is stimulated to produce norepinephrine, which adds its vasopressor effects. All this may lead to an acute neurogenic hypertension,

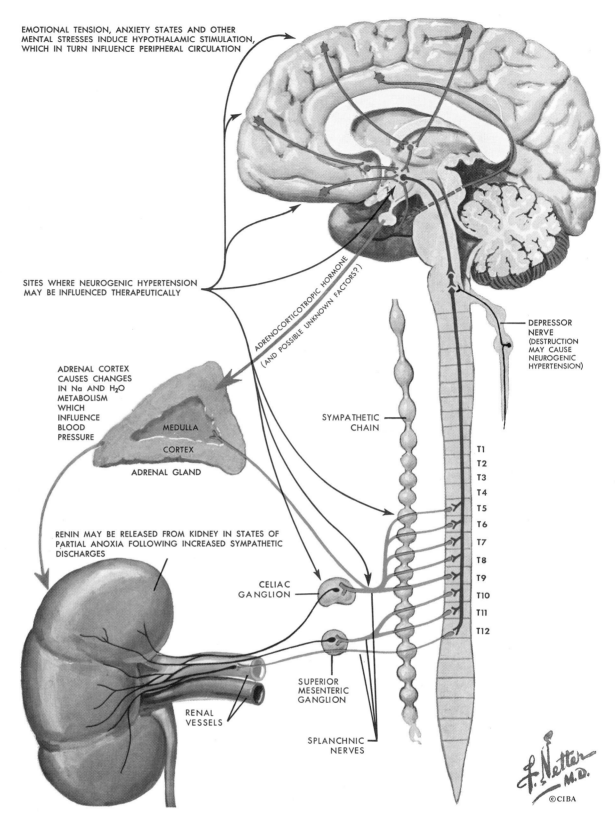

EMOTIONAL TENSION, ANXIETY STATES AND OTHER MENTAL STRESSES INDUCE HYPOTHALAMIC STIMULATION, WHICH IN TURN INFLUENCE PERIPHERAL CIRCULATION

SITES WHERE NEUROGENIC HYPERTENSION MAY BE INFLUENCED THERAPEUTICALLY

ADRENOCORTICOTROPIC HORMONE (AND POSSIBLE UNKNOWN FACTORS?)

DEPRESSOR NERVE (DESTRUCTION MAY CAUSE NEUROGENIC HYPERTENSION)

ADRENAL CORTEX CAUSES CHANGES IN Na AND H$_2$O METABOLISM WHICH INFLUENCE BLOOD PRESSURE

MEDULLA

CORTEX

ADRENAL GLAND

SYMPATHETIC CHAIN

T1 T2 T3 T4 T5 T6 T7 T8 T9 T10 T11 T12

RENIN MAY BE RELEASED FROM KIDNEY IN STATES OF PARTIAL ANOXIA FOLLOWING INCREASED SYMPATHETIC DISCHARGES

CELIAC GANGLION

SUPERIOR MESENTERIC GANGLION

RENAL VESSELS

SPLANCHNIC NERVES

which persists for the duration of the emotional storm.

Other factors are also involved. The hemodynamics of the *kidney* are affected, and under anoxic conditions this organ releases renin, a proteolytic enzyme which acts upon a renin-substrate (hypertensinogen) in the blood plasma to produce angiotonin (also called hypertensin), which is a pressor substance. Many other vaso-active substances have been found in blood and urine, a number of which cause experimentally a rise in blood pressure, but whether these, including renin, have any etiologic or pathogenic connection with clinical hypertension is still a strongly problematic issue.

In normal persons an acute elevation in blood pressure is soon over. In emotionally overwrought, tense, compulsive persons, this hypertension may persist, and for a time may yield to medical treatment with sedatives, tranquilizing drugs and sympathetic block-

ing agents or to surgical treatment involving sympathectomy. If neurogenic hypertension persists, however, with prolonged increased peripheral resistance, the renal circulation may be permanently altered, and the release of abnormal amounts of renin may presumably occur, though this has, however, so far not been demonstrated.

Another still hypothetical factor: The hypothalamus participates in controlling the hormonal output of the anterior lobe of the pituitary. Release of *adrenocorticotropic* (ACTH) and/or other unknown *hormones* can increase the activity of the adrenal cortex to secrete larger amounts of cortical steroid, some of which are known to produce hypertension. Though no direct evidence has yet been made available, the possibility cannot be denied that increased cortical secretion may be a causative or contributive factor in the complex etiology of human hypertension.[17]

PLATE 14

Temperature Regulation

After destruction of the hypothalamus, most mammals can no longer maintain a uniform body temperature. Man is no exception. Many cases have been observed in which tumors or other lesions in the hypothalamus have changed patients from the homothermic to the poikilothermic state. The organization of this hypothalamic mechanism appears, at first glance, to be more simple than it really is. According to current views of neural mechanisms in temperature control, the hypothalamus contains two types of neurons which are primarily devoted to these functions. While these cells have not been histologically differentiated, experimental results point out that one type is affected by elevation in the temperature of the blood, the other by depression in temperature. Many of the neurons susceptible to rising blood temperature are located in the anterior part of the hypothalamus, perhaps extending into the preoptic area. These neurons participate in the mechanisms whereby excess *heat* is *dissipated*. Their descending pathways pass down the *brain stem*, in or near the central gray, and set up connections with respiratory and cardiovascular mechanisms of the brain stem and *spinal cord*.[18] When the blood temperature is elevated, the discharges evoked from these neurons set into play the peripheral processes which contribute to heat loss (respiratory changes, increased peripheral *blood flow* and *perspiration*). It is also possible that heat production may be somewhat inhibited. Since peripheral vasodilation and perspiration are cholinergically regulated functions, some authorities have ascribed primarily a parasympathetic activity to the anterior hypothalamus.

The *neurons affected by falling blood temperature* are scattered in the hypothalamus, mostly below the supra-optic region, and have descending pathways similar to the others. These cells set in motion the complex processes whereby the body temperature is maintained or elevated, including increased production of heat within the body and also conservation of heat by reducing radiation. The latter is accompanied by peripheral vasoconstriction. Heat production is, in part, brought about by the phenomenon of *shivering*, in which *somatic muscles* are brought into play. The neural pat-

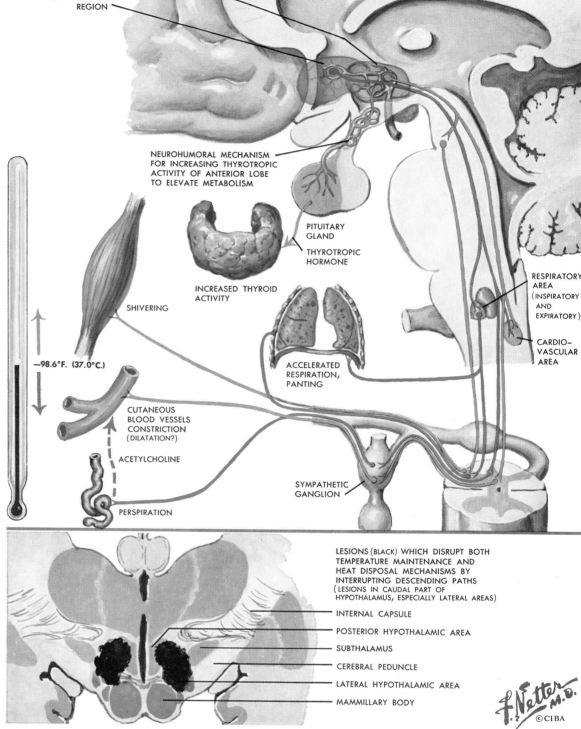

terns responsible for shivering are not well understood. Animals without the hypothalamus do not shiver, and shivering may be modified by hypothalamic stimulation. It is also believed that mechanisms in the midbrain take part. Heat production is also stepped up by a general metabolic speed-up, brought about by increased hypothalamic activity when an individual is exposed to cold. This involves release of the thyrotropic function of the anterior lobe of the pituitary, perhaps through neurohumoral mechanisms, and a resulting increase of *thyroid* activity.

Important from the practical standpoint is that lesions of the anterior hypothalamic areas may result in inability to adjust to high environmental temperatures. In cases of acute trauma or operative injury to this region, the patient may fail to adapt immediately, because the unchecked temperature-maintenance and heat-production mechanisms get out of control. The

result is "neurogenic hyperthermia". This is particularly dangerous if the latter mechanisms are stimulated by infection or by the presence of some pyrogenic substance. Extensive lesions farther caudally, especially in the lateral areas, depress both temperature-control mechanisms in part by interrupting pathways. In such instances poikilothermy ensues.

It will be noted that in the picture no specific nuclei have been allotted exact functions in temperature regulation. The "thermostatic" neurons are not segregated or grouped but are mingled with other types of cells. As a matter of fact, even some intermingling of "heat-production" and "heat-disposal" elements has been observed to an extent which may vary from individual to individual and which accounts for some variation in the effects of lesions. Some evidence has been proffered that these mechanisms are depressed by many antipyretic drugs.

PLATE 15

HYPOTHALAMIC CONTROL OF APPETITE

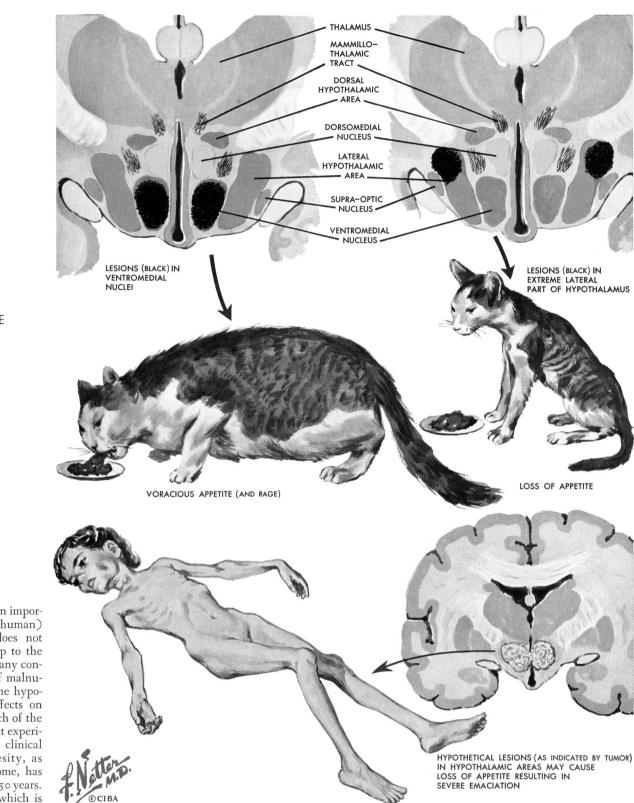

LESIONS (BLACK) IN VENTROMEDIAL NUCLEI

LESIONS (BLACK) IN EXTREME LATERAL PART OF HYPOTHALAMUS

THALAMUS
MAMMILLO-THALAMIC TRACT
DORSAL HYPOTHALAMIC AREA
DORSOMEDIAL NUCLEUS
LATERAL HYPOTHALAMIC AREA
SUPRA-OPTIC NUCLEUS
VENTROMEDIAL NUCLEUS

VORACIOUS APPETITE (AND RAGE)

LOSS OF APPETITE

HYPOTHETICAL LESIONS (AS INDICATED BY TUMOR) IN HYPOTHALAMIC AREAS MAY CAUSE LOSS OF APPETITE RESULTING IN SEVERE EMACIATION

Appetite for food constitutes an important segment of animal (and human) behavior. Although appetite does not necessarily have any relationship to the need for food, it is important in any consideration of obesity and also of malnutrition. That derangements of the hypothalamus may have striking effects on appetite is well established. Much of the evidence is based on rather recent experimental work,[19, 20] although the clinical concept of hypothalamic obesity, as manifested in Fröhlich's syndrome, has attracted attention for more than 50 years.

The experimental evidence, which is much more substantial than the clinical, rests upon the fact that very localized *lesions* involving the ventromedial nuclei of the hypothalamus in animals produce a marked increase in appetite.[20] It would follow, naturally, that the animals with such lesions may be savage. This is true, in general, although not invariably so. An animal may be savage without developing excessive appetite, although the opposite, *i.e.*, excessive appetite without savageness, is, in animals with hypothalamic lesions, very rare. The term "appetite" is used advisedly because of the lack of evidence that these beasts really have hunger. Hunger connotes need for food and is associated with an empty stomach, a low blood sugar, weakness, etc. These animals, however, will eat heartily even when already amply

fed. Their eating behavior is wolfish, and they will even forget an existing animosity for their keeper in their desire for food.

Since these creatures are appreciably less active than normal, if they are given a diet slightly in excess of basic requirements they become obese. The obesity might be promoted by some metabolic changes, which result from suppression of several anterior lobe functions, as attested by a tendency to hypogonadism. As in other types of obesity, this condition can be prevented or relieved by a suitably restricted diet. In rats with similar lesions, a deficiency of somatotropic hormone production is likely, because, while the animals become big and fat, one fails to observe a concomitant growth of bone and muscle. It is also possible that these animals suffer from unrecognized disturbances in the carbohydrate metabolism.

The lesions just described appear to release an

appetite pattern which is ordinarily balanced by a neural mechanism operating in the ventromedial region. A region which apparently plays a key rôle in such an appetite pattern seems to exist in the *lateral hypothalamic area*. *Lesions* such as indicated in the upper right figure abolish the "urge to eat". This is true not only for otherwise normal animals but also for those which have been rendered hyperphagic by the ventromedial lesions.[19]

Besides Fröhlich's syndrome, which has already been mentioned, it is of interest from the clinical point of view that nutritional deficiencies have also been noted in cases of diencephalic lesions. Deficient appetite has been reported in patients with tumors in the region of the *third ventricle,* as indicated hypothetically in the lower right figure. It is a question whether some cases of Simmonds' disease may not be due to hypothalamic involvement.

PLATE 16

SLEEP-WAKING MECHANISMS

If a normal person receives a certain level of stimulation (extrinsic, intrinsic, or both), he will ordinarily remain awake and conscious of his environment, provided he is not overwhelmed by fatigue. When the cortex receives sufficient afferent impulses, it is said to be aroused or activated; that is, a critical number of cortical neurons is brought into the proper patterns of activity to produce a state of consciousness and alertness. Such changes in activity can be recorded electro-encephalographically.[21,22,23] The samples of the *EEG* shown were taken when the subject was drowsy and as she passed into light sleep, which was characterized in part by spindlelike clusters of regular, high-voltage brain waves; then deep sleep, with its random, high-voltage, slow waves. The waking person with eyes closed may show an "alpha" rhythm characterized by regular 10-to-14-per-second waves. The arousal or activation pattern evoked by waking stimuli has low-voltage and high-frequency potentials. Thus, the great afferent systems are important for promoting cortical activity and, hence, wakefulness. However, at relatively low levels of stimulation this is not enough, and the ascending *reticular* activating *system* of the brain stem, which has its upper end in the posterior hypothalamus and lower thalamus, becomes important.[23] The reticular system has a generalized influence upon the cortex. The pathways from its upper extremity to the cortex are not well understood, but impulses are presumably relayed through the thalamic nuclei and through the internal capsule.[23,24] Collaterals from the great afferent pathways feed into the reticular system,[24] and, theoretically, if it receives enough impulses it will discharge to the cortex and produce cortical wakefulness even if the activity of the afferent systems is not in itself strong enough to do so. The reticular system is thus able to maintain wakefulness at levels of visceral and somatic stimulation which would not ordinarily activate the cortex.

After interruption of auditory and spinal afferent paths at high levels, experimental animals may still be awake. However, if the upper reticular system is destroyed in the region of the posterior hypothalamus, somnolence occurs.[22,23] The same is true with extensive midbrain lesions. The sleep produced by lesions of the reticular system is not usually completely irreversible, but an animal with such lesions may be aroused, at least momentarily, by stimuli of very high intensity.

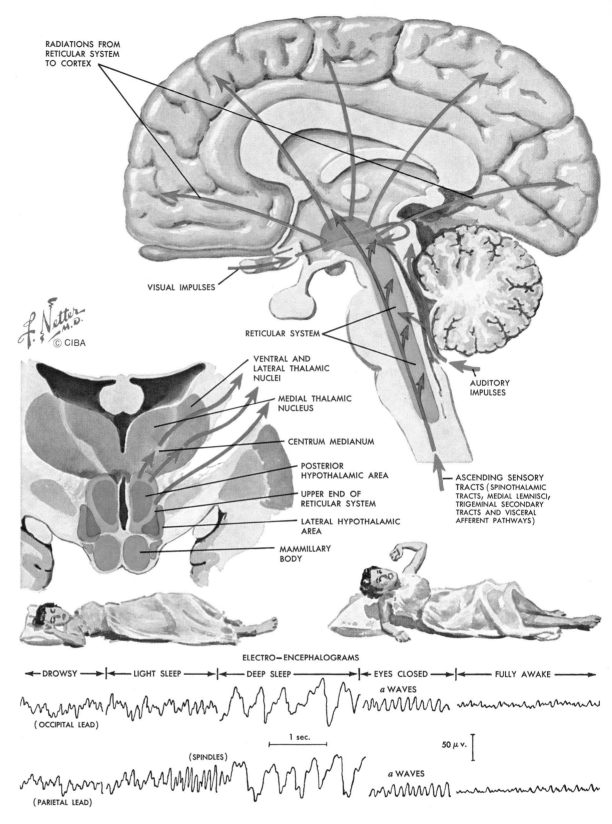

The above ideas are not intended to propose a comprehensive theory of sleep but merely to emphasize the rôle of the brain stem in states of consciousness. The matter is much more complicated than has just been indicated, as is attested by the problems of periodic sleep rhythms, the effects of fatigue and fatigue products, the influence of metabolic changes, etc. Although sleep has been produced with diencephalic lesions, it has also been reported that sleep can be induced by stimulation in the thalamus. If this is true, it might be explained by a disruptive effect of the stimulation on corticipetal conduction, or by a direct effect on cortical and subcortical activity. Another problem is introduced by the fact that an animal deprived of most of its cortex may have periods of what appears to be wakefulness alternating with sleep. It may be that cortical sleep, which seems most important in man, is supplemented by subcortical sleep and

that some form of consciousness, if not awareness, is possible in the absence of the cortex. It is possible that the cortex is capable of activating itself under certain circumstances, which may perhaps be exemplified by a man wrestling with his problems in the dark and quiet of the night, when emotional turmoil rather than sensory stimulation must have the crucial activating effect.

From the practical point of view, it is important that extensive hypothalamic and thalamic lesions may produce somnolence or pathologic sleep in patients. The same is true with large lesions extending through the central reticular formation of the midbrain and pons. The lesions of lethargic encephalitis are most often found in the upper brain stem. All in all, the clinical data support the premise that subcortical, as well as cortical, mechanisms are important for changes in the states of consciousness.

PLATE 17

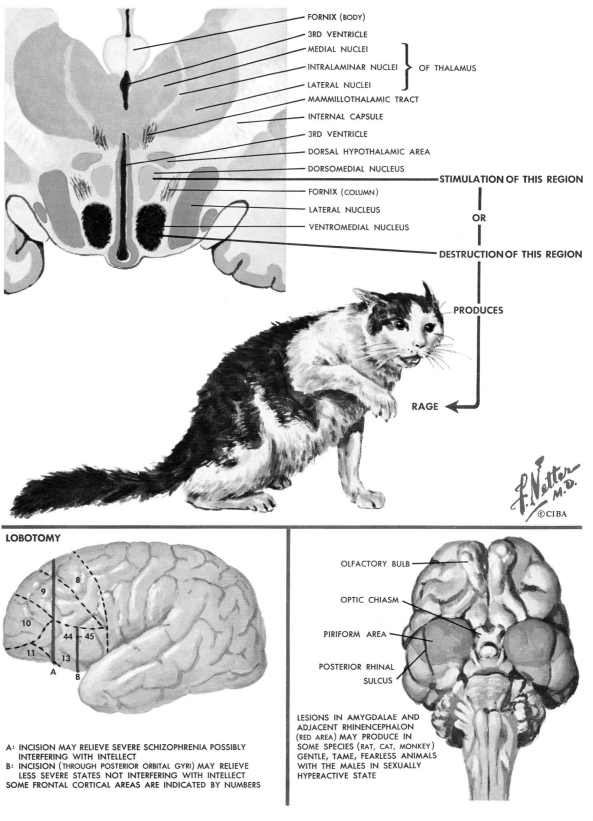

FORNIX (BODY)
3RD VENTRICLE
MEDIAL NUCLEI
INTRALAMINAR NUCLEI } OF THALAMUS
LATERAL NUCLEI
MAMMILLOTHALAMIC TRACT
INTERNAL CAPSULE
3RD VENTRICLE
DORSAL HYPOTHALAMIC AREA
DORSOMEDIAL NUCLEUS
FORNIX (COLUMN)
LATERAL NUCLEUS
VENTROMEDIAL NUCLEUS

STIMULATION OF THIS REGION

OR

DESTRUCTION OF THIS REGION

PRODUCES

RAGE

LOBOTOMY

A: INCISION MAY RELIEVE SEVERE SCHIZOPHRENIA POSSIBLY
INTERFERING WITH INTELLECT
B: INCISION (THROUGH POSTERIOR ORBITAL GYRI) MAY RELIEVE
LESS SEVERE STATES NOT INTERFERING WITH INTELLECT
SOME FRONTAL CORTICAL AREAS ARE INDICATED BY NUMBERS

OLFACTORY BULB
OPTIC CHIASM
PIRIFORM AREA
POSTERIOR RHINAL
SULCUS

LESIONS IN AMYGDALAE AND
ADJACENT RHINENCEPHALON
(RED AREA) MAY PRODUCE IN
SOME SPECIES (RAT, CAT, MONKEY)
GENTLE, TAME, FEARLESS ANIMALS
WITH THE MALES IN SEXUALLY
HYPERACTIVE STATE

HYPOTHALAMIC MECHANISMS IN SOME ASPECTS OF EMOTIONAL BEHAVIOR

This short survey of the available knowledge of the hypothalamus and its relation to emotions and emotional behavior must be restricted to some remarks on certain primitive aspects of behavior which may be interpreted as emotional from the standpoint of observation only. Behavior changes which seem emotional in pattern as the result of lesions or irritation of the hypothalamus have been described in numerous clinical reports. They range from apathy to excitement, manic behavior and uncontrolled expression. The occurrence of impulsive crying or laughing in patients with diencephalic pathologic processes has sometimes been noted. It is known that electrical *stimulation* near the fornix in the lateral and *dorsal regions* of the hypothalamus evokes such physical concomitants of emotion as rise in blood pressure, pupil dilatation, horripilation, rise in blood sugar, defecation, etc., even in anesthetized animals. In unanesthetized animals the stimulation produces the picture of a violent rage which will build up to the point that the animal will attack the observer.

Certain lesions of the hypothalamus will also produce a striking chronic change in behavior.[20] Bilateral *lesions in the region of the ventromedial nuclei* in cats and rats cause previously tame animals to display varying degrees of wildness and savageness. They attempt to escape and, when cornered, growl and hiss, and will often attack savagely if approached. This is an irreversible state and does not respond to taming. General bodily activity is reduced. The gonads are often atrophic, probably owing to a coincidental effect of the lesions upon the hypothalamo-anterior lobe system. Many of these animals show an increased feeding drive which, together with their diminished activity and anterior lobe involvement, leads to obesity (see page 161). Although the food drive is increased, most of these animals will not learn a simple mechanical procedure in order to get their food, whereas normal animals easily learn such tricks. Neither removal of the frontal poles of the hemisphere nor lesions of the *piriform areas* prevent or cure this behavior change.

Removal of cerebral cortex or high decerebration in a cat leaves an animal which responds to innocuous stimulation by apparent fits of senseless rage, called "sham rage". Removal of neocortex is not sufficient; some of the rhinencephalon must also be removed. For maximum appearance of sham rage, some of the hypothalamus must be left intact, although some rage reactions still appear in the absence of the hypothalamus.[25]

Experimental *lesions* of the *piriform area* have produced bland, tame, fearless animals which no longer recognize their natural enemies.[26] In the males these lesions have also been associated with hypersexual behavior, provided androgenic hormone, either endogenous or exogenous, has been present. This behavior pattern has been inhibited by lesions in the ventromedial hypothalamic area.

Hypothalamic mechanisms in emotional behavior tie in with other forebrain activities. Prefrontal lobotomy has been supposed to benefit depressed or withdrawn patients by releasing hypothalamic and other subcortical areas from abnormal cortical inhibition. Thus, incisions severing the connections of the prefrontal areas may relieve some severe schizophrenics, but they may also interfere with intellectual activity. Incisions in the posterior orbital gyri in the ventromedial quadrants of the frontal lobes, however, may relieve such depressed states without altering intellectual capacity.[27]

Larger lesions of the hypothalamus, especially those involving the lateral posterior areas, greatly increase tameness to the point of apathy, with depression of autonomic functions. However, it is necessary to view the effects of hypothalamic lesions as due to the disruption here of circuits which set up the normal patterns of behavior.

PLATE 18

NEUROGENIC AND HORMONAL PATHWAYS IN RAGE REACTION

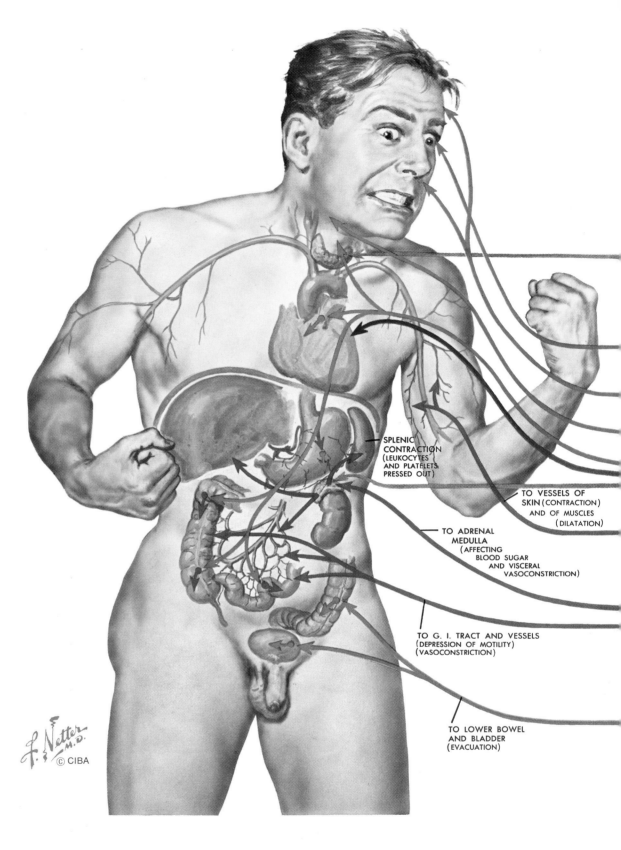

SPLENIC CONTRACTION (LEUKOCYTES AND PLATELETS PRESSED OUT)

TO VESSELS OF SKIN (CONTRACTION) AND OF MUSCLES (DILATATION)

TO ADRENAL MEDULLA (AFFECTING BLOOD SUGAR AND VISCERAL VASOCONSTRICTION)

TO G. I. TRACT AND VESSELS (DEPRESSION OF MOTILITY) (VASOCONSTRICTION)

TO LOWER BOWEL AND BLADDER (EVACUATION)

The complexity of neurogenic and humoral factors in all sorts of human emotions and the many gaps in our knowledge of the working associations of numerous parts of the brain make it impossible to offer a completely satisfactory and scientifically sound explanation of the mechanism of rage reaction or any other behavioral response. In the accompanying plate an attempt has been made to illustrate in a simple, schematic form the numerous sites of origin, the intracerebral and neurohumoral associations participating and the various peripheral organs responding to stimuli and excitation. The picture, unfortunately, has all the shortcomings typical of schematic simplification. It fails

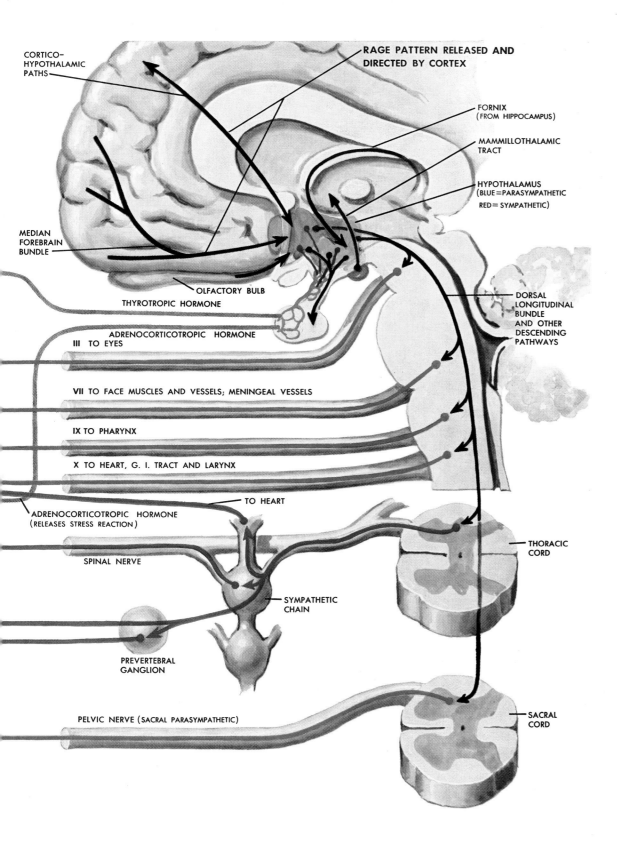

CORTICO-
HYPOTHALAMIC
PATHS

**RAGE PATTERN RELEASED AND
DIRECTED BY CORTEX**

FORNIX
(FROM HIPPOCAMPUS)

MAMMILLOTHALAMIC
TRACT

HYPOTHALAMUS
(BLUE=PARASYMPATHETIC

RED= SYMPATHETIC)

MEDIAN
FOREBRAIN
BUNDLE

OLFACTORY BULB

THYROTROPIC HORMONE

DORSAL
LONGITUDINAL
BUNDLE
AND OTHER
DESCENDING
PATHWAYS

ADRENOCORTICOTROPIC HORMONE

III TO EYES

VII TO FACE MUSCLES AND VESSELS; MENINGEAL VESSELS

IX TO PHARYNX

X TO HEART, G. I. TRACT AND LARYNX

ADRENOCORTICOTROPIC HORMONE
(RELEASES STRESS REACTION)

TO HEART

THORACIC
CORD

SPINAL NERVE

SYMPATHETIC
CHAIN

PREVERTEBRAL
GANGLION

SACRAL
CORD

PELVIC NERVE (SACRAL PARASYMPATHETIC)

particularly to show the timing and dynamic correlations of the many factors involved—those between the determinant origins and resultant effects, etc.

Having dealt in the preceding pages with the anatomy and functional relationships of the hypothalamus and having summarized our still incomplete knowledge of this part of the diencephalon, it should be permissible to give the hypothalamus a quasi central place in this maze of intricate connections, in spite of the fact that scientific evidence supports, but by no means proves, such thoughts. It would be without point to discuss the schematic chart in detail. The picture may well be considered self-explanatory.

ACKNOWLEDGMENTS

Plate 6 is partly based on Pribram and Kruger's paper on the Functions of the "Olfactory Brain" (Ann. N. Y. Acad. Sci., 58:109 [March 24], 1954).

The schematic representations of the blood supply of the hypophysis and hypothalamus (Plate 8) are based upon the work of Professors George B. Wislocki (A. Research Nerv. & Ment. Dis., Proc. [1936], 17:48, 1938), Knox Finley (A. Research Nerv. & Ment. Dis., Proc. [1939], 20:286-309, 1940), and J. D. Green (Amer. J. Anat., 88:225 [March], 1951).

The basic material in Plate 10 is based upon the extensive publications of Drs. E. and B. Scharrer and Professor W. Bargmann (Recent Progress in Hormone Research, 10:183-240, 1954; Das Zwischenhirn - Hypophysensystem, Julius Springer, Berlin, 1954).

Portions of Plate 11 have been adapted from a diagram in Bell, Davidson and Scarborough's Textbook of Physiology and Biochemistry, E. & S. Livingstone, Ltd., Edinburgh, 1950.

The upper figure in Plate 16 is adapted from the diagrams of Professor H. W. Magoun and his co-workers (J. Neurophysiol., 14:479, 1951).

REFERENCES

1. PRIBRAM, K. H., AND KRUGER: Ann. N. Y. Acad. Sci., 58:109 (March 24) 1954.
2. KAADA, B. R.: Acta physiol. scandinav., 24 (Suppl. 83):1, 1951.
3. INGRAM, W. R.: A. Research Nerv. & Ment. Dis., Proc. (1939), 20:195-244, 1940.
4. ARIENS KAPPERS, C. U., HUBER AND CROSBY: The Comparative Anatomy of the Nervous System of Vertebrates, Including Man, The Macmillan Company, New York, 1936.
5. PAPEZ, J. W.: Arch. Neurol. Psychiat., 38:725-743 (Oct.) 1937.
6. WISLOCKI, G. B.: A. Research Nerv. & Ment. Dis., Proc. (1936), 17:48, 1938.
7. GREEN, J. D.: Amer. J. Anat., 88:225 (March) 1951.
8. FINLEY, K. H.: A. Research Nerv. & Ment. Dis., Proc. (1939), 20:286-309, 1940.
9. HARRIS, G. W.: Proc. Soc. Med., 41:661 (Oct.) 1948.
10. ——: Brit. med. J., 1:339 (Feb. 21) 1948.
11. SAWYER, C. H., MARKEE AND HOLLINSHEAD: Endocrinology, 41:395, 1947.
12. EVERETT, J. W., AND SAWYER: Endocrinology, 45:581, 1949.
13. SCHARRER, E., AND SCHARRER: Hormones Produced by Neurosecretory Cells, In: Recent Progress in Hormone Research, 10:183-240, 1954.
14. BARGMANN, W.: Das Zwischenhirn-Hypophysensystem, Julius Springer, Berlin, Göttingen, Heidelberg, 1954.
15. CANNON, W. B.: The Wisdom of the Body, W. W. Norton Company, New York, 1932.
16. WHITE, J. C., SMITHWICK AND SIMEONE: The Autonomic Nervous System, The Macmillan Company, New York, 1952.
17. CIBA FOUNDATION SYMPOSIUM on Hypertension: Humoral and Neurogenic Factors, Little, Brown & Co., Boston, 1954.
18. RANSON, S. W.: A. Research Nerv. & Ment. Dis., Proc. (1939), 20:342, 1940.
19. ANAND, B. K., AND BROBECK: Proc. Soc. exper. Biol. & Med., 77:323, 1951.
20. INGRAM, W. R.: Electroenceph. clin. Neurophysiol., 4:397, 1952.
21. BREMER, F.: Compt. rend. Soc. de biol., 118:1235, 1935.
22. INGRAM, W. R., KNOTT, WHEATLEY AND SUMMERS: Electroenceph. clin. Neurophysiol., 3:37, 1951.
23. MAGOUN, H. W.: A. Research Nerv. & Ment. Dis., Proc. (1950), 30:480, 1952.
24. STARZL, T. E., TAYLOR AND MAGOUN: J. Neurophysiol., 14:479, 1951.
25. BARD, P., AND MOUNTCASTLE: A. Research Nerv. & Ment. Dis., Proc. (1947), 27:362, 1948.
26. SCHREINER, L., AND KLING: J. Neurophysiol., 16:643, 1953.
27. FULTON, J. F.: Frontal Lobotomy and Affective Behavior: A Neurophysiological Analysis, W. W. Norton Company, New York, 1951.

SUBJECT INDEX

(Numerals refer to pages, *not* plates)

INFORMATION ON CIBA COLLECTION VOLUMES

Since publication of its first volume, THE CIBA COLLECTION OF MEDICAL ILLUSTRATIONS has enjoyed an almost "unheard-of" reception from members of the medical community. The remarkable illustrations by Frank H. Netter, M.D. and text discussions by select specialists make these books unprecedented in their educational, clinical, and scientific value.

Volume 1   **NERVOUS SYSTEM**
"... a beautiful bargain ... and handsome reference work."
Psychological Record

Volume 2   **REPRODUCTIVE SYSTEM**
"... a desirable addition to any nursing or medical library."
American Journal of Nursing

Volume 3/I   **DIGESTIVE SYSTEM (Upper Digestive Tract)**
"... a fine example of the high quality of this series."
Pediatrics

Volume 3/II   **DIGESTIVE SYSTEM (Lower Digestive Tract)**
"... a unique and beautiful work, worth much more than its cost."
Journal of the South Carolina Medical Association

Volume 3/III   **DIGESTIVE SYSTEM (Liver, Biliary Tract and Pancreas)**
"... a versatile, multipurpose aid to clinicians, teachers, researchers, and students ..."   *Florida Medical Journal*

Volume 4   **ENDOCRINE SYSTEM and Selected Metabolic Diseases**
"... another in the series of superb contributions made by CIBA ..."
International Journal of Fertility

Volume 5   **HEART**
"The excellence of the volume ... is clearly deserving of highest praise."
Circulation

Volume 6   **KIDNEYS, URETERS, AND URINARY BLADDER**
"... a model of clarity of language and visual presentation ..."
Circulation

In the United States, copies of all CIBA COLLECTION books may be purchased from the Medical Education Division, CIBA Pharmaceutical Company, Division of CIBA-GEIGY Corporation, Summit, New Jersey 07901. In other countries, please direct inquiries to the nearest CIBA-GEIGY office.